CONQUERING AND CURING CANCER

The Cancer Survival Book

Charlene Seaman &
Scott Seaman

CONQUERING AND CURING CANCER

The Cancer Survival Book

Charlene Seaman &
Scott Seaman

Copyright © 2021 by Charlene Seaman & Scott Seaman.

Library of Congress Control Number:		2021920588
ISBN:	Hardcover	978-1-6641-1068-7
	Softcover	978-1-6641-1067-0
	eBook	978-1-6641-1066-3

All rights reserved. No part of this book may be reproduced or transmitted in any form or by any means, electronic or mechanical, including photocopying, recording, or by any information storage and retrieval system, without permission in writing from the copyright owner.

Print information available on the last page.

Rev. date: 10/06/2021

To order additional copies of this book, contact:
Xlibris
844-714-8691
www.Xlibris.com
Orders@Xlibris.com

Contents

Foreword: Leonidas C. Platanias, MD, PhD.. xi
        Henry Chi Hang Fung, MD, FACP, FRCPE....................... xii
        Nicole Liadis, PhD xiv

Acknowledgements: Here's To The Champions Battling Cancer........... xv

Prologue: "You Have Cancer"—The Dreaded Phrase That Too
Many People Hear... xix

Part 1
How Scott Conquered Cancer
(Our Story Of Survivorship)

Chapter 1: Too Many Suffered And Died
(Watching Others Before Us Battle Cancer).. 1

Chapter 2: We're Not Going To Disney World?
("You Have A Tumor The Size Of Two Baseballs In Your Chest")......... 9

Chapter 3: "Honey, I'm A Dead Man"
(The Surgery And Cancer Diagnosis)... 22

Chapter 4: "I'd Rather Have The Tumor In The Pathologist's Jar Than
In My Chest" (Post-Surgery Recovery)... 30

Chapter 5: Re-Emerging In The World
(Getting Up To Speed On Cancer).. 38

Chapter 6: Learning What The Phrase "Sick As A Dog" Really Means
(The Chemotherapy) 44

Chapter 7: The Final Phase Of The Treatment Trilogy
(The Radiation Therapy) 60

Chapter 8: Life Goes On
(Survivorship, Follow-Up, And The Fears Of A Cancer Survivor) 67

Chapter 9: Counting Our Blessings
(Fortunate To Be Alive) 74

Chapter 10: Charlene To The Rescue
(The Caregiver And Advocate) 78

Chapter 11: Putting Our Nation's "Leaders" To Work For Us
(Our Public Policy Advocacy Efforts) 87

Chapter 12: Charlene's Idea Became A Mission
(Fighting Back Through Cancer Fundraising, Awareness, And
Organizing Efforts) 112

Part 2
What You Need To Know And Do To Conquer Cancer
(Your Story Of Survivorship)

Chapter 13: The World's Worst Terrorists Live Within Us
(Developing A Warrior's Mentality And Cogent Battle
Plan To Defeat Cancer) 123

Chapter 14: The Cancer Landscape
(Some Basic Information About Cancer In General And
Blood Cancer In Particular) 131

Chapter 15: Picking The Best Doctors And Assembling Your
Health Care Team
(Choose Your Doctors Wisely) 156

Chapter 16: Hospitals Stays Can Be Scary, But Hospitals
Are Places Of Healing
(Surviving Your Hospital Stay) 168

Chapter 17: Your Survival Rate, Properly Adjusted, May Be 100 Percent (An Illuminating Approach To Conquering Cancer). 179

Chapter 18: Cancer Diagnoses And Staging, Understanding Tests, And Obtaining Second Opinions
(The Importance Of A Prompt And Proper Diagnosis)........................ 185

Chapter 19: An Overview Of Cancer Treatments
(Selecting The Most Effective Treatment For Your Cancer) 198

Chapter 20: Employing A Complementary/ Integrative Approach
(Conventional Medicine Can Use A Helping Hand)............................ 226

Chapter 21: The Superhighway To Curing Cancer
(A Strategy For Curing Cancer And A National Call To Action) 233

Chapter 22: The Impact Of The Covid-19 Pandemic 243

Part 3
Patient's Survival Compendium
Appendices Of Information, Checklists, And A Notebook To Help You Conquer Cancer

Appendix "A" Common Cancer Terms 267

Appendix "B" Cancer Types 272

Appendix "C" Cancer Organizations And Resources Available To You 280

Appendix "D" Questions To Ask Your Doctors 319

Appendix "E" Tips The Doctors May Forget To Tell You 327

Appendix "F" Insurance And Legal Documents 331

Appendix "G" Patient Medical Information Notebook 334

Appendix "H" Patient's Weekly Schedule And Log 353

Appendix "I" Giving Back To Help Others Survive
And To Cure Cancer 361

Appendix "J" A Couple Other Good Cancer Books 362

Appendix "K" Managing Side Effects 364

Appendix "L" Your Key Contacts 371

About The Authors: (we did not set out to be cancer warriors).............373

This book is designed to provide you with information, to demystify the experience of being impacted by cancer, and to help you make more informed decisions on treatments and procedures relating to cancer. It is not intended to be complete or exhaustive, nor is it intended to constitute medical, dietary, exercise, healthcare, business, financial, or legal advice. You should conduct your own research and consult with your physicians, healthcare providers, financial, legal, and other advisors, as appropriate, in order to make the best decisions for you in view of your specific situation and unique circumstances.

Throughout the book, we provide information about cancer and its diagnosis and treatments. We have updated the text and some of the appendices for publication in the fall of 2021. The pace of cancer research and developments has increased substantially in recent years for a variety of reasons including the sea changing Human Genome Project undertaken from 1990 to 2003. In view of the fast pace of cancer research and developments, it is not possible to truly provide up-to-date information about cancer and its treatments in any book format. We encourage patients and caregivers to obtain the most recent and accurate information from reliable websites, sources, and their health care team. Some good sources of information are included throughout this book and in Appendix C.

FOREWORD

Receiving a cancer diagnosis is shocking and a very serious challenge for everyone. Major efforts are required to overcome the initial shock. It is important to understand the disease and work with professionals and family members to develop a support system and create a plan of action. The goal is to control the disease and eventually defeat it completely, when possible. When dealing with cancer, choosing appropriate allies, partners and advisors is of utmost importance. This book is meant to act as a helpful tool and guide, providing important information to help cancer patients during this process. It combines information to facilitate key steps at the beginning of the cancer journey and some practical advice on how to navigate through issues as things evolve.

The authors are true humanitarians and philanthropists who have directly experienced the pain and anxiety of a cancer diagnosis. They have found ways to use their experience to help others, becoming strong advocates for cancer research.

This book reflects the commitment and persistence of the authors in the fight against the pain and devastation of cancer. This commitment has led them through a tremendous effort to collect and provide accurate and up to date information to help others. The book is exceptionally well written and will be helpful to anyone who wants to learn and understand more about cancer, and do something about it.

Leonidas C. Platanias, MD, PhD
Director, Robert H. Lurie Comprehensive Cancer Center of Northwestern University
Jesse, Sara, Andrew, Abigail, Benjamin and Elizabeth Lurie
Professor of Oncology
Professor of Medicine (Hematology-Oncology) and Biochemistry and Molecular Genetics

The National Cancer Institute estimates that there are nearly 17 million cancer survivors in the United States. Indeed, cancers impact almost everybody in this country in one way or another. As lymphoma is one of the most treatable cancers, we are pleased to report that many of the long-term survivors are lymphoma patients. An increasing number of patients are cured of their lymphoma, though some ultimately may relapse. For those who develop recurrent disease, thanks to the advances in medical research, we now have more options available to them. For those who are cured, unfortunately some may develop long-term complications from treatment and may require further medical intervention. Obviously, our ultimate goal is to make lymphoma history, but we are not there yet. Thus, many of our past, current, and future patients need to live with lymphoma.

As a cancer survivor, you can choose to live with sadness, anger, and despair. You can also choose to live the way that Scott and Charlene choose to live—to inspire cancer patients, to promote cancer education, to raise awareness of cancer in general and lymphoma in particular, to fund cancer research, to live with cancer, and to laugh with cancer. Cancer patients and survivors figure prominently in advancing medicine. Participating in clinical trials and raising money and awareness for medical research are examples of the vital role that cancer patients, survivors, and their families play in advancing medical science.

Scott and Charlene have an inspiring story and one that all people impacted by cancer should read. This is an important book that contains helpful information and tips from the perspectives of a cancer survivor and a caregiver who have become champions for people battling cancer. It is our privilege to know Scott and Charlene—the cancer warriors! We thank them for their inspiration, devotion, and leadership!

Henry Chi Hang Fung, MD, FACP, FRCPE
Chair, Departments of Bone Marrow
Transplantation and Cellular Therapies
Fox Chase Cancer Center

Scientists have made tremendous strides in cancer research; however, the sad reality is that curing cancer across the board still is beyond reach. Consequently, newly diagnosed patients and their families can feel emotionally overwhelmed. "Conquering And Curing Cancer" outlines the seemingly enigmatic steps that cancer patients and their caregivers can take to attain the inconceivable – a personalized cure.

Cancer is one of the most feared diseases around the world. Like many, my fear began as a child. I felt concerned that people I love would get cancer and felt sad for those that did. By adulthood, I felt an overwhelming need to jump on the "cancer" bandwagon; the bandwagon destined to understand this devastating disease. As a molecular biologist, I was behind the scenes trying to understand tumor biology responsible for disease progression. I eventually entered the vast cancer world, working on promising clinical trials and connecting with patients whose very own tumors I would dissect. These efforts were made hoping to make sense of their cancer. At times, our findings would be discouraging and eventually my fears turned into rage. This became a defining moment in my life. The rage that I felt inside was combined with helplessness, watching patients ravaged and losing their battle to cancer. Seeing people confront their sad reality motivated me and pushed me onto a brand new bandwagon: one that was destined to help patients "conquer" their cancer. Every night, I went home and carried the stories of cancer patients in my heart, contemplating and wishing to make their lives better. One of the most memorable experiences that I had was meeting a cancer patient who was my age. She, along with her family, was desperate and willing to do anything and go anywhere to cure her cancer. In contrast, another patient that I encountered couldn't grasp the severity of her diagnosis and treatment; naively she was willing to postpone her treatment because she wanted to travel abroad. I took the stance along with others to compassionately fight for her life, educating her about the urgency of NOW. Sadly, I met a father who lost his battle to leukemia and his wife would bring their 4-year-old child to the hospital every day; the little boy couldn't conceive that his father was gone. He would search hospital rooms, even closets for his father. Moments like these and so many more continue to drive my passion to advocate and relentlessly pursue better personalized treatments and outcomes for cancer patients. The authors of this book, Scott and Charlene Seaman, bring to light their own personal story; not only the raw truths about what cancer patients endure but also the obstacles and emotions that caregivers face. Through these accounts, you will comprehend how two people can whole-heartedly come together to be on the same path, but distinct trajectories, each facing different obstacles and emotions. Scott and Charlene's overarching mission was to conquer Scott's cancer.

I first met the authors of the book several years ago through our dear friend Eleni Bousis, founder of the distinguished Hippocratic Cancer Research Foundation. We were drawn to each other because of our common passion to advocate for cancer patients. Over the years, it became clear to me, as I am certain it will be for you, Scott and Charlene are more than just advocates; they are "mentors of advocates." As a cancer advocate and a cancer researcher I have encountered doctors that truly go above and beyond to provide the best care, and treatments for their patients. However, I have also encountered doctors that do not show the same devotion or rise to the occasion. This book comprehensively explains cancer and cancer treatments. It guides cancer patients and caregivers on how to advocate and pursue what they deserve, the best personalized cancer treatment plan. The authors encourage people to not just have any game plan but to "formulate a survival equation." Scott and Charlene show us how this is possible to do, even if you know nothing about cancer or medicine. They give us the reassurance that it is acceptable to ask questions, demand the right information and expect the best care. They inspire us to all be "checkers" like Charlene. Although I am very knowledgeable about cancer, this book taught me more ways to help optimize and individualize treatment plans and I learned new ideas for empowering cancer patients and caregivers. By doing these things, you can transform the cancer journey experience for everybody involved.

The degree of uncertainty and trial in cancer medicine is daunting. This book is timeless, providing insights and hope for the future direction of personalized medicine. Living in a world where GPS can get us easily to a final destination, the book challenges cancer patients to demand the same from their cancer journey and arrive cancer-free. Scott's and Charlene's invincible spirit will not be suppressed by cancer. They continue to be outstanding advocates for cancer patients. Their altruistic stance is not only of faith, but of knowing that it is possible to "live" after cancer.

    Nicole Liadis, PhD
    Educator, molecular biologist, cancer
    researcher, cancer foundation board
    member, cancer patient advocate, mother,
    daughter, wife, sister, and aunt

ACKNOWLEDGEMENTS

HERE'S TO THE CHAMPIONS BATTLING CANCER

There are numerous people that we wish to acknowledge and thank. Out of respect for people's privacy, we rarely will refer to any living person by name elsewhere in this book. We send our heart-felt thanks to the wonderful doctors, nurses, and medical professionals who provided us with outstanding health care. We are truly blessed to have world-class physicians and healthcare centers right here in the Chicagoland area and across our nation. We thank those who are committed to providing the best possible care to their patients, taking the health and well-being of their patients personally, and befriending their patients—treating them as important individuals, not transient patients or hospital room numbers. Thanks to those researchers committed to finding better cancer treatments and dedicated to curing cancer.

There are some physicians we have to mention by name because they personify the above standards. Thanks to Dr. Stephanie Gregory and Dr. Henry Fung (who wrote one of the forewords) for helping so many people impacted by lymphoma, leukemia, and myeloma. They are outstanding physicians and educators who genuinely care about their patients and are fully committed to curing cancer.

The august surgeon we write about in our book graciously gave us permission to disclose his identity. There is no way to express adequately our appreciation to Dr. L. Penfield Faber. Dr. Faber is the finest thoracic surgeon in the world. Moreover, he has trained and educated so many doctors over the years, instilling in them cutting edge surgical skills, professionalism, and unwavering standards.

For nearly a quarter of a century, we have been on the front lines in the war against cancer. We are particularly proud of our current efforts through the Hippocratic Cancer Resource Foundation ("HCRF") in supporting the world class research of Leonidas C. Platanias MD, PhD, Director of the Robert H. Lurie Comprehensive Cancer Center of Northwestern University and his amazing team of scientists. HCRF proudly supports his team's out-of-the-box, cutting edge, impactful research seeking treatments and cures for all types of cancer.

Dr. Platanias is a warm, kind, and wonderful man as well as a world renown clinician, researcher, and leader. No one is more committed to his patients and to curing cancer than Dr. Platanias. We are honored that Dr. Platanias wrote a foreword for this book. He stands at the top of the world of cancer research and oncology.

In Chapter 21 we discuss the superhighway to curing cancer. It is because of the doctors and researches such as those mentioned here and the late Dr. Janet Rowley that we say confidently that the superhighway runs through Chicago.

Special thanks to our dear friends Eleni Bousis (who founded, drives, and is the Chair of HCRF), Jimmy Bousis (a rock star), Vonita Reescer (Chicago's First Lady of Philanthropy), Dr. Nicole Liadis (a brilliant medical researcher who graciously wrote one of the forewords for this book), Mr. Elias Boufis, Kristine Farra, and to all of our fellow Founding Board members as well as all of the wonderful people supporting the efforts of HCRF.

We are very appreciative of those family members, friends, partners, and clients who provided love, support, comfort, prayer, and inspiration to us over all of these years and through all of our cancer initiatives and adventures and other philanthropic activities.

Charlene has committed us to turning our tragedy into a blessing for others. As laypeople, we cannot cure cancer or develop more efficacious treatments ourselves. We can raise money and put it in the hands of outstanding medical researchers. We can promote public awareness about cancer. We can educate patients, medical professionals, and family members. We can talk with, comfort, and provide support to patients and families. We can share our experiences with others battling cancer to provide encouragement and pointers to them and their families. We have been able to do these things as part of our mission to eradicate cancer, but we have not done enough. What little we have accomplished has been because of the efforts and generosity of so many. We are very grateful to: the volunteers serving on non-profit boards; the team captains, walkers, runners, bike riders, and donors, sponsors and event volunteers who have supported galas, fundraisers and educational events; media partners; healthcare professionals; and to all who have contributed so much along the way. To all of you—and you know who you are—please accept our heart-felt thanks and appreciation!

We dedicate this book to all of the people who have lost their battle to cancer and to their families and loved ones. Sadly, this includes members of the HCRF family Julie Platanias, Dr. Christina Mantis, Cheryl Rabine, and Jay Michael. We often think about the wonderful people that cancer has taken from us and they strengthen our resolve to defeat cancer. We also dedicate this book to people who are battling cancer and other health problems and to those people who care for them and advocate on their behalf.

The COVID-19 pandemic has hit cancer patients and the cancer community particularly hard. We mourn those who lost their lives from COVID-19 and are grateful to those who helped save lives during the pandemic. The COVID-19 pandemic has been the most profound adverse event in recent memory. The response to the pandemic has demonstrated the power of the human spirit, the positive impact of a large and cogent commitment of funds by the government, and the importance of private/public partnerships in defeating disease. It is important to remember that it was cancer research that provided the platform for the COVID-19 vaccines that have saved many lives and for important therapeutics as well. It is long past time for our country to make a more substantial commitment to curing cancer in all of its forms similar in scope to Operation Warp Speed.

We urge those impacted by cancer—and those not yet impacted directly or indirectly by cancer—to join the mission of eradicating cancer and serving those impacted by the disease in its many horrible manifestations. This is a national – indeed an international – call to action to eradicate cancer. There is something that each one of us can do to help!

PROLOGUE

"YOU HAVE CANCER"—THE DREADED PHRASE THAT TOO MANY PEOPLE HEAR

This book is intended for anybody battling cancer or who has been touched by cancer in any way. This includes cancer patients, cancer survivors, and caregivers, family, friends, and colleagues of those with cancer. Doctors and healthcare providers should read the book as well. A deeper understanding of the perspectives of patients and caregivers will make medical treatment better and more patient friendly. In view of the incidence rate of cancer, we are catering to a very large audience. The statistics tell us that approximately one of every two men in America will get some form of cancer during their lifetime and more than one of every three women will develop cancer during their lifetime (and these numbers do not even include non-melanoma skin cancers). These are staggering figures. Only a healthy hermit can avoid being impacted by cancer.

Yes, cancer is an indiscriminate killer. It attacks people of all political parties, all social-economic classes, the educated and the illiterate, all races, creeds, and colors, men, women, and children, and even our pets. It passes through the gates of the good, the bad, and the ugly. The amount spent seeking better treatments and cures pales by comparison to the economic costs of cancer to society, not to mention the tremendous humanomic costs cancer exacts on patients and their families. We address some of the global issues of conquering beating cancer because they are important. But for us to be longterm warriors in the critical mission to cure cancer, we have to beat the disease ourselves. Accordingly, conquering cancer is the focus of this book.

Everyone knows cancer is prevalent and horrific at some level. When it strikes you or someone you love, cancer can be an overwhelming, devastating, life-altering, and life-threatening reality. It can hit you like a ton of bricks. It can frighten the bravest of us and make the most controlling of us feel out of control of our own lives. You may feel alone, but you are not alone. The statistics and the waiting time at the oncologists' offices are proof enough to make the point.

Now more than ever there are better treatments available. There are remedies and preventatives for many of the side effects of treatment. For many patients, cancer treatments not only extend life during the period that the treatment is effective, they provide a bridge to the next treatment to become available. Ultimately, it is about curing your cancer. Until your cancer is cured, however, it is about living long and well with cancer.

Most of the cancer information that patients read about today refers to cancer generally or addresses a particular type of cancer. The reality is that each person's cancer is unique, treatment response can vary and so can outcomes. Further, the same person's cancer may evolve over time. The Human Genome Project has provided immense opportunities for the development of targeted therapies, ushering in the age of personalized or precision medicine. More and more, cancer patients and their doctors should put together an individualized treatment plan for the patient with the focus on their specific cancer and the treatments that will get the patient the best outcome. As the characterization of cancer becomes more complex, the methods used to assess cancer and treatments are becoming more elaborate. With the explosion in modern capabilities to address a patient's specific cancer there has been an explosion in data volume and data type. For that reason, we will see how cancer knowledge, patient diagnoses, and treatments will be optimized with new technologies, including artificial intelligence and platforms to benefit an individual patient's outcome. Although far too little is spent on cancer research, there is an enormous effort put into research and significant progress has been made by many wonderful people invested in finding better treatments and cures. This means there are many people and researchers out there to help you. There are also several organizations, materials, and websites. And we believe this book will help you as well.

Part 1 of the book tells our personal story. It is not a biography—we focus our story on our relationship with cancer. It is our subjective view of cancer, Scott's diagnosis and treatment, Charlene's role as a wife and caregiver, our individual and collective experiences, what cancer did to us and what we did to cancer. We think there will be many feelings and experiences to which you can relate. We were comforted, informed, and encouraged by hearing other cancer survivors' stories and want to pass that on to you.

There may be things that you cannot relate to or do not agree with, but we retain our individuality and unique responses notwithstanding all of us receiving the unwanted label of "cancer patient" or "caregiver." We have different experiences, approaches, and views. We go into the experience in our unique way, we will get through it in our own way, and we emerge from it as individuals. All of our lives will be changed in some manner by virtue of this unwanted experience. We hope that Part 1 of this book will make you laugh, cry, nod, shake your head, or move you in some way. For those just entering the journey, we hope it will demystify the process and provide you with some insights. If nothing else, you should be comforted to know that, if someone with Scott's low pain threshold and numerous frailties as a patient can beat cancer, you too will beat cancer. Beating cancer is your goal and our mission.

Part 2 of the book is about you and what you will do to survive. Someone on the patient's team needs to have information and knowledge about cancer. Whether it is the patient, family, friend, or any other advocate, information and knowledge represent power in beating cancer. Ignorance may be bliss, but it does not increase the chances of a good outcome (that's medical speak for living). There are many things you need to do to ensure that you are on the "surviving" side of the statistics, including: obtaining a prompt and accurate diagnosis; getting the best doctors and healthcare providers available to you; knowing your treatment options (conventional and clinical trials); selecting the proper treatment for you and your cancer; employing complementary techniques to bolster your body, mind, and immunity; and taking advantage of available resources. Part 2 purports to be the objective part of the book, but it also is quite subjective. For those of you just becoming embroiled in the world of medicine and beginning the process of converting from "person" to "patient," we should disabuse you promptly of the notion that medicine is pure science. Of course, there are substantial scientific components to medicine. Yet, there is a lot more "art" and "instinct" involved in this "science" than we ever imagined prior to beginning our journey.

Part 3 is loaded with checklists and useful resources. It also provides space for you to write questions, take notes, and record pertinent medical and insurance information. It is your personal cancer survival resource center. In fact, the book contains a Patient Medical Information Notebook in the back. You can carry the book with you so that you have your health information available on demand when you need it.

Some additional information about us is contained in the "About The Author" section at the end. All you need to know about Scott is that he is a Chicago-based trial lawyer who represents companies in commercial, business, and insurance litigation on a nation-wide basis. He is a problem solver for his clients, but often the problems are solved through litigation, trial, appeal, and arbitration. He loves his wife, family, friends, he is committed to his clients and practicing law, and he loves pets and Frank Sinatra music. He has a low pain threshold and hates being sick and never thought that he could survive any surgery—not even having his tonsils taken out. One more thing – Scott is a 23-year survivor of non-Hodgkin lymphoma.

Charlene, his better half and co-author, is a warm, loving, nurturing, motherly, brilliant, direct, strong, passionate, impatient, and truly one-of-a-kind lady. While Scott is a doctor of law, Charlene is as knowledgeable as a lot of medical doctors even though she never went to medical school. She has been invited to speak at medical conferences around the world. Like most wives, she keeps track of her husband's mistakes and makes Scott do things that he does not want to do. In his case, the list includes chemotherapy, radiation, talking to patients, and charitable work.

We have written this book jointly and it includes both of our memories, views, and perceptions. Much of the book is written by us in the third person so that you can appreciate our separate thoughts and actions. A couple of chapters are written in the first person with separate sections by each of us so that you can see the viewpoints of both patient and caregiver.

We hope that you will understand that we know the seriousness of the subject matter and we assure you no one hates cancer more than us. When confronting cancer, however, we find it difficult to believe anyone can prevail without a sense of humor.

The fundamental point of this book is surviving—conquering and curing cancer. Most people actually do survive and you should be one of them. Once you get over the initial shock of the diagnosis, you have to go into motion and educate yourself about the disease and your options. Being a knowledgeable and active patient makes a significant difference.

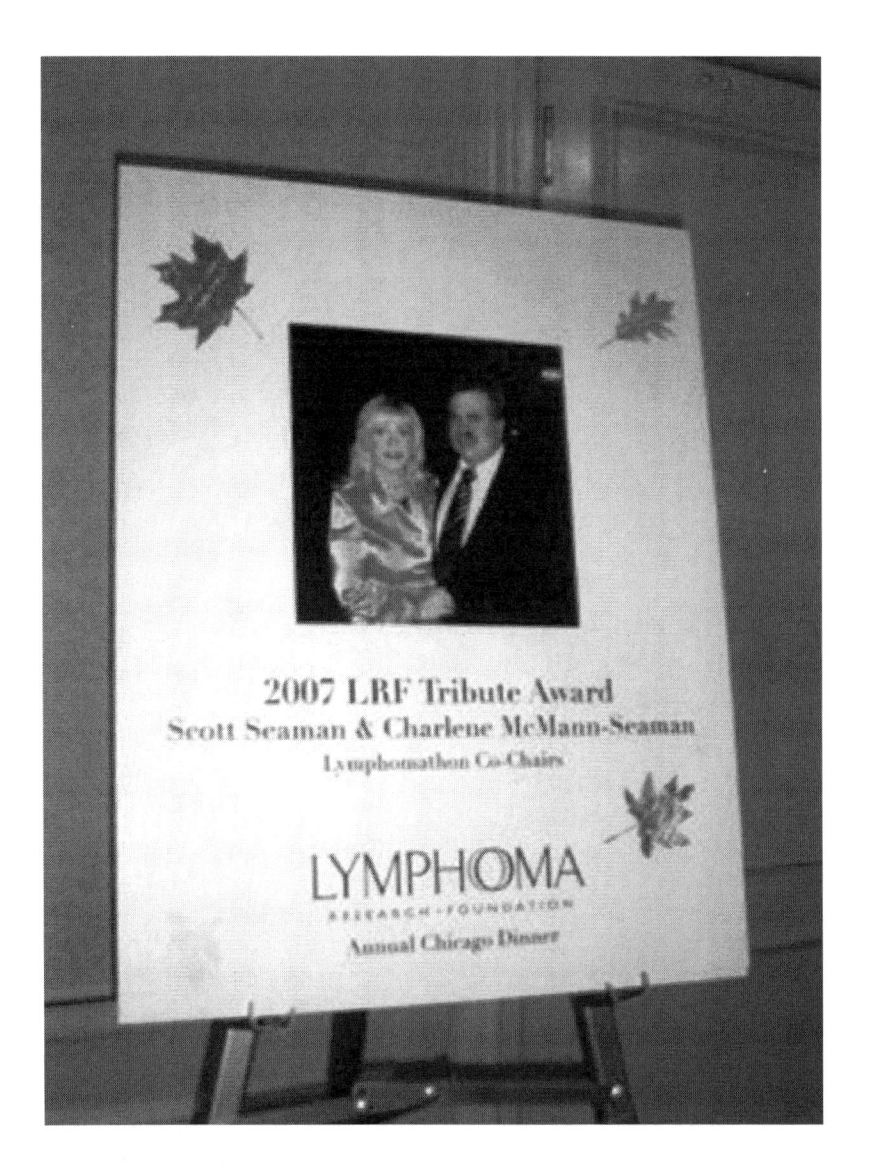

2007 LRF Tribute Award
Scott Seaman & Charlene McMann-Seaman
Lymphomathon Co-Chairs

LYMPHOMA
RESEARCH FOUNDATION
Annual Chicago Dinner

PART 1

HOW SCOTT CONQUERED CANCER (OUR STORY OF SURVIVORSHIP)

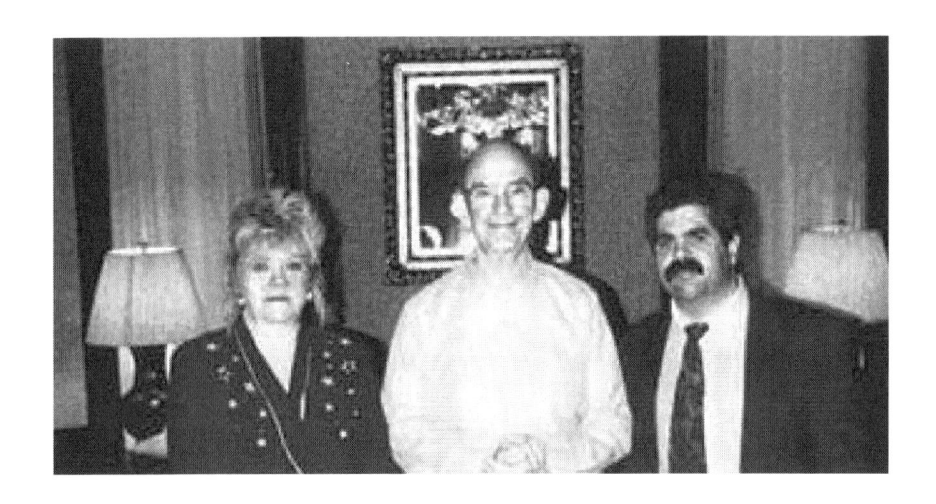

Charlene and Scott with Chicago's beloved Joseph Cardinal Bernardin.

CHAPTER 1

TOO MANY SUFFERED AND DIED (WATCHING OTHERS BEFORE US BATTLE CANCER)

Cancer can be a difficult or uncomfortable subject for the person with cancer, their family, and people around them. Sometimes there is denial on the part of the patient or others, but generally, at least after a while, it becomes part of their life. It is a part of many of our lives, and we have to deal with it. Better to live with it than to die from it! There are many articles on things to say or not to say to people with cancer, but the main point is to be a good listener and to be supportive.

When in doubt, take the lead from the person with cancer as to whether, when, and how to discuss the subject. Some people like to discuss it. Others do not. When you are the person with cancer, you should set the tone. How people react to you as someone with cancer may depend upon how you are dealing with it yourself. Sometimes you have to help people feel comfortable with the subject. Other times, peoples' own fears or feelings impact how they deal with you or may cause some people to be distant or even to ignore you.

What we originally learned about cancer came from the experiences of the people we knew who had it. That experience was unfortunate as it often took one of two forms. The first paradigm was that people we knew got cancer and died within a short period of time. The second is that people got cancer, underwent treatment (usually surgery or chemotherapy), suffered, withered away, and then died. Fortunately, we learned later through our own experience that living also was a possible—indeed probable—outcome.

We have vivid memories about some people close to us who had cancer. For example, there was our friend Pat, a smart, fun-loving woman who we met because she ran the parent company of the company for which

Charlene was the Vice President and Chief Operating Officer. She ruled with an iron fist – fair but firm. She and Charlene saw a lot of themselves in each other. Pat had metastasized cancer that she did not discover until it spread to her bones. We sent her medical records and scans to leading doctors across the country. They all came back with the same answer, which was a prognosis we refused to hear.

Now we turn to our friend and Chicago's beloved Joseph Cardinal Bernardin. The Cardinal had pancreatic cancer and was being treated at Loyola University of Chicago Medical Center at the cancer center that later would bear his name. Charlene is Catholic and we both always respected Cardinal Bernardin because he was a religious leader in the best sense of the word. He was someone who brought people of all religions together.

When Charlene cares about you, she will do anything she can for you. In fact, she has gone to extraordinary lengths for many people she does not even know. Charlene was getting frustrated because Pat was not getting better. We saw Cardinal Bernardin on the news. They reported on him spending a lot of time in the cancer center talking to and getting to know all of the many patients undergoing treatment who sought him out. The Cardinal's cancer was put in remission and Charlene thought that it would give Pat (who was a devout Catholic) a boost to get a note of encouragement and prayer from the Cardinal. So Charlene called the archdiocese. She left a message and explained Pat's circumstances.

A night or two later, we were sitting on our living room couch watching television and the phone rang. This was before the days of caller identification and "do not call" lists. Charlene answered it abruptly because we received a couple of unsolicited marketing calls a few minutes before. "Hello Cardinal Bernardin," said Charlene while motioning Scott to silence the television. The Cardinal called to ask how Pat was doing and to find out where Pat lived. Charlene told him Pat's condition and where she lived (about 50 minutes outside of the city) and the Cardinal said he was not up to going on that long of a drive yet. The Cardinal said that he would like to write Pat a letter. Charlene handed Scott the phone while she dashed off to get Pat's address.

As Scott remembers it, his end of the conversation went like this: "Hello Cardinal. I am Charlene's husband. I am so glad that you are in remission. You are the best Cardinal in the country and we need to keep you healthy. I am a lawyer and if you ever need anything, do not hesitate to contact me." The Cardinal said he was giving his first post-cancer mass

Sunday at his residence on State Parkway and asked whether Scott thought Pat was up to attending. Scott said, "I don't know, but if there is any way possible for her to come, she will be there." The Cardinal added that we should come and bring Charlene's mother Mary (also a cancer survivor) as well. When Scott hung up he was smiling as he told Charlene the deal he had just negotiated. In the interest of full disclosure, Scott told the Cardinal he was not 100 percent Catholic and inquired as to whether he was still invited. Cardinal Bernardin responded, "of course, nobody's perfect."

We were both excited because we knew that this would mean a lot to Pat. Charlene was hoping that this might start Pat down the road to recovery. Charlene called Pat and she sounded very excited. We think Pat was hoping the same thing.

On that Sunday morning, we arrived at the Cardinal's residence along with Mary. The Cardinal gave us a tour of the residence, it was beautiful. Scott asked him about his health (the Cardinal was optimistic and feeling well that day), about being a cardinal (looking for the obvious similarities in their professions), and about prayer. It does not matter what religion you are, when you were in Cardinal Bernardin's presence, you knew that you were in the presence of a holy man. He was not only a holy man, but a loving, humble, and generous man. In response to Scott's inquiries, the Cardinal described his daily routine. Scott asked the Cardinal how he was able to keep his concentration during prayer. The Cardinal readily admitted that his mind sometimes would wander and he would have to re-focus. He explained his prayer routine to Scott in greater detail. The Cardinal then went upstairs and emerged with a few items that he would share later. He said over the years he had collected numerous items, but he gave them all away. He did not like the fact that he seemed to value material things.

Soon Pat arrived along with some members of her family. She was in a wheel chair that extended out like a bed so that she was lying almost flat. We carried her up the stairs and we all went into the cathedral in the Cardinal's residence. The Cardinal's niece and nephew were there along with a couple of nuns and another well-known priest. They were all so gracious and it truly was an enriching experience. The Cardinal said a touching prayer for Pat and for Mary. When the Cardinal finished, Scott got up and approached the altar. Charlene's mouth opened and she reached out to try to stop Scott. According to Charlene, "you are not supposed to go on the altar." Charlene did not know it, but Scott had cleared this with the other priest ahead of time. Scott proceeded to say a 3 or 4 minute heart-felt prayer for the Cardinal. Although we will not attempt to recreate the prayer here, Charlene agrees that it actually was appropriate and moving. Cardinal Bernardin and Scott embraced afterwards. Charlene offered to make a donation to the church, but the Cardinal flatly refused to accept any donation. The Cardinal said he wanted to do this for Pat because he was touched by Charlene having reached out to him on behalf of her friend.

Before we left, the Cardinal passed out rosary beads that were blessed personally by Pope John Paul II when the Cardinal was last in the Vatican. He gave Pat and Charlene a special relic from Saint Peregrine, the patron saint of cancer patients. Charlene later bought Pat a special chain for the relic and put it around her neck to comfort her. The Cardinal spoke with Pat and, while he was looking at her, both of us had the feeling that the Cardinal was wondering whether he would be in a similar condition down the road. Whether we picked up on something the Cardinal was thinking or not, we don't know. Little did we know – and we never imagined – that a couple of years later Scott would be battling cancer and would be treated at the Cardinal Bernardin Cancer Center!

We would speak with Cardinal Bernardin periodically and Charlene would send him fruit baskets because she knew that he loved fruit. We were very moved by the experience and grateful that we had the Cardinal's friendship for the remainder of his life. We called him the evening after he announced that his cancer had returned. He talked about his deep faith and said he knew he would be going to a better place. But he also said that he was scared. Many people say Pope John Paul II taught people how to die, but actually Cardinal Bernardin taught those of us in the Chicagoland area that lesson several years earlier.

Sadly, Pat already had lost her battle. When people are battling cancer or other hardships, it is common to turn to prayer or even to grasp at straws. Charlene really believed that prayer would help Pat and was somewhat depressed and disillusioned when the prayers did not accomplish what we wanted. But we realized that we are not in charge of the world. This is the part where we are supposed to write that the Lord works in mysterious ways and sometimes we do not have a full appreciation for his plans. Nonetheless, the seeds were planted for an approach that we would use down the road. We would do whatever we could to help people with cancer and to cure cancer during our lifetime. Although many things are beyond our control, it should not prevent us from trying.

Scott's grandmother lived in Florida. She had lung cancer and had a lung removed. She neglected to tell anyone about her diagnosis or about her surgery until after the operation. We guess it was her way of dealing with cancer "without being a burden." Of course, we were shocked to learn about this after the fact and can tell you that this was not the best approach for dealing with cancer. We went to Florida to visit Grandma Rose and her sister, Scott's Aunt Bess. The "Golden Girls" lived together for the last few years of their lives and looked out for each other after Scott's grandfather and uncle (a former Warner Brothers executive responsible for bringing *My Fair Lady* to the big screen) died. Aunt Bess was a few years older (an elegant and lovely lady then in her early 90s), but she always looked a couple of decades younger than her biological age. We spent a couple of warm and wonderful days with them and had some "quality one-on-one time" as Grandma Rose called it. We learned the importance of getting to the restaurant by 4:30 p.m. so that we could eat dinner promptly at 5:00 p.m. This was reality, not just a *Seinfeld* scene.

We got married a few months later. Grandma Rose and Aunt Bess were not up to making the trip to Chicago for our wedding, so we planned to go see them on our honeymoon. Grandma Rose told us to bring pictures, which we did. We arrived and Aunt Bess said that Grandma Rose was in the hospital. We visited with Aunt Bess for a while, but she did not want to accompany us to the hospital. As soon as we drove up we could see the hospital actually was a hospice. Grandma Rose was in terrible pain and was being treated with the indifference, disregard, incompetence, and lack of compassion that many patients can expect, particularly elderly patients without an advocate at their side. You bet we advocated, provided some comfort to her, and we did get her some pain relief. But this would be the last time that we would see her. She was in her mid-80s, but once again cancer took its toll.

We knew many others who died from cancer. Charlene's father died from cancer after living the majority of his life in the VA hospital after being injured in World War II. He was shot in his head and never really recovered. He was diagnosed with lung cancer and died one year later. Charlene's aunt died at the age of 48 from ovarian cancer. Scott was very close to his uncle Al who died in his 50s from adrenaline cancer. Scott remembers that chemotherapy was very rough on his uncle and unsuccessful.

We remember kids dying from leukemia. We know so many people with breast cancer. And the list goes on. Our hatred of cancer long preceded Scott's diagnosis. Years after our cancer journey, Scott's mother, Elaine, was diagnosed with ovarian cancer. She died within a year or so of her diagnosis and after enduring a difficult surgery and chemotherapy. We tried to have her benefit from the lessons we learned over the years, but she was resistant to obtaining a second opinion and would not follow our advice. She went to a local doctor and underwent the treatment he recommended even though there were better options available to her. We believe she could have lived much longer and Scott deeply regrets that he was unable to alter her course. Our suggestions, however, were met with stone cold resistance from her husband and we realized ultimately that we had little choice but to simply provide unwavering support and love — which we did. Unfortunately, too many cancer patients limit their options and fail to obtain optimal treatment.

Those battling cancer often are characterized as "fighters," "champions," "tough," "survivors," or even "heroes." Perhaps the characterizations are entirely fair, as cancer patients are fighting for their lives. Yet, sometimes we think they go too far or mischaracterize the reality. After all, this is not a battle we enlisted in and the alternative to fighting is not an attractive one. No matter how strong one's religious beliefs or how wonderful heaven may be, few of us are ready to leave the people we love and our missions on earth. So whatever labels are placed on cancer patients, most of us are just trying to live. The unfortunate flip-side to the positive terms to describe cancer survivors sometimes is the implication that those who did not survive or did not live long with cancer were not "fighters" or somehow were weak. Such suggestions are unfair. For some of the world's strongest, most religious, patriotic, and productive members of society have died from cancer. We just mentioned some of them. To be sure, losing wonderful people to the disease as well as knowing how they suffered was the main thing we knew about cancer.

Since Scott's cancer diagnosis, we have encountered, befriended, and have been befriended by many people with cancer. It is incredible how many people are living with cancer and have beaten the disease. Even people battling a form of cancer that is not yet curable have every reason to be hopeful. By staying alive, you are buying time for treatments to extend your remission until the next treatment or breakthrough. We used to think everyone with cancer ultimately succumbs to the disease. Our eyes have been opened. Most people actually beat cancer or at least live many, many years after being diagnosed. We are providing our pre-warrior mindset in this opening chapter, but don't despair. Our previous mindset was not accurate. Scott made the mistake of initially assessing his chances of surviving based upon a few people he knew who died from cancer and our vision was clouded by the traditional feeling of gloom associated with cancer. Cancer may have been a virtual death sentence in the early 1900s when the chances for long-term survival were very low or even in the 1940s when only one in four survived. But things have changed considerably. The overall 5-year cancer survival rate today is above 67 percent and still on the rise. Moreover, about 77% of all cancers are diagnosed in people 55 and older. The aging population does impact the rate of incidence of cancer.

Even we had positive examples of people who beat cancer. Charlene's mother, Mary, was diagnosed with breast cancer. She found a lump in her breast, had a mastectomy, and beat the disease. Fortunately, she did not need chemotherapy. But five years later, she was diagnosed with colon cancer. The surgery was very hard on her, but she pulled through. We do not know anyone tougher than Mary. For years, her doctor said that her heart could not hold out very long. Through the courtesy of her powerful will to live, she beat the odds multiple times and continued to live. In fact, she ultimately succumbed to hospital infections and her heart was the last organ to fail.

One of Charlene's friends since they were teenagers was diagnosed with a rare bone cancer in her mid-20s. Most people died from the type of cancer that she had. She had to be admitted to the hospital for her chemotherapy—that was back in the 1970s. Charlene remembers visiting her and thinking "she is so young and has two little girls." She was afraid her friend was dying and cried when she saw her in the hospital (her patient advocacy skills have come a long way since then). Charlene's friend said to her that she wasn't going to die and she didn't. She was the only survivor of her cohort and went on have another child, grandchildren, and we remained close friends until she passed away a couple of years ago from an infection. We now could easily list hundreds of people we know who beat cancer and are alive because of the marvels of modern medicine and research.

The overall message of this book is one of optimism because there is so much for people impacted by cancer to be optimistic about. If you are a "glass half full" person, you already are optimistic. If you are a "glass half empty" person in general or scared about confronting cancer, our main point is that you will survive even though you are scared and may have known others who died from cancer. We both tell patients and their families about being positive and will share that with you throughout the book. Scott generally is optimistic, positive, and energetic. But he was not a good patient and Charlene had to supply the optimism during that chapter of our lives. Scott did retain his quiet inner strength and that, combined with his dumb sense of humor and his smart wife, got him through.

According to Charlene

I wanted to write this book with Scott for everyone who has been touched by cancer. I insisted that the first several chapters be mostly about Scott, so he could express what he was feeling as he battled cancer. I asked him to be totally honest with his feelings. He describes things in an honest (and sometimes raw) way, while adding a little sarcasm and humor to explain his feelings. Hopefully, it will help you realize that you are not alone. I always have said that I was his caregiver, but I was not the patient and never truly felt what he felt. I admire his strength and willingness to share feelings and thoughts to help others even though I know he would have preferred to keep many of these things private.

CHAPTER 2

WE'RE NOT GOING TO DISNEY WORLD? ("YOU HAVE A TUMOR THE SIZE OF TWO BASEBALLS IN YOUR CHEST")

According to Scott

Charlene and I were set to go on vacation in Florida. I was in good general health (or so I thought). But for a couple of days before we were scheduled to leave, I had been experiencing an unusual feeling in my chest. Not so much pain as discomfort and heaviness—some unusual type of indigestion. The heaviness grew to the point that I felt I had about 20 pounds of weight on my chest. The night before we were to leave for Florida, Charlene told me to go to the local convenient care facility in the morning, if I was not feeling better. She thought I may have pulled a muscle in my chest or was just pulling her leg to get out of going on vacation. But she insisted that we would not leave until I got checked out.

I awoke to a sunny, mid-May morning. I still felt the weight on my chest so I dashed over to the nearby convenient care facility to get checked out quickly in compliance with Charlene's instructions. Sometimes it is easier to listen to your wife, especially when she is right. I got there, filled out a form, and told the nurse my symptoms. There were several people ahead of me, but they took me back to see an attending physician immediately. You have to know how to fill out a form properly to get to the front of the line. They hooked me up for an EKG. They were moving with too much urgency for my liking. Someone said that my description of the feeling of weight on my chest could be a sign of a heart attack. Men in their 30s do not do well with heart attacks. I was not particularly concerned because I did not feel like there was anything wrong with my heart. I reminded the doctor that I was a lawyer and the chance of me having a heart, much less a heart attack, was quite remote. He laughed, but did not seem amused. I recall becoming impatient and thinking that I should just go home.

The doctor had other plans for me. An ambulance arrived, a couple of EMT men appeared, and they were set to take me to the local hospital. I declined to go in the ambulance, and thought strongly about not going at all. But in view of the doctor's insistence, I went to the hospital. I drove to the hospital in my car being led by the ambulance.

As soon as I entered the emergency room, they swarmed me. It seemed like the movie *Groundhog Day* at first—providing the same history and hearing them express the same concerns as at the convenient care facility. An attendant took some blood, my history was taken by one of the doctors, and an intense discussion ensued about my symptoms. There was a lot of commotion and doctors all around. A nice young nurse took me for a chest x-ray. Once it was taken, I asked the technician whether the x-ray was normal. I did not receive a satisfactory answer. I was waiting for what seemed like an eternity. I have read many x-rays in my day and knew it did not take long. At one point, I asked for the x-ray film so I could review it myself, but they never got around to providing it to me.

It was getting late so I called Charlene to tell her I was all right, but went to the hospital for an x-ray and would be on my way home soon. There is nothing like being cross-examined by your wife. As I was explaining to Charlene on the phone what had transpired, a doctor came in and told me that I had "a mass the size of baseballs" in my chest. It was largely a blur after that, but I handed the phone to Charlene to speak directly with the doctor. Before the emergency room doctor placed me in the hands of other doctors, he said that I likely had cancer of some form. He wished me well.

I felt cold and clammy and started pacing back and forth. The next thing I knew, Charlene was with me at the hospital. Again, I was surrounded by a swarm of doctors, nurses, and various other unidentified people. It was a feeding frenzy. One doctor arrived on the scene and tried to take control. I think he was a thoracic surgeon, but he got off to a very bad start. He said that it might cause some discomfort, but he wanted to palpate my testicles, explaining that chest tumors are a common site for tumors secondary to testicular cancer and that form of cancer is fairly common in men my age. I declined in no uncertain terms.

"Mr. Seaman, we will need to admit you to the hospital and do several tests, it is important that we do this right away." I did not want to be admitted to the hospital. Charlene shared my discomfort about being admitted, but insisted that I have the scans and tests done. So I agreed to get the tests done, but only as an outpatient. I was not admitted, but they arranged to have a room for me as a place to stay between tests and to act as our central theatre of operations. I checked my voicemail numerous times, but unfortunately nothing required immediate attention as I had cleared the slate expecting to be on an airplane flight.

We embarked upon a day of extensive medical testing. I had much more medical testing done this day than in my entire life up to that point. There is much that I do not remember and that I probably did not even perceive. It was overwhelming and all seemed surreal. What I do remember is going for various tests and scans, but I recall only one at the moment—an ultrasound of the testicular area. The test proved to be negative. Of course, as Charlene says, the doctor was entirely correct to order this test as part of the work-up. I did not feel that way at the time and already decided he would not be my doctor on a going forward basis—that is assuming that I was indeed going forward.

While waiting in this hospital room between tests, a hospital staff person came into the room. She seemed friendly enough. She asked me if I would like something to drink. I thanked her and said I would like a Dr. Pepper. About forty-five or fifty minutes later, this young lady returned and said "Mr. Simons, here is your Sprite." Needless to say, she did not deserve a tip. You may be wondering why I recall these details, but cannot recall all of the tests I took? I don't know. But I do recall thinking, "since these people can't get my name right and they brought me the wrong soft drink, how can I trust them to give me the correct medications and to diagnose me correctly."

After the day of testing, the doctors had a lot to say, but no firm diagnosis. They tried mightily to get me to agree to be admitted to the hospital. My only mission at this point was to get out of this hospital. Charlene did not want me to be admitted (occasionally even she will agree with me) and she thought that we should get another opinion, consult, or at least have some time to determine the proper course of action. They were mulling around too long in the hospital so I expedited the discharge process, uttering something like, "thank you doctors, I am leaving now." One of the doctors said something like, "Mr. Seaman, you really need to stay here and . . . ." Charlene asked the doctors whether I would be endangering my life by leaving now. They said no, but we would need to make decisions in a day or two. Fortunately, Charlene had the presence of mind to get copies of the medical records and test results. Out we went, with no diagnosis other than a tumor the size of two baseballs in my chest, which likely was some type of cancer.

Notwithstanding the candid recitation of my contemporaneous feelings, the doctors and staff in the hospital did exactly what they were supposed to do. We did reach out to them subsequently to thank them.

We were physically and mentally drained when we left. There were things Charlene thought she heard that I did not hear. There were things I thought I heard that Charlene did not hear. Neither of us really knew what to do or where to turn. We probably stopped for something to eat, but neither of us can remember where. Arguably, I may be somewhat germophobic. To make matters worse, a few months earlier we watched someone die in the hospital during the course of a single day from what they said was a blood infection.

When we got home, I gave firm instructions to Charlene: "don't call anybody and don't say anything to anyone about this." I needed time to get my arms around things and did not want events to get ahead of me. I went upstairs and took a shower to rid myself of any hospital germs. By the time I returned downstairs a few minutes later, Charlene had called my mother and our daughter and a doctor was standing in our living room. Our neighbor and friend, a resident surgeon, was reading the records Charlene brought home. He said that I needed to see a thoracic surgeon immediately and he knew the top thoracic surgeon in the country.

He called his surgeon's office and set up an appointment for 11:00 a.m. the next morning. The surgeon's office said that medical records were not enough, we needed to bring the actual CT scans and x-ray film. I just reminded myself that I had CT scans of the chest, abdomen, and pelvis taken earlier that day. I was amazed (and displeased at the time) that we were able to be seen by the leading thoracic surgeon in the country the next day, when it can take months to get an appointment with an internist. Sometimes, it is who you know.

As I recall, I agreed reluctantly to see the doctor and find out what he had to say. It would be just an office visit, not a visit to schedule surgery. I thought it would buy me some time to think things over.

The next morning we headed back to the hospital to get the scans. Charlene spent a lot of time the evening before making the arrangements. Many of you know the hoops you have to go through to get your own medical records and we went through all of those hoops. Even so, when we arrived the next morning, the records department people claimed that they needed a minimum of three days to get copies of the scans for me. I was persistent and refused to leave without the scans. After some heated dialogue, they emerged with the scans, handed them to me, and I left.

Even though our friend vouched for the surgeon, we needed more information. Charlene called around. After we picked up the films, we went straight to the surgeon's office. On our way to the surgeon's office, we spoke to an out of state thoracic surgeon who was very nice and took the time to speak with us at the request of one of my partners. He gave us a lot of information and some questions to ask. He confirmed that this doctor was not only a preeminent thoracic surgeon, but the best in the world. He told us how the surgeon we were going to see was revered by other thoracic surgeons. This gentleman ended by saying he thought I had better than a fifty-fifty chance of survival. I am sure he intended that to be comforting, but I have lost a lot of coin flips in my life. So have the Chicago Bears.

We arrived at the surgeon's office on time. We filled out forms, gave the receptionist the medical records, the x-ray film, and the CT scans. We had to wait a few minutes, but not as long as the usual waiting period. We saw a tall, distinguished, white-haired man walk into the office wearing blue scrubs. He reminded us of General Waverly from the old Bing Crosby movie *White Christmas*. We admired the way he seemed to flow from surgery into the office without skipping a beat. Charlene and I like *White Christmas*, but I was thinking that I had seen my last Chicago winter.

Next, we were escorted into an examination room. Both Charlene and I were impressed that the room was impeccably clean. The tile floor was shining, everything was in its place, and it looked like you could eat off the floor. Since he was dealing with a germaphobe, the surgeon was off to a good start. A few minutes later, he entered the room and introduced himself by providing his full name. He had a voice that was both commanding and soothing. We shook hands and I confirmed he had a good grip and learned he was a quarterback in college. He took my history. He said he had just read all of the records we provided. He flipped the CT scan films right on the clips on the lighted board in his office. He did it with flair and the scans stuck right where they were supposed to stick. This would be the case in every follow-up examination. Remember, never use a surgeon that does not look at the films himself or does not have the "flip and clip" down pat. This is just a sample of the cogent advice we will be providing you throughout this book.

While pointing to the scans, the surgeon showed us exactly where the tumor was and pointed out its large size. The surgeon told us there were six potential causes of the huge mass in my chest, all but one were cancer. It is possible that it was a benign thymoma, but he doubted it. I forget what all of the menu items were but they included germ cell carcinoma and lymphoma. He said if it was lymphoma, the standard procedure would be to close me up without removing it and send me to the oncologist for chemotherapy. Nonetheless, he said that he was going to remove it surgically even if it was lymphoma. The mass appeared to be invading my heart on one end and the lung on the other. He said he performed surgery a couple of years earlier on the wife of a prominent doctor at another leading medical institution who had lymphoma. He said it caused some controversy, but the outcome was very good. He warned that, if the tumor was impacting the phrenic nerve (the nerve that controls breathing), it was possible that I would lose that nerve and the ability to breathe from the right side. He said I would live, breathe only from the other side, and adapt to it.

Next, the surgeon started to explain the potential for the tumor to be secondary to testicular cancer. I am now reminded that this was one of the menu items as was lung cancer. I told him that I had an ultrasound done and everything was alright. Suspecting this issue might raise its ugly head again, I had the report in my pocket. He looked at the report I handed him and was satisfied without the need for further examination.

This doctor was old school, had a commanding presence, and obviously knew exactly what he was doing. I immediately had complete confidence in him. Charlene felt the same way. Charlene asked what other doctors the surgeon was going to have me see. The other hospital was trying to set me up with a cardiologist, pulmonologist, and several other doctors in addition to a thoracic surgeon. The surgeon said he reviewed all the tests and records and did not see any evidence of a cardiac problem. He asked whether I had any heart conditions or complaints. I said no and Charlene explained what the other hospital intended to do. He just laughed confidently and said that he was the only doctor that I would need. There are times and cases in which a multidisciplinary approach is appropriate, but this was not one of them. He said that he would operate the following Tuesday. He then gave us explicit directions about when and where we should go, and about what to do and not to do the night before surgery. We asked some other questions which he answered. I don't recall all of the questions or answers. I do vividly remember him telling us confidently and without qualification that I would survive the surgery. The receptionist gave us lots of papers to read on our way out of the office.

While we were waiting outside for the valet to get our car, I called my office and spoke to one of my partners. I briefly told him about the strange thing that happened to us on the way to our vacation. I alerted him to the fact that contingent plans must be made promptly for all of my cases and I would be in to begin that process.

As fate would have it, I was diagnosed with cancer the same day that Frank Sinatra died. This did not improve my mental state. I thought the death of the Chairman of the Board did not auger well for my long-term survival. Later that day and over the course of the next several days, I was inundated with phone calls, cards, letters, and voice messages from across the country with people expressing condolences on Frank's death. This was before email and social media. Word had not yet leaked out about my diagnosis.

During the less than a week between my visit to the convenient care center and the impending surgery, a lot of things happened and I had a lot of things to do. Keeping busy was better than just sitting around and worrying. Besides, I was able to do enough worrying anyway. To my mind, I had less than a week to live, not including any period for lingering and suffering. Surely dying in surgery would be more noble (and less torture) than dying from chemotherapy. To the outside world, I was in good spirits, laughing, telling jokes, and projecting complete confidence that I would fully recover in short order. I hate the word "short," so the fact I used the phrase suggests that I was not in my normal state of mind. Of course, on the inside, I was preparing to die and was taking the appropriate steps. I made sure my personal papers were in order. I filled out a health care power of attorney form, a living will, and a general power of attorney in favor of Charlene. I revised my will to take out the unworthy.

The next day, I went to the office and started implementing my plan to reassign cases and make sure that our clients' interests were protected. The firm and my partners were very supportive. I had to confront the issue of what to tell clients. I thought my health was a private matter and my personal preference would have been to say nothing or simply indicate that I would be extending my vacation by a couple of weeks. But our clients' interests overrode my own preferences. I had been entrusted to handle multi-million dollar matters and matters implicating serious portfolio interests of our clients. Accordingly, I needed to assure them that contingency plans have been made and make sure that they felt comfortable with those plans. The approach was simple and clear. Tell them the truth and provide them with as many or few details as they wanted. Not only was this the right thing to do, it turned out to be a blessing. I was truly touched by the genuine concern and interest of these wonderful professionals who had entrusted us to handle their cases. Although respectful of my privacy, most wanted to know all of the gory details. Notwithstanding my statements here about thinking I would die, there was a part of me that had faith that somehow I eventually would be alright. My private predictions of the outcome did vacillate considerably, but my public declarations were consistently positive. I suppose that I was suffering from a condition known as "pre-surgery schizophrenia."

Apart from getting my personal and professional affairs in order, I had to say my goodbyes to family and friends without actually saying goodbye. I had to convey final thoughts and words of advice without indicating finality or evoking sadness in others. The hardest thing was realizing that I might be saying goodbye to Charlene and our daughter. In the final analysis, I knew that I needed treatment to live. I was very worried about what would happen to Charlene if I died. I am hardly the perfect husband, but I do try to look after Charlene. In convincing me (or forcing me) to have treatment, Charlene made two major arguments. I had to do it for myself. And she made the much more powerful argument that I had to do it for her and our daughter. Charlene emphasized that cancer would not kill me, but she would kill me if I did not get whatever treatment was necessary.

I did take a modicum of comfort from something my grandfather introduced me to as a young boy, a copy of which still hangs in my office to this day:

> Go placidly amid the noise and haste,
> and remember what peace there may be in silence.
> As far as possible without surrender
> be on good terms with all persons.
> Speak your truth quietly and clearly;
> and listen to others,
> even the dull and the ignorant;
> they too have their story.

Avoid loud and aggressive persons,
they are vexations to the spirit.
If you compare yourself with others,
you may become vain and bitter;
for always there will be greater and lesser persons than yourself.
Enjoy your achievements as well as your plans.

Keep interested in your own career, however humble;
it is a real possession in the changing fortunes of time.
Exercise caution in your business affairs;
for the world is full of trickery.
But let this not blind you to what virtue there is;
many persons strive for high ideals;
and everywhere life is full of heroism.

Be yourself.
Especially, do not feign affection.
Neither be cynical about love;
for in the face of all aridity and disenchantment
it is as perennial as the grass.

Take kindly the counsel of the years,
gracefully surrendering the things of youth.
Nurture strength of spirit to shield you in sudden misfortune.
But do not distress yourself with dark imaginings.
Many fears are born of fatigue and loneliness.
Beyond a wholesome discipline,
be gentle with yourself.

You are a child of the universe,
no less than the trees and the stars;
you have a right to be here.
And whether or not it is clear to you,
no doubt the universe is unfolding as it should.

Therefore be at peace with God,
whatever you conceive Him to be,
and whatever your labors and aspirations,

in the noisy confusion of life keep peace with your soul.
With all its sham, drudgery, and broken dreams,
it is still a beautiful world.
Be cheerful.
Strive to be happy.

Desiderata—Max Ehrmann—1927

I was quite busy the few days before surgery. Still, on one level, my mind was in a reflective and assessment mode: Who had been good to me during my life? Who had cheated me? What did I accomplish? What will I miss? What should I do during my last few days on this planet? What will heaven be like? Will I be able to look down and see what's happening or have any influence on things? Naturally, I had more questions than answers. Regrets . . . I had a few. I wondered what I could do for my friends and allies before surgery. I prayed a little and Charlene prayed a lot.

The night before my surgery, Charlene and I stayed at a hotel downtown. This made it easier for us to get to the hospital at the early hour we had to arrive. Before dinner, we went outside for a walk. We saw a group of priests stirring and starting to vacate a gathering. Perhaps they were there to administer my last rites? Charlene looked over and said, "there is Francis Cardinal George." She called him over, introduced us, and told him about my impending surgery. Cardinal George knew we were friends with Cardinal Bernardin and could not have been nicer. He wished me the best and promised to pray for me. Charlene took seeing Cardinal George as a sign from God that everything would be alright.

We had dinner and attempted to have a good time, but it was impossible given what I faced the next morning. When Charlene and I returned to our room, we watched a tape of Sinatra in concert—it seemed like an appropriate way to end things. Although we were going through this together, we also were going through this separately. Here is how Charlene saw things.

According to Charlene

Talk about a change in plans. We were going to Disney World, my favorite place on the planet. Everyone I know could testify that it is my favorite place. Usually I would drag Scott there once or twice a year. No matter how busy our schedules, we had to find the time to go. He had these pains and I thought he was trying to get out of going to Disney World. To be safe, I made him go to the convenient care facility to get checked. Honestly, I thought he would come home with some muscle relaxers and that would be the end of it. I really thought it was just from carrying around those big briefcases that lawyers use. He didn't seem to have heart attack symptoms or I would have rushed him to the hospital. Still, I wanted to make sure he was alright before we left.

Scott called me from the hospital and said he was okay, but they were doing more tests. While I was speaking with him on the phone, a doctor came in and said to Scott, "you have a large mass in your chest!" The doctor got on the telephone with me. The emergency room doctor reiterated to me that he had a huge mass in his chest. I asked what it was and he said it could be many things, most likely cancer—maybe lymphoma, maybe a thymoma (which could be benign), maybe metastasized testicular or lung cancer. Everything that had to be ruled out was a cancerous tumor, except a benign thymoma. I headed straight to the hospital. My heart was in my hand.

When I arrived at the hospital, I took one look at Scott and knew that I had to take charge and be as strong as I could. He was hooked up to equipment and just pacing back and forth. Though his demeanor generally is calm during challenges, that was not the case today. He was a completely uncooperative patient. He was extremely impatient with the doctors. There were plenty of doctors with whom to be impatient. They seemed to come out of the woodwork—a cardiologist, a pulmonologist, an internist, an oncologist, and others that I cannot remember or never knew who they were. They were talking fast and I just kept hearing bad things. This was not Disney World and it was the opposite of fun and relaxation. I thought this was turning into a nightmare and I wanted to wake up.

I remember telling Scott that I had to go to the bathroom. I went to the bathroom to try to comprehend what was taking place. I threw water on my face and started hyperventilating. I was crying in the paper towels trying to muffle the sound. I actually had a panic attack and had to try to gain control. I had to try to compose myself because I could not let Scott know I was freaking out. I went back in the emergency room area and tried to comfort Scott saying, "it is not going to be cancer, don't worry!"

Scott was refusing a testicular ultrasound. I told him it was important to see if there was a tumor or cancer in that area and that the test would eliminate this as a possibility. We had to start ruling things out to find out the cause of the mass. Scott had a stress test, CT scans, extensive blood work, and he saw all the doctors they wanted him to see. All Scott wanted to do was get out of the hospital. I insisted he have the tests done, but thought we needed a second opinion and time to absorb what was happening. The doctors were pushing us to stay. I asked the doctors whether Scott was in any kind of immediate jeopardy if he left and they said he could leave, but we needed to act immediately.

I did break the "order" that Scott issued about not talking to anyone about the unfolding events. This should not have come as a surprise to him. When we got married I promised to love and honor him, but I refused to include the words "and obey" in our vows. I needed to talk to someone because I was so scared. Yet, I could not show Scott. I had to be tough for him and tell him no matter what we were dealing with he was going to be alright. While at the hospital, I used the public phone to cancel our reservations for the flight and Disney World resort reservations. I remember telling the girl at the Disney resort we wouldn't be coming. There was a 24-hour cancellation period and she said my credit card would be charged. I told her my husband was in the hospital and he had a mass in his chest that could be cancer. I was crying softly. She was very nice and said they would cancel the reservation and told me to call back when we wanted to rebook. I told her I did not know if we would ever be back. Our whole life changed in minutes and I did not know what the future would bring.

I called our daughter and told her. Next, I called Scott's mother and I was crying. She was shocked and I told her we would call back later. I then called Scott's firm and spoke with the executive director. I told him that Scott had a large mass in his chest and it might be cancer. I was crying and he got very quiet. He assured me that the insurance was very good and everything would be okay. It was time for me to wipe the tears and go back to being tough and not showing my fear and the horrible feeling inside thinking Scott may die.

I called our daughter and Scott's mother again when we got home. Scott did not know that I called them from the hospital. Our neighbor was a good friend and a resident surgeon. Within a couple of minutes, our friend was at our door. Soon after he arrived, Scott came downstairs and he was correct—I did have a doctor in the living room. I made sure to bring home copies of all the test results. The doctor studied everything and called the thoracic surgeon who we saw the next morning. We were just starting on our horrific adventure.

The one bright spot was we had the best surgeon and Scott and I knew it. This turned out to be so important not only because of his skills, but because if it were any other doctor I am not sure that I would have been able to convince Scott to have any treatment for cancer. He did not want to have surgery. He generally is open-minded and logical. But when he does not want to do something, he can be intractable. After we met with the surgeon, Scott realized that he needed to undergo surgery. Once we made up his mind, there was no vacillating on the subject. We both were preparing ourselves and each other.

Scott did what he felt he needed to do in terms of preparing papers and documents. We had the discussions I suppose all couples have at these times. In terms of health care wishes, he made it clear that he did not want to be a vegetable. He gave me the health care power of attorney, but did not provide any more instructions despite my pressing him. He said "I trust you to make the decisions that you think are best, you are the doctor in the family."

I was strong on the outside, but on the inside I was very scared and nervous. Scott is the love of my life and I could not imagine living without him.

CHAPTER 3

"HONEY, I'M A DEAD MAN" (THE SURGERY AND CANCER DIAGNOSIS)

According to Scott

Naturally, I did not sleep well, if I even slept a wink the night before the surgery. It did not matter because soon I would be under the knife and might have the rest of eternity to sleep. About 4:30 a.m., I took a shower, using extra amounts of anti-bacteria soap, and got ready to head to the hospital. We hopped in a cab and I filled the cab driver with many deep thoughts on the brief cab ride. Unfortunately for him, he spoke little English and likely received little of the wisdom I provided. His eyes lit up when I gave him a $100 dollar bill for a ten dollar cab ride and told him to keep the change. Charlene sometimes complained (erroneously) that I was a light tipper. I remember Frank Sinatra would always instruct his people to "duke 'em a c-note." So I thought my final tip on earth should be a c-note. It seemed both appropriate and ironic that I was thinking about Bill Zehme's book *Frank Sinatra And The Lost Art Of Livin'* as my own art of livin' was about to be lost.

We arrived at the hospital and began the admission process. I filled out various papers and signed consent forms. These are forms that no rational person, particularly a lawyer, should ever sign. But you either sign the forms or they won't operate. At this point, not being operated on was an appealing option to me. I had some specific instructions that I wrote out and made my consents expressly contingent upon them being followed. Among my instructions were that Charlene must be allowed to be with me at all times after surgery regardless of where I am. There is no better advocate than Charlene and I wanted her around at all times. Also, there must be a television in the recovery room tuned to the Chicago Bulls basketball game. It was the NBA finals. It was billed as the Bulls last dance and it could be mine. I turned in the completed forms and was instructed to take a seat.

Before I knew it, they called my name and I was ushered to the back. This was all new to me, I had never had surgery before. I went into surgery sooner than I expected. My surgeon liked to operate early when the staff was fresh. He had seniority and got his choice of operating times and staff. I looked around and saw other poor souls starting to get prepared for surgery. Now gurneys were beginning to line up behind me. This was one parade I was not happy to be leading. As I was laying on the gurney, I could not help but think this may be the last time I am conscious. Well, I didn't have much time to think about what my final thoughts should be because they quickly rolled me into the operating room and started pumping anesthetics in me. I looked up and saw a bunch of people in masks, just like on *ER*. I saw the face of the surgeon that I wanted to see. I told a quality joke or two, and Charlene will have to pick up the story from here because I am now out cold . . . .

According to Charlene

After Scott went into surgery, I walked around the hospital nervously trying to stop thinking about what was going on. I thought the surgery would take about three hours and I had to try to keep my mind free from all the things that could go wrong. I called our daughter to tell her that her dad was in surgery. She was taking care of a bunch of errands for us, including putting one of our dogs – who was 17 and sick – to sleep. It was too much for us to handle at the time. I then called Scott's mother to tell her. She was going to come up to the hospital later in the day. I was alone with no one to talk to about what was going on. I just walked around because I could not sit still. Time dragged on and on. After two hours, I started going to the surgery waiting room because I knew the doctor would be out soon. I got there and asked the receptionist if Scott still was in surgery. She called back to the operating area and she told me that he was not out of surgery yet. So I sat and waited and waited. When you are in a surgery waiting room it is horrible because every time that phone rings people jump up and are waiting for the news about their loved one knowing their life and well-being are hanging in the balance. I had experienced this horrible waiting before with my mother. It is nerve racking and going through it never gets better. After three hours of surgery, there still was no call. Four hours and there still was no call from the surgeon. I kept going to the receptionist and asking for the status. The surgeon had said he expected the surgery to take about three hours and it has now been four hours. I felt something must be wrong. I feared maybe Scott had died and they were trying to revive him. I wanted to be someone else so I did not have to think of all of these terrible thoughts. I just tried not to think of the bad stuff. It was going on five hours and I was a nervous wreck.

After five and one half hours, the phone rang and the receptionist called me in and told me that the surgeon was coming out. She escorted me to a small room. I knew it was not good that she was taking me to a room to be alone with the surgeon. I did not know what the doctor was going to tell me. The room had a couch, a chair, and a table with a lamp and a telephone. I still can picture this vividly. The surgeon walked into the room, I stood up, and the surgeon told me to sit down. As I was in the process of sitting down, he also started to sit and he said, "Scott has cancer." My heart fell to the ground. I started crying and the doctor just sat and did not say anything. I was just crying and tried to compose myself so I could ask him questions. I remember apologizing for crying. I asked, "How is Scott now? Is he going to die?" I was so scared.

The doctor started explaining how the surgery went and I remember him saying he worked very hard to remove all of the cancer that he could and he worked until he saw pink tissue. He said "I worked all the way to my elbows to get out all I could." He said the tumor was in his right lung, in his pericardium (the covering around his heart) and it was wrapped around his phrenic nerve and the phrenic nerve had to be removed. He also removed the pericardium and part of Scott's right lung. He said the initial frozen biopsy report indicated that the tumor was a germ cell cancer, but he said they will not have a clear diagnosis until the full and final pathology report came back. He explained it could be another cancer and that, of course, it could be lymphoma, but so far the tests said germ cell. I asked him how bad is a germ cell tumor and he said it was not the best type of cancer to have. Other cancers would have a better survival percentage.

Now everything depended on the grade, stage, and type of the cancer with which we were dealing. The surgeon was very nice and sat with me and explained as much as he could. The tumor was around 10 cm x 8 cm and it was very invasive. One good thing was that the tumor was all in the same area (albeit a broad area) and they did not see any masses anywhere else. He told me that Scott would have to learn to breathe a little differently and that his breathing would diminish on his lower lobe of his right lung and the left lung would have to compensate. He said the most important thing now is to identify the tumor and then determine what chemotherapy or radiation would be appropriate. He said I could stay in the room if I wanted and make some calls. I asked when I could see Scott and he said Scott was still in recovery. He said they would call me back to see him in a few minutes. He left, shut the door, and I just started crying uncontrollably.

I picked up the phone and called our daughter and she said she was on her way. Next, I called Scott's secretary to tell her. I was crying as I told her Scott had cancer. She was real quiet on the phone and she handed the phone to one of Scott's partners. He got on the phone and I told him Scott had cancer and he asked me where I was in the hospital. He said, "I will be right there." I hung the phone up and didn't know what to do with myself. I was so upset. The door opened and it was Scott's mother. I just told her immediately that he had cancer and she started saying, "damn it, damn it." I remember her anger. We both started crying and hugging each other. The door opened again and it was Scott's law partner. I couldn't believe how fast he got there. He showed up almost immediately. The three of us were all in the room and hugging each other and crying. Now, of course, his partner was not crying like Scott's mother and me, but there were tears coming down.

According to Scott

Either I am in hell or heaven is not living up to its billing. Hold on a minute . . . to my surprise, it appears that I may have survived the surgery. I have no memory of the surgery itself. My first post-surgical memory is laying in the gurney after the surgery. I think I was in the hall outside of the operating room, but I could have been in the grocery store parking lot for all I knew. I asked whether the surgery was over and how it went. Some man in green scrubs told me that I was out of surgery and provided me with some standard form of assurance. I remember seeing our friend, the resident surgeon, after the surgery and he told me that surgery went well. I took it as a good sign that he was joking with me about several things that I will not get into here.

Although the medication certainly numbed the pain, I felt a deep soreness all over and in a way I had never felt before. I must have been run over by a truck. I heard clanging noises as they banged my gurney against others on the way to or from the recovery area. Those gurney drivers seemed to bang into everything and everyone around. I vaguely remember seeing one of my partners while I was in the recovery area. This was in spite of my instructions for no one to come, but the violation was alright because it reminded me that I actually may be alive or at least had the nucleus to form a law firm in heaven.

Eventually, I made it to the intensive care area. I remember seeing Charlene when I was rolled into intensive care. I wanted to grab her hand, but was unable to move my hand for some reason. She asked me how I felt and I lied and said fine. I asked her how she was and she said she was fine. She told me that the surgeon said he worked his fingers to the bone to remove the entire tumor. I figured the surgery was going to be expensive since the doctor already was marketing his work. Charlene told me that I was going to be okay. I did not believe her, but I did not have the energy to argue. I was in and out of consciousness all night—it actually was all afternoon and night. I do remember being introduced to my nurse and thinking that I needed to be nice to her because she easily could kill me. Later, another nurse introduced herself to me and told me that she was taking over for the other nurse. One of them was named Michelle. Either their shifts were unusually brief or I was knocked out for a while.

At some point, I noticed that they did not have the Bulls basketball game on in direct contravention of my orders. They claimed they could not get the channel. I likely was sleeping through most of the game anyway. Later, when I expressed my irritation over their failure to follow my instructions, they wheeled in a television set and I saw the highlights on the late night news. The Bulls won.

I noticed that I had various tubes in me. In particular, there was a drainage tube in the abdominal area. We had made arrangements ahead of time for Charlene and my mother to stay at a hotel just a couple of blocks away from the hospital. I did not have a phone in intensive care, but the nurse told me Charlene kept calling to check on me. I told the nurse to tell Charlene that I was okay and wanted her to sleep. I asked the nurse to get the surgeon so I could get the straight story on my expiration date. She said he would be in to see me in the morning. I asked her to get my medical records and to read the surgery report and post-operation report to me line by line. I don't know whether she even attempted to humor me by reading the report to me because I was sleeping much of the time.

Later that night or the next morning they moved me again. I remember being given a sponge bath by a large, elderly, and very nice lady. I did not like the helplessness that I felt. I was lying flat on the bed and could hardly see a thing. Bells were ringing, alarms were sounding, frantic movements and conversations were emanating from surrounding areas. I had no way of knowing the time and I was in and out of consciousness. Back to the nice lady who was bathing me with a sponge. She was singing religious hymns in a soft and sweet tone. I was impressed by her gentleness and her taking the effort to be reassuring. I am sure this was not unique to me, but rather her wonderful way of approaching her job. I thanked her and she said I would be okay.

Afterwards, I was starting to get agitated and impatient—I guess the meds were wearing off. I was feeling more discomfort, and my natural nasty personality was starting to reemerge. I was complaining about the noise and told the nurse or whoever was trying to poke me to go away.

Charlene arrived. She started reassuring me and trying to make me feel better. I was still out of it, but was starting to orientate myself to my curtained partition area of the intensive care unit. Shortly after Charlene arrived, the surgeon showed up. He towered over my bed dressed in his scrubs. He must have finished his surgeries for the morning. He asked how I was doing. "You're the doctor, you tell me" was my response. I knew that it was a bad sign that the surgeon came to give me the news directly. As I lawyer, I would often allow attorneys working with me to report to clients on favorable developments, but I would always deliver any bad news myself.

The surgeon looked at me and said "well, it's cancer." I turned to Charlene and said "Honey, I'm a dead man!" The surgeon continued to talk, but I tuned him out. I heard all I needed to hear. He did say that the tumor was very invasive, but they worked hard and he was confident that they got everything out. He said he made sure that there was a healthy margin of pink tissue (non-cancerous tissue) everywhere. He said that the phrenic nerve was heavily incased in the tumor and it was removed. I imagine that a surgeon has to be able to pour on the bad news without taking a breath. "Doctor, you could have been a lawyer," I mumbled. I remember thinking, I might not be able to breathe properly for my remaining days.

The surgeon stated that the preliminary "frozen section" biopsy taken during surgery showed that it was a "germ cell" tumor. I did not know what a "germ cell" cancer was, but it was cancer and I hate germs. He tried to emphasize the "good news," that he was confident that he removed all of the cancer. I asked the surgeon what was next. He said that they needed to get the final pathology report back. Once he had the final report, he would be able to tell me more about the prognosis and what, if any, additional treatment I would need. I thanked the doctor. He had no control over what it was he removed and at least he was able to remove the entire tumor. Moreover, thanking the surgeon was proper form. The surgeon instructed me to rest and told us that he would be sending me to a room later in the day. He wanted me up and walking as soon as possible.

When he left, Charlene told me that the key was that the doctor removed all of the cancer and I was going to recover. She told me that I had to be strong and fight for her. She was strong for me and I knew that this fight was just beginning. She told me that my mother was here and my daughter and brothers were coming to see me later. One had come in from out of town. I told her that I did not want to see or talk to anyone. I am not quite sure why I felt so depressed and devastated. I had presumed going into surgery that I had cancer. Yet, when the surgeon told me it was cancer, it hit me. It is human nature to hold out hope for the best even while fearing the worst. I was not out of the woods yet, I was not even out of the hospital. The diagnosis was cancer. I did not like it. It scared the hell out of me. But I was going to have to come to terms with it. I was under the care of the best surgeon in the world. I would have to fight through this and tough it out. With my daughter, mother, and brothers coming to see me, I had to try to collect myself and put on a positive face. No problem, as a lawyer I probably should not have feelings anyway and there was no need for me actually to believe the sunny picture that I would try to paint.

It was not until I left the hospital and looked at the medical records that I realized just how extensive my surgery actually had been. Had I known this earlier, the raw power of my mind would have caused me to die instantaneously. The records confirmed that the surgeon did a masterful job in removing the entire tumor and underscored the importance of being in the hands of a fine surgeon.

According to Charlene

The surgery and recovery were physically and emotionally draining for me. I really was concerned that Scott would die in surgery. One of Scott's partners (whose husband was a doctor) reassured me that Scott would do fine in the surgery. Post-surgery was the more dangerous time. Still, I knew that it was going to be a very invasive and difficult surgery. I did not want to leave the hospital at all the night of the surgery, but they did not want me to stay in the intensive care area overnight. I also knew that I needed to try to get some sleep and had to be back very early in the morning. Scott did not know he had cancer and I knew the doctor would arrive early and tell him. I wanted to get there before the doctor so that I could tell him in as gentle way as possible that he had cancer and to reassure him that everything was going to be okay. Needless to say, I was not able to sleep. I kept calling intensive care to check on Scott. I kept tossing and turning and did not sleep at all. I had been undergoing surgery of the mind.

I got up and headed back to the hospital first thing in the morning. Scott still was in intensive care. He saw me and smiled. We hugged as best as we could, considering all the equipment hooked up to him and his limited mobility. He asked me how I was feeling. Just as I thought, I was not there but a couple of minutes and the surgeon arrived. Before I could tell Scott in my way, the doctor blurted out to Scott that he had cancer. Having to see Scott learn the news this way was painful.

Our roller coaster ride was just beginning and there was much to be sad and scared about. But there was one huge silver lining. Scott survived surgery and was alive. We would have our battles ahead, but this was far better than what I feared: never seeing him alive again. At least, he was here to battle and we could battle things through together. And that's the way we will tell the rest of our story—together.

CHAPTER 4

"I'D RATHER HAVE THE TUMOR IN THE PATHOLOGIST'S JAR THAN IN MY CHEST" (POST-SURGERY RECOVERY)

Scott was still highly medicated, but starting to come around. He saw his visitors and actually was glad that they came. He was weak, but spoke with everyone for a few minutes. Just knowing they were there and cared made things better as we were beginning the recovery and damage assessment stage of our unwanted adventure. Scott attempted to put a positive spin on things for our family. He said the surgeon did a fabulous job. He does remember telling them that the surgeon removed the entire tumor and "I'd rather have the tumor in the pathologist's jar than in my chest." He liked that line and used it a lot over the next few days.

Scott's time in the intensive care unit was about to come to an end. For some strange reason, he did not want to leave the custody of the intensive care unit. He was starting to realize just how invasive the surgery had been and that his recovery was not going to be easy assuming he would recover at all. He was in the intensive care unit for less than a day and felt entitled to at least two or three days of intensive care as part of his deluxe hospital stay package. He could not move much and he had a lot of difficulty breathing.

He wanted privacy and did not want to deal with any other patient or their germs or problems since there was no doubt in his mind that he was now the sickest person in the world. They moved him to a private room. The next couple of days were a blur, but here is what we do recall. At some point during the first night in the room, Scott was able to talk Charlene into leaving for the night to get some rest. Once she left, Scott remembered that he was a lawyer with clients and cases. For the first time since law school, he had not thought about that for 24 hours. In his defense, he was sedated most of that time.

Suddenly, the compulsion came over him to check his voicemail. There was a phone on a nightstand about a foot away from the bed. He could not move well and when he moved even a little, he could feel his heart actually move and bang against his chest. He was exhausted after his futile attempts to move a few inches. After about 30 minutes of maneuvering, twisting, wiggling, losing his breath and resting, he finally got close to the phone and struggled to pick it up. It took every ounce of energy that he could muster to reach and dial the phone. This was before I-phones. He dialed his voicemail and, after all of that effort, was denied access to the voicemail system. The firm's executive director, in collusion with others including Charlene, decided it would be best if Scott did not start making calls or checking messages until after he recovered from surgery. His efforts to retrieve voicemails were thwarted, at least for the time being. He was displeased.

The next day, the surgeon came in with "good news." The frozen section biopsy report was not correct. The final pathology showed lymphoma, not germ cell cancer. The surgeon said that Scott would need chemotherapy and possibly radiation. "Where is the good news," Scott asked. He said, "lymphoma is cancer. I can't breathe. Every time I move even a little my heart rolls around in my chest like a bowling ball. There is no way that I am going through chemotherapy or radiation. Where is the good news?" The doctor said the exact type of lymphoma that he had, but we only remembered "non-Hodgkin." The surgeon said that the good news was that this meant a better prognosis. It turns out that a germ cell tumor of the size and location as the one in Scott would have meant a poor prognosis. Scott failed to gleam a scintilla of good news from the surgeon's words, but Charlene did. She knew that lymphoma meant a better prognosis based upon what the doctor told her previously and her research.

The surgeon was a task master, he told us not to worry about any of the follow-up treatment now. Scott's tasks were: start getting up and walking; start coughing to clear his lungs; and start breathing into a spirometer, which the surgeon handed him. In response to Charlene's questioning, the surgeon said Scott would be okay, his breathing would come around to a large extent in time, but he had to start moving, walking, and coughing. With those words, the tall, distinguished surgeon left the room.

Now it was time to assess the doctor's recovery plan. First, we had seen a spirometer before, as Mary had it after some of her surgeries. We did not know its name. As to getting up and walking, Scott thought that was out of the question for at least a month or two. Finally, there was no way he was going to try to cough. Even with the morphine, it was painful as his ribs had been sawed and his chest opened as though he had open heart surgery. He no longer had two functioning lungs. Now he was reduced to one functional lung and parts of another lung that was paralyzed.

By this time, Scott noticed a more "pressing danger." He had a drainage tube and stuff was leaking from his abdomen. He wanted to speak with the surgeon immediately. The surgeon was gone, but the nurse paged his fellow who assisted during the surgery. The fellow was a fine young surgeon who was honing his skills (on Scott) by learning from the best in the business. At the time he was the younger doctor who Scott thought he could trick into telling him the truth.

The medication and pain temporarily dulled Scott's acumen as an interrogator, but he proceeded to poise questions to the young surgeon. First, some background. What are your credentials? How many surgeries like this have you done? What was your role in the surgery? Was the main surgeon there directing you? Next, Scott launched into what he called the substantive questions. How long do I have to live? How much cancer was there? What was left when you finished? Why was the frozen section wrong and how do we know what cancer I really have? What is the difference between lymphoma and germ cell cancer? What is my prognosis? How can I breathe? What about my heart rolling around—that can't be good? The young surgeon did the best he could to answer our questions, but Scott generally was not satisfied with the answers.

Now we had the name "lymphoma" tossed out there. What is this exactly? Scott did not like the way the word sounded or how it was spelled. He was too tired, whacked out, and now in too much pain to be able to put much mind power into it. The surgeon said he got it all out. Scott figured if it stays gone, he will fight this through and live. If the surgeon did not get all of the cancer or it comes back, he can at least say that he attempted treatment.

* * *

We briefly skip ahead to demonstrate "It's a Small World After All." Moving forward, 15 or 16 years later when Scott was hospitalized at a different hospital for a heart attack we ultimately learned was caused by his chemotherapy and radiation treatment for lymphoma, a general surgeon came into Scott's room to evaluate whether he was a candidate for bypass surgery. The doctor looked at Scott and said that, due to his prior cancer surgery, he was not a candidate for bypass surgery. Scott appeared to be completely ignoring what the doctor was saying, instead focusing all of his attention on the doctor's name tag. Apparently he actually heard what the doctor was saying because he looked at the doctor, laughed, and asked the doctor whether he recognized him. The doctor gave a blank stare. Scott told the doctor "I wouldn't complain about the prior surgery too much if I were you because you were involved in the surgery." The general surgeon was the fellow who assisted Dr. Faber with the surgery. He was the young doctor Scott was interrogating above. Scott refreshed the doctor's recollection and we all talked about the surgery, Scott's subsequent course, and Dr. Faber. Scott was glad to see the doctor was now an accomplished surgeon and held a prominent position. He actually took this news about not being a candidate for bypass surgery quiet well because he preferred stents to bypass surgery. Back to our cancer story.

* * *

While Scott was contemplating a graceful exit from the planet, Charlene got to work learning all she could about lymphoma. She spoke with a husband of one of Scott's partners. He is an obstetrician and one hell of a good guy. Charlene asked him what the treatment would be and about Scott's prognosis. He gave Charlene a checklist of information to obtain: exactly what type of lymphoma; the precise location; how many lymph nodes were involved; and how bulky was the tumor? These were staging questions. Charlene demanded information from the hospital. It was very late at night. The nurses did not have any information and no doctors were around. Charlene asked a nurse to wake up an intern who was trying to get an hour or two of sleep. The intern knew less than we did, but was kind enough to go to the medical library and bring Charlene a couple of medical books. While Scott was sleeping and complaining, Charlene was reading.

Scott may have known he had an abdomen, but claims he certainly did not know he had a mediastinum until they broke it open. He now was beginning to feel the area intensively and had to hit that morphine pump often. He was becoming a big fan of morphine. Unfortunately, there was a limit as to how much he could get from the pump.

To make matters worse, the hospital staff, in cahoots with Charlene, was trying to force him to get up and walk. "You have to get up and move around to start recovering and to prevent pneumonia." Charlene became a trader by joining the hospital staff in urging Scott to move. She would not relent until Scott got up and started to move around. He still was connected to all these drains and drips. It was a major production to get up, much less walk. The nurse pointed out that, in a couple of days, he would be walking around the floor.

It appears that, since the surgery, getting up to walk around has become an Olympic event. Keeping his balance, holding back nausea, putting one foot in front of the other, now took on a degree of difficulty sufficient to warrant at least a bronze metal. Walking a quarter of the way around the hospital floor seemed like an endurance test. He could feel his heart moving and banging against his chest since the removal of the pericardium.

Over the next couple of days, the routine consisted of multiple walks a day, breathing into the spirometer, and coughing. Scott was like Humpty Dumpty, put back together with wire mesh. It was painful to cough because he had been carved, gutted, and re-engineered. When he coughed, it felt like he was being stabbed in the chest. So what steps did they take to help him as his pain level was increasing? They took away the morphine pump and gave him pain pills. Pain pills were not a welcome substitution for morphine. Now they started pushing him to eat. He was not hungry, had no appetite whatsoever, and absolutely would not eat hospital food. To coax him into eating, Charlene brought some food in from the outside world. He had a bite or two of something along the way, but that was the extent of his eating. We ordered food for the staff several times.

With the loss of the morphine, it became clear to Scott that the hospital accommodations were completely unsatisfactory. It was a private room, but too small. The bed was not comfortable. The television did not get the good stations. He still had no voicemail access. Yet, he did not feel ready to go home. He was on oxygen and still not breathing properly. He would lose his breath just by turning slightly. You get the idea that Scott was not using the power of positive thinking to his advantage.

Charlene and our daughter stayed by his side. Scott had a lot of heart to heart talks with them. He did not want any other visitors to see him when he was not in "game shape." Charlene did not allow visitors after the first day. Scott needed his rest and she knew he would exert too much energy entertaining people. Scott could hear Charlene talking on the phone and giving updates as he faded in and out. Her familiar voice in the background reminded him that he was alive. Many relatives and friends were unhappy about Charlene's "no visitor" mandate, but she had to do what was best for Scott.

Without the morphine, it seemed harder to sleep and with the increasing pain Scott wanted to sleep more. He was at a teaching hospital, but he was not invaded by medical students making the rounds. We were fortunate enough to have an old school surgeon who recognized the health of his patients was the main priority. Also, Scott was not badgered by the nurses the way people usually are in hospitals. Charlene was always there and would call on a nurse whenever we wanted something. There was the standard call button he could use. The nurses came in occasionally unannounced, but we don't remember Scott being disturbed every couple of hours to be poked at. We are grateful for the excellent care he received at this first-rate institution. We also noted that the entire staff was more professional and less intrusive than at other hospitals. There were few of the flaws we found in visiting others in the hospital. We attribute a lot of this to the surgeon. He was demanding of his staff, unwavering in his standards, and commanded the respect of the staff. They did not want to mess up on his watch.

As soon as he was able to function, Scott traded in the hospital attire for sweats. They were more comfortable. The next morning, he talked the nurses into letting him go down the hall to take a shower. He thought he would surprise Charlene by being clean and ambulatory for a change. He probably should not have attempted to shower at that point, but he knew he had to start pushing himself to recover.

Scott still was having difficulty breathing. He was no longer breathing from his right side and his heart was physically relocating itself each time he moved even slightly, further causing him to lose his breath.

Charlene was spending a lot of time learning about lymphoma: the best doctors; the treatments; the prognoses; and the staging. She read a lot, talked to organizations, patients, nurses, and doctors. She shared a lot of information with Scott, but she filtered many things because she knew that Scott could not deal with everything. Scott picked up on some things, but ignored most of it.

The surgeon was trying to get Scott out of the hospital. At the time, we thought this must be an insurance thing. It might have been a consideration, but the main reason was he wanted Scott up and out without contracting any hospital infections. Scott's hospital stay lasted a couple of days less than scheduled, but a day longer than we think the surgeon wanted him to stay. Scott was just too tired and weak to leave. But he was starting to think about his cases which was a good sign—he was returning to the land of the living. He even was complying with the doctor's orders—breathing and walking—and was making progress. The next day, the surgeon came in and said that Scott would need to see an oncologist. Charlene asked a lot of questions. Scott took away only a couple of points. First, he would need both chemotherapy and radiation therapy and that scared the hell out of him. Second, the surgeon was very specific about the oncologist he must see. Charlene had narrowed her list down to three outstanding oncologists who specialized in lymphoma. But the surgeon was insistent that we see this doctor (who was on her list) because of a good outcome with a patient with a similar presentation.

The surgeon asked whether Scott felt ready to go home. Scott said "yes." He was determined to leave the hospital that day regardless of whether or not he was feeling better because the next day was his birthday. He thought it probably was going to be his last birthday and he certainly was not going to spend it in the hospital. Charlene asked a lot of questions about what Scott should and should not do, what to expect, what to watch for, and how to reach the surgeon in case of emergency. The surgeon was patient and answered all of her questions. He saw Scott was more receptive to receiving information now and he provided him with assurances and told him what to expect and what to do to improve his breathing and to live with his newly designed body.

The surgeon said that he would have the staff put together the hospital records and film because the oncologist would need them. He said Scott should see him in two weeks and make an appointment to see the oncologist shortly after the follow-up with the surgeon. He said Scott needed to recover from the surgery and improve his breathing before he went to the oncologist. The surgeon said that he would prepare a letter to the oncologist providing the essential information so that the oncologist would have it before seeing Scott. The surgeon said that he would give us a copy when we saw him in two weeks.

The process of leaving the hospital seemed complex, time-consuming, and frustrating to Scott. He was not participating in the process because he was "a sick man." He was just waiting as Charlene, our daughter, nurses, and other hospital personnel scrambled.

Scott was released with medications (antibiotics, pain pills, and whatever else), gauze for his wounds, instructions that he did not pay attention to, and an oxygen tank he did not intend to use and never did use. He was concerned that he could not function for a couple of weeks without the doctor around and with all these issues and limitations. Still, he was anxious to leave and he had Charlene to care for him. He wondered aloud how cancer patients could go home without someone there to take care of them. He was fortunate to have Charlene and she was confident that she could take care of Scott and also was anxious to get him home.

Scott felt every bump on the drive home. After we pulled onto the driveway, Charlene went into the house and put our dogs away. Scott wanted to see them, but he knew that, if they jumped on him (which they would), they could kill him. He also knew that one of our dogs would not be there. He started to climb the flight of stairs. It took so long that Scott lost patience with himself. He wound up spending the next couple of days and nights on the main floor. The house began to fill up with baskets of flowers and gifts. We were overwhelmed by the well wishes from family, friends, lawyers, partners, business leaders, and clients. We could not believe the outpouring of support. Dozens of packages came from people Charlene had never met or even heard of before. Many of them were co-counsel or opposing counsel on Scott's cases and other people Scott apparently touched over the years. She thought that was a tremendous sign of respect.

His favorite gift was a large and beautiful basket of chocolate covered fruit. For a couple of days, he was on a self-prescribed chocolate covered fruit diet. He would eat nothing else. Charlene let him get away with it because she was just glad that he finally was eating something. Coughing, pain, walking, and not breathing properly became Scott's routine. He much preferred practicing law than practicing patientry. We were inundated with phone calls as more people learned of his surgery and Charlene did most of the talking to people.

CHAPTER 5

RE-EMERGING IN THE WORLD (GETTING UP TO SPEED ON CANCER)

It took a while to recover somewhat (not completely) from the surgery. Recovery consisted of Scott quickly weaning himself off pain medication, walking, starting to eat real food to build up his strength, trying to improve his breathing, and informing the public that he was still alive. The latter task involved two critical trips and many telephone calls.

The first trip would be to see Mary. We did not tell Charlene's mother Mary that Scott had cancer or that he had surgery. We felt that she would worry too much. Scott reports that it was no easy task keeping this from Mary because Charlene must have acquired her "nosiness" from Mary. Charlene, a master in deception, was able to keep Mary in the dark. Charlene tells everyone that there were two reasons Scott married her. First, she shares Frank Sinatra's birthday (December 12). Second, she is a good driver. Charlene's chauffeur skills were tested during this time as she did the driving.

When Scott felt up to it, we drove over to Mary's. We walked in, went into her living room, and sat on the couch. Charlene distracted her so she could not perceive Scott's slow and awkward gait. We engaged in some small talk, Scott told Mary he was feeling alright and Mary said that she was as well. Then Charlene told Mary that Scott had cancer, went to the hospital, and had surgery. She quickly added that Scott was going to be alright. We realized at that moment that telling Mary after the fact was the correct decision. Mary could see Scott for herself. By this time, she had had surgery for cancer herself (a mastectomy). Mary asked questions, we told her the details, and she satisfied herself that Scott was alright. Then she started laughing, "Scott, I can't believe you had surgery. I thought that, if you ever needed surgery, you would die first." Over the years, we had talked about Mary's high threshold for physical pain and medical treatments and compared it against Scott's low tolerance.

The second trip was downtown to Scott's office. Charlene placed three restrictions on the trip, each of which generally was unacceptable. First, Charlene would come with Scott. Although Scott enjoys her company, Charlene usually wants to sit in Scott's chair when she comes to his office for a visit and has a tendency to take over. Second, Scott could not carry anything including his briefcase. This was unacceptable because a briefcase is important equipment to a trial lawyer. Third, Scott could only stay a couple of hours. Scott is old school and stays until the job is finished. Still, Scott agreed to the terms because he wanted to check his mail, messages, and review the critical upcoming events in his cases.

We attempted to enter quietly so that Scott could get a little work done. Word got out that Scott was in the office and people kept coming in to see us. It was not a productive couple of hours, but a wonderful couple of hours for Scott. He was back in the office and it was heartwarming to see everyone. Some of his female partners and associates cried. Scott thought he must look even scarier than usual, although everyone said he "looked great." His time in the office would be sparse the next week or two as he had lots of medical tests and appointments scheduled and was still recovering. Charlene was a strict time-keeper and after two or three hours declared that we were leaving. Charlene still was able to overpower Scott and he was getting a bit tired anyway, so we left. One of Scott's partners helped him pack up a box of documents and brought it out to the car. Nothing is more comforting to a lawyer than a box of documents.

Scott was starting to get back among the living. Scott called in daily, checked messages frequently, returned calls, and read mail and pleadings that were sent by messenger to our home. Within a week Scott was directing his cases again, much of the time from his office.

Now we were still in the phase of learning as much as we could about lymphoma. Actually, it would be more correct to say Charlene was learning. She continued to read medical articles and materials and spoke to lots of people. Before seeing the surgeon for the scheduled follow-up appointment, Charlene made an appointment with the oncologist. We knew the surgeon would inquire as to whether we already had an appointment scheduled. Charlene knew the type of lymphoma and, based upon her research, staged Scott. She also predicted his treatment. She read a very recent study on the exact type of lymphoma that Scott had and that study was conducted by doctors in multiple medical institutions, including the oncologist that we were scheduled to see.

We went to see the surgeon. He looked at the surgical site, did a physical examination, and asked how Scott was feeling. He was pleased Scott was not taking pain pills any longer and that the surgical site was healing well. He inquired about our appointment with the oncologist. He gave us a copy of the letter he sent to the oncologist. He asked how often Scott was breathing into the spirometer. Scott told him that he wasn't doing that anymore. The surgeon gave him a new one, scolded him, and told him to use it 8 to 10 times a day. He said it would help clear his chest, improve his breathing, and get him used to breathing without his right side fully functioning. Scott and the surgeon were laughing and sharing stories. After spending a few minutes talking it was clear that, under the surgeon's stern exterior, was a big heart. It seems surgeons and trial lawyers have many things in common. We would continue to see the surgeon periodically for the next couple of years. Being under his care was very comforting to us because we had such confidence in him.

There was an educational event about lymphoma in downtown Chicago that Charlene had learned about from her investigation. Several leading doctors from the Chicagoland area were scheduled to speak. She arranged for us to go. Most of the questions were asked by patients with indolent forms of lymphoma that did not pertain to Scott. During a break, we provided some information to one of the oncologists and asked about recommended treatment. The answer was six to eight rounds of chemotherapy followed by radiation. Scott immediately determined we would not be seeing this oncologist. The study we mentioned earlier suggested that as little as three or four rounds of chemotherapy may be required. Charlene asked a lot of questions to the doctors. Charlene felt this was a great opportunity to get information and insights. Scott couldn't wait to leave. He found the whole thing depressing. He asked only about the side effects from chemotherapy, which was his current fixation.

Things were getting crazy. Scott felt he still was not in control of his life. He was subject to the will and whim of doctors, hospitals, appointments, and tests. "This is my life and I must take control back," he said. Scott read enough to know that there were too many risks and symptoms from chemotherapy for his tastes. He did not want any chemotherapy. Since the surgeon said he got all the cancer, maybe he did not need it. Charlene did not share Scott's view. "You are going to have the chemotherapy whether you want to or not. I will help you get through it, but you are going to do it." Scott did not find this persuasive. Charlene was relentless and finally convinced him. She pointed out that it was not just Scott's life, but her life too. Similar to surgery, Scott ultimately realized that he had to make a decision that was best for his family. He had to make sure that he was giving himself the best chance to survive. He began mentally preparing himself for the punishment of chemotherapy. Still, he intended to limit the punishment. Going through six or eight rounds of chemotherapy was overwhelming. But he felt that he could make it through three rounds. If more were required, he would deal with it at the time.

As we will discuss in more detail in Part 2, it is very important that the patient have an advocate (be it a spouse, family member, or friend) and that the team of patient and advocate be well educated on all of the treatment options, potential side effects, and the steps needed to make it through. As educated professionals, we needed to be knowledgeable and participate in an active manner. Yet, as a patient and someone who is not good at dealing with medical procedures, Scott knew that he could not fixate on the medical issues or he would psyche himself out of having any treatment. Fortunately, he had Charlene who is knowledgeable about medicine and a first-rate caregiver and patient advocate. He says he would not have made it through the treatments without her. Scott relied on Charlene to know all of the details, to ask all of the right questions, and to make sure that the treatments, medicines, and dosages were correct. Charlene is a "checker" and she confirmed and verified everything. When you are sick and going through the rigors of treatment, you need to have a "checker" on your team. Some patients are more involved and read more than Scott did—others much less. The point is that the team of patient and advocate must have the information and take the steps to protect and advance the interests of the patient all the way through the process. The mix will depend upon the feelings, knowledge, and interests of the team members.

We also will talk in Part 2 about selecting doctors. Suffice it to say, the recommendation of Scott's surgeon was the most important factor in our choice of oncologist. Not just because a doctor made the referral, but because we had tremendous respect for the doctor who made the referral and because the doctor expressed solid reasons for making the recommendation, including direct experience with the oncologist. But Charlene also spoke with cancer and lymphoma groups to learn about the leading lymphoma oncologists in our area and about the recommended oncologist and medical center in particular. We also spoke with patients. If it had been a few years later, we would have turned to the internet. Before we went to the oncologist, we knew a lot about his background, training, and education. Thanks to Charlene, we had obtained and read his recent study on lymphoma and other publications he authored and co-authored. Going into the initial consultation, we had confirmed that he was one of the top lymphoma oncologists in the country. The only thing we lacked was a good sense of his demeanor and personality.

We (mostly Charlene) had also done research about the type of lymphoma that Scott had and the treatment options. We also determined preliminarily that Scott's cancer would be treated with a conventional regimen and did not think we would need to go outside the greater Chicagoland area for confirmation of the diagnosis or for treatment. Had other treatments or facilities offered a better chance for success, we would not have hesitated to travel for treatment. We still did not have all of the information needed for staging and prognosis and we would keep all options on the table as we moved forward. We were going into the appointment with the oncologist under the assumption that Scott would be under his care, provided that we felt comfortable with him. We also knew that we would obtain a second opinion regarding the diagnosis, staging, and treatment recommendation regardless of how the initial appointment went. Scott was dreading what was in store for him. He was still recovering from the surgery. He tried to take a one-step-at-a-time approach as he often told his clients.

Charlene always says that you have to give credit where credit is due. Although this may be lost on you due to Scott's complaining and his self-deprecating humor, Scott actually amazed Charlene (and himself) while going through the surgery and recovery process. He did not like it, it was not in his nature to be a patient, but he called upon his inner strength to have the surgery and he pushed himself hard to recover. Until now, no one other than Charlene knew what Scott was going through because he did divulge anything to the outside world and he made it a point to have his "game face" on when dealing with anyone. He would need to draw upon the same strength to get through the chemotherapy.

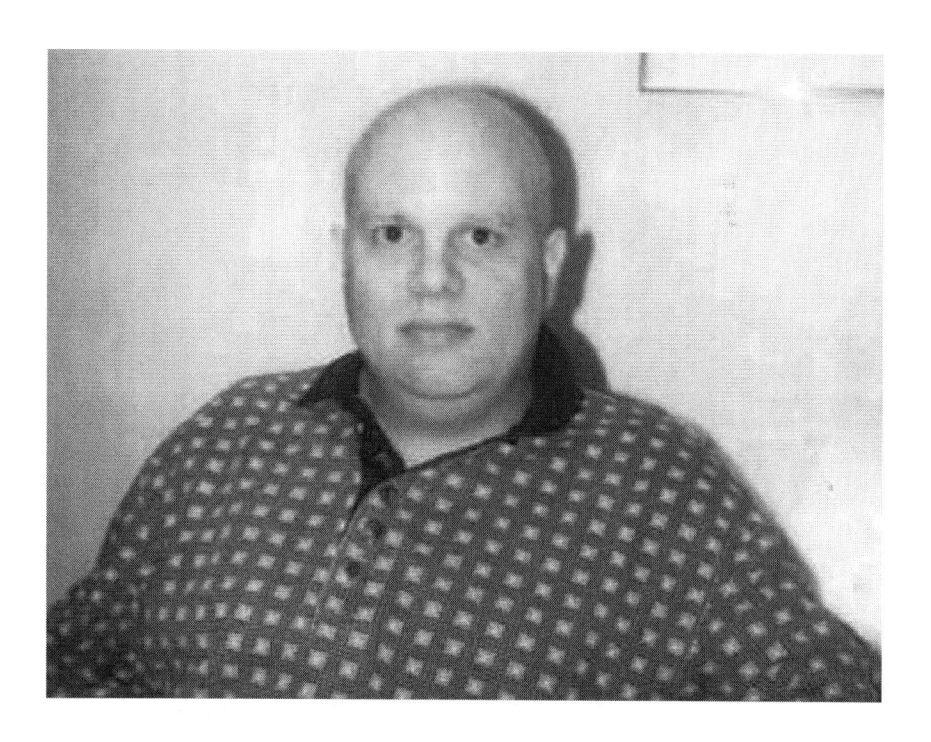

Scott during the dog days of chemotherapy.

CHAPTER 6

LEARNING WHAT THE PHRASE "SICK AS A DOG" REALLY MEANS (THE CHEMOTHERAPY)

We were getting ready to visit the oncologist. Scott already felt agitated and nauseated. Charlene reminded him that chemotherapy cannot cause nausea before it is administered and that Scott would not be starting any chemotherapy that day. Charlene was prepared. She had a list of questions written out. As for Scott, he had read a couple of the articles Charlene had assembled and had two questions and one demand: (1) what are my chances of surviving?; (2) what are the treatment options and the side effects?; and (3) I will agree only to a maximum of three rounds of chemotherapy and absolutely no more! For some reason, Scott was more nervous about the chemotherapy in some respects than the surgery. We had gone through surgeries before with Mary so maybe there was greater apprehension about chemotherapy because he had less knowledge about it. Also, he was still recovering from the surgery and his mental and physical strength was not at its usual level. For whatever reason, it is an understatement to say that Scott was not happy to be confronting an oncologist.

By the time we arrived at the treatment center, most of the paper work was completed. Charlene took care of that in advance. Scott had some blood work done. We waited to be called into the office. This would become a routine for the next couple of years. The nurse comes in, takes Scott's temperature, weight, and height (never mind how tall he is), obtains a brief history, a list of medications and allergies, and asks about his complaints. Scott had a lot of complaints and the chemotherapy had not even begun. It turns out the nurse was not really interested in his complaints, only his physical condition.

Next, the fellow came into the examination room. The fellow palpated the lymph nodes throughout Scott's body. Lymph nodes are bean shaped structures located throughout the body through which blood passes. The fellow took a more detailed history. Scott says Charlene knew more about lymphoma than the fellow did. Charlene certainly had more questions than he had answers. She was trying to pin him down on the stage of Scott's lymphoma. She kept telling Scott this is important to know so we can determine his survival chances and the treatment. Stage 1 estimated the fellow. Charlene said at least stage 2. She turned out to be closer than the fellow was in assessing the stage. Scott's demeanor was pleasant, but he was put off by having a fellow examine him and "waste his time." He was waiting for the "regular doctor."

The oncologist finally arrived. He spoke with us, answered some of Charlene's questions, and balked at others for now. There are two major categories of lymphoma—Hodgkin and non-Hodgkin. Those two types can be broken down into over 80 forms now (about three dozen then). Scott had non-Hodgkin (large, diffuse, B-cell if you are interested). The overall 5-year survival rate for Hodgkin is over 85%. The overall 5-year survival rate for non-Hodgkin is about 73% now (about 57% then). There are variances within the various forms of non-Hodgkin. Scott's type of cancer was fairly aggressive. At first, we thought this was a bad thing. By this time we were starting to learn that it may be a good thing in terms of survival, at least now that it was diagnosed and surgically removed.

Charlene's inability to completely stage Scott was understandable. Even the oncologist was unable to do so until further tests were done. We needed to get all of the blood work back and to get the actual tumor from the hospital where Scott had surgery so that the pathologists at this center could look at it. We were glad the doctor said this because we would have insisted on a second review by another pathologist in any event. Scott needed more CT scans and a bone marrow biopsy. Like Charlene, the oncologist knew enough to say it was at least stage 2 and likely stage 3. The oncologist would not commit to a treatment plan until all the results came back, but suspected it would be a chemotherapy regimen known as CHOP to be followed by radiation therapy.

We discussed the oncologist's article at length since it was the latest study on the type of lymphoma that Scott had. Basically, there were two findings that we took away from the study. First, a combination of chemotherapy and radiation worked better than chemotherapy alone (even more rounds of chemotherapy). Second, CHOP was as effective as another regimen of chemotherapy that had more side effects. The doctor explained that previously he had been an advocate of the more toxic chemotherapy because his own experience suggested it was more effective. He was quick to add that the study was a solid study and, in view of the findings, he was now using CHOP for his patients. We were impressed that he would alter his approach and abide by what the science showed even though it meant he was changing course. The oncologist definitely scored points for that approach.

Scott was a unique case because he had the bulky tumors removed surgically, which is very rare for lymphoma patients. The bulky nature of his disease (big tumor) was not a favorable factor in terms of his prognosis. But there were no studies (including the recent study) that addressed the impact of the surgery and whether or not removing the mass surgically should alter the treatment plan or prognosis.

Scott offered his medical opinion that the surgical removal of the tumor increased his chances of beating this disease. Further, Scott opined that, because the mass was removed, he should not need any chemotherapy or radiation whatsoever. The doctor also suspected removal of the mass was helpful. He emphasized that lymphoma is a blood cancer and there likely were cancer cells throughout his body, which may or may not be detectable by testing at this point. He was confident that Scott needed chemotherapy. He also acknowledged that the surgery was not a variable in his study or in any study assessing the benefits of the combination of radiation and chemotherapy. The oncologist needed to see all of the test results, but believed that he would recommend both radiation and chemotherapy for Scott. Scott had a fallback position that, because of the surgery, at most he would need a round or two of chemotherapy. He wanted to leave some negotiating room to land on three rounds.

Scott thought that additional CT scans were unnecessary as he had the scans done three weeks earlier and brought the scans and films for the doctor to view. The oncologist stated we needed post-surgery scans. He disliked swallowing barium, but he could handle CT scans easily so he did not make this a point of protest. Besides, Charlene concurred that another set of scans was in order.

"What exactly is the bone marrow biopsy and how is that done," we asked. The doctor said it was a simple procedure that they would do right there in the office. The doctor offered some encouragement, ordered tests, and scheduled an appointment to talk once the results were back. He knew Scott was a lawyer and was sure to include a host of disclaimers, emphasizing the seriousness of the disease and the risks of treatment.

At least Scott did not have a lot of time to worry about the bone marrow sample. We were ushered into a larger examination room that was set up for small surgical procedures. There were three or four needles about 8 to 12 inches long and a three-foot long corkscrew. The young doctor explained to Scott that the shots were to numb him up and the corkscrew (he called it something else) was what he would use to extract a bone marrow sample. We had already figured that out. First, the fellow stabbed Scott with the needles. Next, he started turning the corkscrew. Scott was bent over on the table at the time so he did not see exactly how the fellow was doing it. It only took a moment or two to get the sample. But once it was over, there was not much pain. There was some minor residual discomfort in the area for a couple of days. Actually, Scott was somewhat fortunate because the young doctor who did the procedure was particularly adept at bone marrow biopsies, we later would learn.

By our next appointment all of Scott's test results were back. The results were somewhat mixed. There was no evidence of cancer in the bone marrow, which was good. The CT scans showed enlarged lymph nodes in the abdomen, which meant the lymphoma was both above and below the diaphragm. Not good. The CT scans taken prior to the surgery did not show those nodes enlarged. Charlene asked the oncologist whether the enlarged lymph nodes could be a result of the surgery, rather than disease. The oncologist did not rule out that possibility, but pointed out that his CT scans were better than those from the other hospital (something to do with smaller cuts and greater sensitivity). We were fighting for a diagnosis of stage 2. The doctor was diagnosing stage 3. The oncologist stated that he was going to treat the cancer the same way regardless of the staging, so Scott could consider himself stage 2 if that made him feel better. Of course, it made him feel better as it increased his survival percentages. But it was difficult to feel much better because the doctor reiterated that Scott actually was stage 3.

Scott still had one major issue to address with the doctor regarding his treatment. "I will only have one or two rounds of chemotherapy, correct doctor?" The doctor tried to avoid the question. Scott would not let him off the hook and pressed for an answer. The doctor stated that he intended to give Scott six rounds of CHOP for a variety of reasons, including the bulky nature of his disease and the fact that he was a lawyer. After Scott pressed further, the doctor stated that we would do testing and scans after three rounds and we would see where things stood. We knew that the doctor was only humoring Scott and was going to sell him six rounds whether he wanted them or not. The doctor laughed and reaffirmed that he thought six rounds were appropriate. But he agreed to reassess after three rounds. The doctor scheduled the chemotherapy.

We told him that we needed to take the scans and reports with us because we were going for a second opinion that we had scheduled and we wanted to have that done right away so that the chemotherapy started on schedule. Actually, the timing was at Charlene's insistence. Scott would have preferred to schedule chemotherapy a year or two down the road. The doctor stated that we did not need a second opinion because he wrote the book on the subject. We went anyway and, of course, the oncologist was professional about our obtaining a second opinion.

We went to another leading institution in the area for a second opinion. It was one of the doctors that we heard speak at the educational event a couple of weeks earlier. We brought the records and the actual scans. The doctor met with us and said he read all of the records and results that we provided to him and said that he thought he had everything he needed. He came up with the same diagnosis and recommended treatment plan as our first oncologist. We both noted that the doctor did not do much of a physical examination. Scott asked him whether he looked at the actual scans or just read the radiologist's reports. He admitted that he just read the reports. Scott told him to go back and look at the scans personally. He hoped this would throw the doctor off balance and get him to reduce his recommendation regarding the number of rounds of chemotherapy.

The doctor returned after purporting to examine the scans and stated his opinion remained the same. We were confident in the basic diagnosis (though Scott was still a stage 2 advocate) and the treatment. Scott was pushing hard to cap the chemotherapy at three rounds and offered this doctor the business if he would agree to do no more than three rounds. The doctor reiterated that he also felt that it was in Scott's best interest to have six rounds and maybe even eight rounds of chemotherapy. When he said eight, Charlene looked at Scott and knew the doctor just flunked the interview. Scott wanted to doctor shop some more in search of three or less rounds of chemotherapy.

The proper course was to have six rounds to ensure all the cancer was gone. Charlene always felt this way and so that was what would be done back with the first oncologist. We went back to the surgeon because Scott wanted him to see the latest CT scan and get his take on the "new" lymph nodes. The surgeon looked at the CT scan and stated he was "not impressed" by the lymph nodes. We were not either. The surgeon assured us that Scott was ready for the chemotherapy.

Within a month of surgery, Scott was set to start his chemotherapy. Scott was apprehensive to say the least. Although he wanted to return to work the day after each of his chemotherapy treatments, he prepared for the possibility that he would be out a few days and brought a lot of work home.

With the surgeon's clearance, we were about to enter the "dog days of chemotherapy" as Scott called it. We arrived at the medical center and began, as usual, with the blood work. Next, one of the oncology nurses took us to the patient consultation room. This was a room next to the examination rooms, but it contained chairs and materials regarding various forms of cancer. She asked us to read several pieces of paper and provided consent forms for the chemotherapy. For each of the separate drugs that made up his chemotherapy regimen there were multiple sheets of fine print disclosing potential side effects of the drug. Scott started reading the first sheet and it was clear that this drug could adversely impact every part of his body and cause every medical condition imaginable up to and including death. Charlene discouraged Scott from reading the rest of them. She already had read this information as part of her prior research and she knew that no good could come from planting more ideas about side effects in Scott's mind. Charlene was correct as usual—reading this served only to add to Scott's apprehension. Scott stalled for a while, but ultimately signed the consent forms.

The nurse returned with an unfamiliar face wearing a white coat. We now learned for the first time that the oncologist had a new fellow who started the day before. It looks like we have to break in a new doctor just as Scott was starting chemotherapy. We asked the fellow questions about some of the potential side effects, including the likelihood of actually experiencing them.

The young doctor broke things down into three categories. The first category was side effects that Scott was likely to experience to one degree or another. These included nausea, gastrointestinal and flu-like symptoms (vomiting, diarrhea, constipation, weakness, soreness, fatigue, and low grade fever). The length of time and severity of these symptoms vary considerably from patient to patient. The doctor said that there were medications to help ease these symptoms. Mouth sores also were possible. Loss of hair and periodic difficulty in focusing were likely as well. Scott also could expect to experience some "moon face." There were no medicines to prevent these side effects, but they were all expected to be short term. Scott's hair would grow back after the chemotherapy.

The second category was serious potential side effects, including heart damage and developing other cancers from the drugs, in particular, leukemia. These were not likely side effects, but needed to be disclosed because of their gravity.

The final category was all of the other things listed in the informational sheets that were so remote that the doctor felt they were not worth discussing.

The young doctor assured us that he would be available any time we needed him. A major concern was that we take all necessary precautions to avoid infections because Scott's immune system would be low to non-existent at times. In response to Charlene's questions, the doctor went over the typical chemotherapy cycle and what Scott's blood counts were likely to be at various times. Basically during each cycle Scott's counts should start out normal, drop thereafter (particularly white blood cells), and then start to rebound. By the time the counts approach their normal level, the doctors would beat them back down with the next round of chemotherapy. After a couple of rounds, it may be harder to get the blood counts back up. The counts would have to reach a certain level in order for them to proceed with the next round of chemotherapy. They would be monitoring Scott's blood counts closely during the entire course of chemotherapy treatments. The doctor did not say anything that Charlene had not already told Scott. More important, Charlene already had a plan in place to deal with many of these issues, in particular "Operation No Infection."

Scott suggested it would make sense for him to take a week or two to digest all of the information before starting the chemotherapy. Charlene and the young doctor denied Scott's request to delay the treatment.

Although we were concerned about the timing of the fellow transition and being in the hands of a new fellow, we really came to appreciate this young doctor. He was available whenever we needed him, whether day or night, weekend or weekday. He helped us get through the chemotherapy, which was very difficult for Scott and he helped Charlene cope with Scott. In fact, during some tough times Charlene and the doctor talked at various times including overnight and weekends to help Scott make it through. The chemotherapy, for Scott, would prove to be as bad as he had feared.

We expected to meet next with the oncologist as was the procedure that we followed every time, except for this time. However, we were told that the oncologist was out this week. We just looked at each other in disbelief. Had we known this in advance, we would have delayed the start of chemotherapy until the oncologist returned.

Charlene caught an error in the chemotherapy scheduling. The hospital was scheduling the sessions four weeks apart, instead of the three weeks apart called for by the chemotherapy regimen as reflected in the oncologist's recent article. After Charlene pointed this out, the hospital initially denied that the schedule was incorrect. After checking, they realized the error and adjusted the scheduling. Scott had noticed this as well, but did not point it out thinking he was entitled to an extra week between sessions.

Our next stop was the cancer center's "drug store." There were no magazines, candy, or the other items that you would expect any fine quality drug store to carry. This one only had bags of chemicals, jars of pills, and ancillary medical items. They would get the drugs for Scott's regimen, Charlene would double-check them carefully, and a nurse would come and take us to have the drugs administered. Usually, there was unwanted waiting time. Knowing that he could not get out of the treatment, Scott wanted to get it done.

While waiting in the pharmacy area, we met a nice 21-year old girl who was getting chemotherapy for a recurrence of breast cancer. How terrible that a young lady had to go through this two times! We tried to comfort her, even though Scott was afraid of what awaited him. Although Scott felt like he was the only person in the world with cancer and being tortured by chemotherapy, by looking around the cancer center he could tell business was booming and there were lots of people going through what we were. Many were less fortunate. We were always taken aback when we saw babies and young children going through treatment. Scott learned at the moment we met the young lady how important it was to rise above his condition and help others. Charlene already knew that lesson. By helping others get through, you are helping yourself. There is a special bond that develops between people battling cancer, similar to warriors fighting on the front lines of any war.

Now it was time for the chemotherapy. They pre-medicated Scott for nausea and with a mild tranquilizer. We went into the chemotherapy area, which is a large room with curtained sub-divisions. Some sections had reclining chairs, others had beds. Scott selected one with a chair and a television. He was given some of the chemicals intravenously. These drugs were in bags that hung from a stand with wheels, just like the ones they use in hospitals to administer fluids. The drugs dripped down and went through an IV line. One chemical was given to Scott as a shot in a two-foot long tube. The chemical was bright red. As the nurse was administering the red agent, Scott told her that he was feeling very warm, nauseous, and was about to vomit. Scott asked for a bag or bucket. The nurse told him to relax and not to worry, the feeling would go away and he was not going to vomit. As an experienced oncology nurse, she reiterated that the nausea would soon dissipate. Just as she completed her reassurance, Scott started spewing volumes like never seen before or since. According to Charlene, it looked like the Linda Blair scene from the *Exorcist*. He was embarrassed, but too concerned about his fleeting mortality to focus on that now. As most cancer patients will tell you, the nurses and staff are extremely important. They do most of the work and deliver most of the care to the patients. Ironically, this was the chemical that – along with the radiation – caused Scott's heart attack more than fifteen years later.

Typically, Scott would be at the cancer center for five or six hours during each chemotherapy session. Two or three hours involved the actual administering of the drugs. The rest of the time was spent getting blood work, getting the drugs, getting examined, and of course waiting. Charlene was there with and for Scott during every moment of every treatment. Scott found the first round of chemotherapy to be extremely disagreeable. He was "as sick as a dog" for two or three days. When we got home, he still was vomiting severely, running a fever, and feeling terrible. Charlene was concerned because the vomiting was putting further strain on his chest and surgical area. Charlene learned that, although Scott was given medication for nausea, there was a much better medicine available that Scott was not given.

Charlene contacted the oncology nurse on call and was furious to learn that they had given Scott a less effective anti-nausea medication rather than other available options out of concern that the insurance company may not want to pay for Zofran—a much more effective (then more expensive) medicine. Charlene demanded that a prescription for Zofran be called into the pharmacy immediately. She thought that sending Scott home with a medicine that was not working made no sense to put it charitably. Our advice: make sure you get Zofran.

Actually, today there are several medications available that help with nausea caused by chemotherapy treatments, including: Emend (aprepitant), Zofran (ondansetron), Kytril (granisetron), Anzemet (dolasetron), and Aloxi (palonosetron). Zofran is available today in generic form.

We were not pleased with the first round of chemotherapy and, after Scott was out of the woods, Charlene let the oncologist know about it. It was a good thing he was a hematologist-oncologist because Charlene's blood was boiling. The oncologist apologized for these mix-ups and asked us to give them another chance. He promised things would get better.

The chemotherapy lasted about six months and we will not bore you with a long chronology. Instead, we will provide an overview and hit some of the highlights and lowlights. People react differently to chemotherapy. Even people with the same regimen and same disease react differently. In Scott's case, he did not do particularly well with chemotherapy acutely. He suffered from nausea, aches and pains, difficulty sleeping, and other symptoms that fell under the first category described by the oncologist fellow. It was cyclical, as he had chemotherapy every three weeks or so. He was really sick for the first couple of days, nauseous, uncomfortable, weak, and his output system was not operating correctly. Some days it was a struggle to try and do the basics such as forcing some food down. The week before Scott's next chemotherapy, he generally felt fairly good. He was able to eat, concentrate, and felt nearly normal. But just when you are feeling better, boom – they knock you back down with more chemotherapy. That's how it works, at least that is how it was for Scott.

For the most part, Scott was able to work. The hours sometimes were unconventional, but he was able to do what he had to do to fulfill his obligations to his clients and firm. He did not go to work the day of the chemotherapy. Sometimes, he would not go in the next day or would go in a little late. When he was overly tired, he went home. He could not sleep most of the time so often he would work in the middle of the night. Scott preferred not to fly during this period due to the poor air quality on planes and the risk of infection. Regardless of his preferences, Charlene and the doctor ordered him not to fly. He participated by telephone conference in a couple of meetings that he otherwise may have attended in person. He really was able to handle his work load. In fact, work was a good thing for him. It was a release to be able to focus on clients and cases instead of on how bad he was feeling.

Although his team – which he calls "the A Team" – consists of excellent attorneys and professionals, there were some decisions on matters that only he could make, some advice and strategy decisions clients would only accept from him, and some tactical matters that only he could handle and demanded his personal attention. It is corporate America, the matters are high stakes, and executives needed his input or sign off on some things to satisfy officers and directors. No matter how bad he felt, Scott would always deliver and his clients and partners knew it.

Scott was fairly effective in putting his best foot forward and keeping from people (other than Charlene) just how bad he felt at times. At work and with others, he went out of his way to be upbeat and appear healthy. He felt people do not want to hear complaints or be around someone who is sick. Sometimes acting normal took a toll on him internally. Other times pretending to feel alright actually made him feel better. At any rate, he believed it was best to maintain his "game face" as much as possible. And there was no way he would allow his adversaries to sense any weakness whatsoever. Fortunately, Scott could complain and let his guard down at home around Charlene. We both maintained our senses of humor throughout. At times, it took extra effort for Scott to maintain his focus. But his ability to read, write, watch television, listen to the radio, and maintain a conversation at the same time probably served him well and helped him fight through any fog associated with "chemotherapy brain."

Scott does not believe that he experienced any – or any significant – "chemobrain" or "brain fog." However, some studies show that at least 25% of people with cancer reports memory and attention problems after chemotherapy. This may lead to problems paying attention, focusing, finding the right word, or remembering things. Chemobrain may begin during treatment or not until a significant time passes after treatment concludes. It usually resides fairly quickly, but not always. More research still needs to be conducted on this subject.

One important thing was to avoid germs, getting sick, and infections. Many people die from the side effects of the chemotherapy and other treatments. When your immune system is down, your body lacks the weapons necessary to fight infection. Chemotherapy, by design, weakens the immune system. At times, Scott's white blood counts were barely measurable. Once again, Charlene's talents came into prominence.

Charlene took every precaution to make sure that he did not get sick and was not exposed to people who were sick. She kept people away from Scott whenever she could. She kept him and the house clean. She wiped him down with antibacterial wipes. We carried antibacterial wipes and hand gel with us at all times. We washed our hands and faces constantly. When Scott took the train to and from work, Charlene suggested that he wear a mask. Scott was self-conscious about this and resisted at first. Later on, he liked being the "masked lawyer." He always had his own seat on the train because no one wanted to sit next to him. This probably sounds more normal (and manageable) now in view of the pandemic than it seemed at the time.

When you are battling for your life, there are more important things than physical appearance. Yet, most patients are concerned about whether they will lose their hair from the chemotherapy and about other effects on their appearance. Some people lose their hair, others do not. Some people look sick, other people do not show any discernable signs that they are undergoing treatment. It depends upon the chemotherapy regimen and the person. In his case, Scott had a lot of hair going in and wanted to keep it. The chemotherapy had a different plan.

Scott had completed the first round of chemotherapy and was a couple of days away from the next round of punishment. He was walking with a couple of his partners on the way to a meeting with a client. He scratched his head and a clump of hair fell out. He just kept on walking, but knew that meant he was about to lose all of his hair. He went the next day to get a buzz cut. Over the next day or two he lost all of his hair. He did not like it, but had more important things to worry about. He knew that, if he survived, his hair would grow back. Over the next several weeks, Scott got a collection of caps and hats from friends and clients. There is no denying that the chemotherapy took its toll on Scott's appearance. He saw someone that we had known for years at a store. He approached this woman and started talking to her. After a few seconds, it became clear to him that she had no clue who he was or from whence he came. When Scott got home, he took a long look in the mirror and decided that he did not even recognize himself.

Part of his chemotherapy regimen included steroids. So he developed "moon face" as well as the bald look. Not a particularly attractive look. Scott points out that generally people are not beating down the door to take pictures of him. But he steadfastly avoided having his picture taken during the chemotherapy. The hospital did manage to take one picture of Scott.

You have already seen the picture, which was included in this book over Scott's objection. When Scott looks at that picture, he does not see himself. He sees a creature from outer space. The picture makes him realize that, just when you think you cannot look any worse, the chemotherapy can make you look a lot worse. Scott is not a fan of revisionist history, but one of the lines he often uses could be considered revisionist history. He often tells people that, before cancer, he was "six foot two with eyes of blue and a face for GQ."

Let's cover a few more points about the dog days of chemotherapy. The first is the great infection scare. Scott had red spots on his skin in the area near the surgical incision on his chest. He noticed this one morning and pointed it out to Charlene. He thought very little of it and went to work.

Charlene called the oncologist fellow and described the surgical area to him. The oncologist fellow panicked and told Charlene to call the surgeon immediately. He told her that Scott's immune system was very low and the infection could quickly spread to his heart and kill him. Charlene called the surgeon who demanded that Scott come into his office immediately. Needless to say, Charlene was worried.

Meanwhile, Scott was at work preparing for a routine status hearing. Charlene called and told him that he needed to see the surgeon immediately because he could have a skin infection. Scott asked her to try to make an appointment for the next day. Charlene insisted that Scott leave and head straight for the surgeon's office, where she would meet him. She would not tell him why. Scott was puzzled, but knew something was going on that Charlene was not disclosing. So he got one of his partners to cover the status conference and obtain a continuance. Scott met Charlene at the surgeon's office. The surgeon took a look and was visibly relieved. He said that the way the oncologist fellow was speaking about "an infection," he was concerned that the mesh they used to reassemble Scott was infected. If that were the case, it would have been a serious matter because they would have to go in surgically to remove the mesh, address the infection, and reassemble Scott. The surgeon said what Charlene had said—it was a simple skin irritation. The surgeon felt the young doctor's alarmism was "inappropriate." Charlene called the oncologist fellow back after we left the surgeon's office and told him everything was alright. She said nothing further because we both realized the young doctor genuinely was concerned for Scott's well-being and we both appreciated that very much.

Most of the time, Scott did not have an appetite. He often had to force himself to eat. There were some strange exceptions. For example, on the ride home from the cancer center after receiving chemotherapy he would get very hungry (this was not the case after the first round). There were only two things that he wanted to eat: either chili or pasta. The oncologist encouraged Scott to eat red meat while undergoing chemotherapy. He said this suggestion may sound strange coming from a doctor, but it was important that Scott kept his red blood count up.

While on chemotherapy Scott hated food and the thought of eating usually made him nauseous. When he had to eat, his preferred items were peanut butter and crackers and cream cheese. Those were his cravings. In terms of drinks, the only thing that he could tolerate on a consistent basis was a specific brand of peach ice tea. He still likes it. Sure, it is best to eat healthy at all times, including when you are on chemotherapy. Still, it is better to eat something than nothing at all, even if what you are eating is neither a balanced nor a particularly healthy diet. It is important to keep your strength up. Charlene did not like his dietary choices and tried to supplement Scott's diet where she could. We made all of the appropriate inquiries regarding diet, but Scott would eat only what he could eat and keep down.

We also asked about vitamins and supplements. Our oncologist said it was alright to take one multi-vitamin a day, but nothing else. He pointed out that, if there were any magic vitamins, minerals, or supplements, he would be prescribing them. He also said that part of the intended cycle of the chemotherapy involved lowering the immune system and he did not want any large volumes of vitamins interfering. The take away point is to advise your doctor of any vitamins, minerals, or supplements that you are taking or intend to take.

After the first three rounds of chemotherapy, Scott went for scans. We were both on pins and needles waiting for the results. What if the chemotherapy was not working? It took multiple calls to get the results. The doctor finally called and read the results over the phone. He said there is no evidence of tumors depicted by the scans. Scott has blood cancer, so this certainly is good news, but does not rule out the potential for the presence of cancer cells. But we finally heard the words we were waiting to hear "there is no evidence of cancer—you are cancer-free." Charlene asked him to repeat it three times.

A couple of days later, we met with the oncologist. The doctor said good progress was made, but he believed that Scott should have three more rounds of chemotherapy. Three more rounds was not the answer Scott wanted to hear, but it was what we both expected to hear. Charlene always felt that was the proper course. Scott protested, but also knew that undergoing the additional rounds of chemotherapy was the prudent approach. It was better to take the additional steps to make sure all the cancer cells were dead so we did not have to confront lymphoma again.

The last couple of rounds of chemotherapy were particularly hard on Scott. It seems that his instinct to limit the chemotherapy to three rounds had some validity. Scott's immune system was very low. His blood counts were on the margin of being too low for him to be given more chemotherapy. As Scott puts it, "it was a race to see whether the chemotherapy or the cancer would kill me first." There were times when Scott questioned whether he would survive and had some heart to heart talks with Charlene about living without him. Charlene also was worried by the toll the chemotherapy was taking on Scott.

In order to continue the chemotherapy, Scott had to take shots to boost his white blood count. Charlene administered them. These shots are another example of important progress in recent years that accrues to the benefit of cancer patients and reduces deaths due to cancer and its treatments. You should keep in mind that today there are medications available to boost white blood cell, red blood cell, and platelet counts.

In these darkest hours when we were both afraid he may succumb to the chemotherapy before the cancer was gone, there were two signs that gave us hope that Scott might outlive the chemotherapy. The first sign occurred before chemotherapy round number six. Scott looked in the mirror as part of his routine of watching for swollen lymph nodes and he noticed something. He had hair on his head. His hair started to grow back a couple of times before, but had fallen out by this point in the chemotherapy cycle. He took the "return of hair" as a good omen. Charlene found the surge in Scott's spirits to be heartening.

The more important sign, however, appeared a couple of days later, when we were driving in the car. We had the sunroof open. We stuck our hands out of the sunroof and were holding hands. Suddenly, we both experienced a warm, tingling, wonderful feeling. A feeling neither of us felt before. It was a feeling of peace, serenity, and that everything was going to be alright. You may be thinking that it is time to put us in a rubber room, but we both felt the same thing at the same time. We got to the driveway and Charlene did not want to say anything because she thought Scott would think she was crazy. Charlene asked Scott whether he had just felt something. Scott said yes and described the feeling. Charlene felt the same thing. We truly felt that it was someone or something telling us that everything was going to be okay. It was the best feeling either of us ever experienced. It only lasted for a moment, but it was unforgettable and amazing. Charlene thought "if this is what heaven feels like, it is beautiful." Charlene said that someone is trying to touch us whether it is God or Pat or an angel. We tried to replicate this feeling by holding hands through the sun roof subsequently, but we never could.

Chemotherapy was hard on Scott. But it is important to point out that many people go through chemotherapy and do quite well and experience very little in the way of symptoms. Also, newer treatments such as immunotherapies often do not cause the same types of side effects. For you, chemotherapy may well be less difficult. But either way, with a proper game plan you will get through it and the cancer will not! Appendix "K" contains some tips for dealing with side effects of treatment. Scott would survive the chemotherapy and live to fight other battles. The next battle was coming around the radioactive bend.

CHAPTER 7

THE FINAL PHASE OF THE TREATMENT TRILOGY (THE RADIATION THERAPY)

Another one of Scott's standard jokes is that he went through surgery, chemotherapy, and radiation and when the doctors learned that he was a lawyer, they wanted to try electrocution. He came up with that line while looking at a couple of fabulous oncologists as we were delivering a speech at the First Annual Lymphoma Dinner. The line was well received so Charlene has now heard that line a few more times. Well, they did not resort to electrocution with Scott, but the radiation part was not a joke.

Although we were concerned about the radiation, Scott's concern and anxiety level was nowhere near the level that it was with respect to the chemotherapy or the surgery. Actually, Scott thought compared to the chemotherapy, the radiation would be a walk in the park. Part of him was starting to think that maybe he actually would beat this cancer thing. Despite several requests by Charlene, the oncologist provided us with very little information about the radiology aspect of the treatment in the preceding months. Whether it was because the oncologist did not know much about it or did not want to deal with it, we do not know. Charlene did not make it easy for the doctor to avoid answering questions. On many occasions, Charlene would physically block the door so that the doctor literally could not leave the examination room until her questions were answered.

True to form, we tried to eliminate radiation from Scott's treatment plan at the outset. Charlene forcefully argued that there was no scientific proof that the radiation would be of any benefit to him in view of the absence of studies on patients that underwent surgery. The oncologist felt strongly that the best course was for him to have radiation and relied upon the studies showing that a combination of chemotherapy and radiation produced the best results. Charlene pushed the oncologist for answers and more information.

There are at least three types of radiologists. The first type read and interpret scans and films. The second type are intervention radiologists. These doctors perform procedures and surgeries using imaging tools. The third type are radiologist-oncologists. They oversee the radiation given to cancer patients as treatment as opposed to for diagnostic purposes. They are skilled clinicians who are also very qualified at reading and interpreting scans.

Consistent with our practice, Charlene did our research on the radiologist-oncologist. The oncologist recommended him because he was the radiologist-oncologist on their staff that handled lymphoma patients. The oncologist did not know much about him because the radiologist was brand new to the hospital. This recommendation simply was not good enough for us because the basis for the recommendation seemed flimsy. We requested the radiologist's curriculum vitae (the fancy term for a doctor's biography or resume). He was well-trained at Mayo. We were not sure what a radiologist-oncologist would be doing to Scott, but we were concerned.

Our first encounter with the radiologist did not inspire our confidence. We went to the dungeon of the hospital—that is where the radiologist-oncologists usually are housed. The doctor was late, but that was no surprise and by this time we were not even upset. When he arrived, the doctor shook Scott's hand, apologized, and stated he was seeing a patient that they suspect might have a specific type of contagious condition. Charlene was concerned about Scott being exposed to any infectious agent, particularly given that Scott had just completed chemotherapy. Remember, Charlene is the General in charge of "Operation No Infection." The doctor assured us that he had protective gear on when seeing the other patient and had scrubbed twice before entering the examination room. Scott still was not convinced that he would benefit from radiation. Charlene was more concerned about the radiation dosage. We left unconvinced that either this doctor or the radiation was a good fit for us. In retrospect, we should have followed our instincts to avoid radiation as we would later learn that it caused his heart attack several years down the road. But we went with the best information available at the time.

We called the surgeon to get recommendations for other radiologist-oncologists. We turned to the surgeon whenever there was any issue or doubt regarding Scott's treatment because of the tremendous respect we had for him. Scott really bonded with the surgeon and valued his opinion regardless of the medical subject matter. Before we went to see any other radiologist-oncologist, Charlene got a call from the office of the radiologist-oncologist that we had seen a few days earlier. They said the doctor had Scott's radiation plan prepared and wanted us to come in the next day. We decided to go and at least see the plan.

The radiologist-oncologist began by performing a very detailed physical examination of Scott. Actually, he impressed both of us with his mastery of Scott's history and the comprehensive nature of his physical examination. It was unquestionably more thorough than the oncologist's examinations. The radiologist-oncologist showed us a three-dimensional colored picture that he said was prepared by a physicist. He explained the radiation plan, the entire process, the side effects that he thought Scott would experience, the side effects that he was confident that Scott would not experience but he had to advise us about, and the basis for his assessment.

We had a lengthy discussion of the benefits of the treatment and the impact of Scott's surgery on the equation. He actually agreed with our assessment that, from the standpoint of recurrence, Scott was better off than had he not had surgery. He conceded the absence of studies on lymphoma patients like Scott who underwent surgery to have a bulky tumor removed. The radiologist-oncologist explained in detail how chemotherapy can kill cancer cells that were released prior to and perhaps during the surgery and how radiation could cover things that the chemotherapy may have missed. His conclusion was that the benefits of fully treating Scott's disease at the outset as opposed to at a time of a recurrence outweighed the risks. What he said made sense, even though we realized he was peddling his product. The doctor also pointed out that he had state of the art equipment—three-dimensional radiation equipment that would maximize the radiation to the site of the initial tumors in a targeted way and that would minimize unwanted radiation to nearby areas and organs. This was long before proton radiation was used.

It is worth mentioning that there have been meaningful improvements and refinements with respect to radiation therapy. Thus, when evaluating options and looking at long-term studies with respect to survival rates and side effects, the data can be difficult to compare and evaluate. One area of interest, for example, is whether a young lady with Hodgkin lymphoma should be given radiation, which may make a very favorable prognosis even a bit more favorable. The concern is a higher rate of breast cancer. So these are some of the considerations that come into play in weighing treatment options. You should also discuss with your physician ways to minimize any unwarranted radiation.

To that point, Charlene was concerned about the amount of radiation that would be going to Scott's vital organs, such as the heart and lungs. Charlene articulated the concerns and the doctor did not dismiss them. Charlene thought we should tailor the radiation as much as possible. The radiologist took notes on Charlene's concerns, suggested some improvements, and said he would have the physicist alter the plan. He told Charlene he would minimize the amount of rams to the extent possible. The radiologist-oncologist returned with a new three dimensional colored chart showing exactly how many rams of radiation would be received in each area of Scott's chest. We entered the appointment with doubts about radiology and about this doctor, but left very confident in the doctor and somewhat more confident that undergoing the treatment was in our best interests. The radiation plan was formulated as improved by Charlene and that was the first step.

The next step was getting a mold made for Scott to lay in while undergoing the radiation, which was done in a subsequent appointment. The radiologist-oncologist had Scott lay on a big steel table, focused some equipment on him, and made some bright colored marks on Scott's chest at precise locations. He fit Scott for a cast that he would use during the radiation treatments. The marks would be reference points for the administering of the radiation. The goal was simple: Scott needed to be in a precise position for each radiation treatment so that the radiation went exactly where it needed to go. Scott was not impressed with the artistic quality of the doctor's markings. He told the doctor that he must have gone into medicine because he lacked artistic flair. Charlene noted the same could be said about Scott's career choice.

The couple of appointments for the mold were at an adjoining Veterans Administration facility. Charlene spoke to many of the patients along the way as she would often do. Scott was unusually talkative with the patients because they were veterans and he has tremendous respect for them. We both made it a point to thank all of them for their service to our country.

Starting the following week, Scott would go every weekday for six weeks for radiation treatments. The hospital accommodated Scott's schedule by scheduling him for late afternoons. This way Scott could go to work early in the morning and work until mid-afternoon. We were concerned that the daily treatment would be inconvenient and take its toll on both of us. Knowing that doctors and hospitals notoriously run late and later (except on a days where you are delayed in traffic, in which case they seem to be precisely on time), we thought daily radiation would be a scheduling nightmare. There were a couple of times of inordinate delay, but for the most part, Scott was in and out within two hours or so. Still, it was tiring and a grind—but thankfully the end of our ordeal was in sight. The first session took the longest because the radiation-oncologist was present and checked the fit of the mold to ensure that the radiation beam was hitting the precise areas.

The radiation room was about the only place (other than the operating room and restroom) where Charlene did not accompany Scott. The routine was simple. Scott entered the room and climbed up on a large metal table. Next, the technicians put the mold on the table and Scott would then get into position in the mold. They made sure that the mold was in the correct position on the table and that Scott was in the correct position in the mold. Then they lock in Scott. They aim the machine in an appropriate spot by reference to the marks the radiologist penned on Scott's chest. They run and hide in a safe area that protects them from the radiation. Then it was time for them to deliver the radiation. You hear a noise that sounds like the circuit breaker box in a house is blowing, the lights flicker, and they leave the machine on for a couple of minutes. They repeat this routine three or four times, directing the radiation to other locations. The session then is complete. Obviously, the routine and side effects vary depending upon the area of the body receiving the radiation. Some patients even get full body radiation. Scott estimates that he was in the room for a total of about twenty to thirty minutes each time and that about six to eight minutes was actual radiation. Most of the time, the radiologist-oncologist was not present. Two or three times he was present and looked into the eye of the machine to make sure the plan that Charlene and the physicist designed was being implemented properly. The radiation routine was the same every day for six weeks.

We became friendly with a man suffering from esophageal cancer and his wife. Our chemotherapy sessions had lined up two or three times and we had a lot of time to talk. This man's father had died from esophageal cancer a few years earlier. The couple had young kids. He seemed optimistic about his outcome, even though his dad had died from the same type of cancer and he admitted this weighed on his mind. He had a lot to live for. Our radiation sessions also were close together for a couple of weeks in a row. They were glad his chemotherapy was complete because he was experiencing severe numbing and tingling in his lower extremities and they were concerned it would become permanent if he required another round or two of chemotherapy. Midway through Scott's radiation treatments, we did not see the couple any more. We learned that the man had died. We both felt bad. Scott was reluctant to admit it, but this depressed him. He had to fight through it.

There were side effects from the radiation. There were some minor skin burns in the area of the radiation. They gave Scott some creams and the burns were manageable. There was some fatigue and weakness from the treatment. The schedule worked out well because he would be home by early evening. He would take another shower to kill any hospital germs and sometimes a brief nap. He was able to rebound from the radiation treatments fairly well. After a couple of weeks, he was having severe difficulty swallowing. This was due to the location of the radiation. The radiologist-oncologist provided Scott with medication, which he dubbed a "cocktail" to ease the pain and difficulty in swallowing. It might have worked, except that it made Scott very sick to his stomach and reminded him of chemotherapy.

Ultimately, Scott decided that not being able to swallow properly was the lesser of the two problems. Accordingly, he stopped taking the cocktails and toughed it out for two or three weeks. He went on a self-prescribed liquid and soft food diet. Fortunately, the symptoms resolved after the completion of his treatments. For a day or two toward the end of the treatments, Scott had some sharp chest pains. We never received a satisfactory explanation for these pains, but they stopped shortly after the radiation treatments were completed. As with the chemotherapy, at the mid-point and conclusion of the treatments they took CT scans. Still no signs of cancer!

With the insight that some time and distance can bring and all the acumen he could muster, Scott describes the ordeal this way: "they gutted me (surgery), poisoned me (chemotherapy), and nuked me (radiation therapy) and somehow, like a rat, I survived." Now, Scott was being followed up monthly by the oncologist and by the radiologist-oncologist. He still saw the surgeon occasionally. The radiologist-oncologist left to take a position at another hospital. Scott was assigned to a young radiologist-oncologist.

We knew her as she had been the radiologist's fellow and she was a very nice young doctor.

After a few months, we determined that follow-ups by a radiologist-oncologist were no longer needed. We continued seeing the oncologist regularly. Charlene would accompany Scott on most of the follow-up visits. There was one time when Charlene did not go with Scott. After the oncologist did the physical examination, he handed Scott a some papers. Scott asked, "what are these?" The doctor responded, "these are your blood test results, I know Charlene will want to see them." Scott responded, "Charlene trained you well, doctor."

The treatments that started in early spring concluded the day before Thanksgiving. We were very thankful that Scott was alive and that the active treatment was concluded. There have been some scares and bumps along the way and Scott has some residual issues, but he has been able to function for the most part over these several years. About 15 years later Scott would suffer a heart attack as a result of the chemotherapy and radiation treatments.

Scott resented having cancer, having to go through the treatments, and having to put aspects of our lives on hold while being subject to the dictates of doctors and healthcare providers. We have met so many people with prognoses that are more grim, treatments more punishing and debilitating, and we have admired the courage, strength, and toughness of so many cancer survivors that we have been privileged to know over the past several years. Cancer and its treatments leave their physical and emotional scars, even if a person ultimately is cured.

Scott was excited to not be undergoing active treatment and happy to be alive and reasonably well. Scott credits Charlene for saving him and caring for him. Charlene reminded him that he owed her a Disney vacation and, like the Super Bowl winner he wishes he was, he said "honey we're going to Disney World!" We went and it was the best vacation that we ever had. Scott actually enjoyed Disney World and we both knew how fortunate we were to be there together and to pick up where we left off.

Only this time, we looked at life differently. We noticed nature and things we used to take for granted. We had a new understanding and appreciation for how precious life is and how important it is to show the people you love how much you love them because things can change in a second and you may never have that opportunity again.

CHAPTER 8

LIFE GOES ON (SURVIVORSHIP, FOLLOW-UP, AND THE FEARS OF A CANCER SURVIVOR)

Throughout his life, Scott always knew that he would not be a good patient and that he could never go through major surgery or treatment. He was just not cut out for that stuff. So he just hoped he would never need to have surgery. He never gave much thought about dying because he was always too busy living.

Charlene always feared that she would get cancer. Cancer runs rampant in her family and sometimes she says she feels like it is just a matter of time before she is diagnosed with cancer of some type. We both hope and pray that day never comes and that Charlene lives a long and healthy life. Neither of us ever imagined that Scott would be the one diagnosed with cancer and certainly not in his 30s. The point is that cancer impacts so many people and we all should feel a vested interest in curing cancer.

Scott supported sick friends and family members, but never got overly involved in health matters. He did not truly realize how fortunate that he had been to avoid major health problems. After all, his role in the universe is to work and be productive, his calling is the law and his passion has always been the practice of law. He worked extremely hard and still does. He recalls one of the books on success listing good health as one of the common traits of highly successful people. He now has a fundamental understanding of why good health is listed among various leadership qualities and how poor health or disabilities can present major obstacles to success in the professional or business world. He also understands the power of the mind and human spirit and how people often can excel in spite of health challenges. He has a healthy respect for accomplishments of people with health challenges and an understanding for those limited by health restraints in a way, and at a level, he never had before.

Charlene already was in tune with these matters. She had taken care of many people with cancer and other conditions, advocated for patients' rights, helped people who were sick, and did a lot of charitable work. As Scott says, "Charlene is my angel and one that I am happy to share with other people."

We have all had conversations about the deceased. Often someone will point out that "life goes on." The statement is true enough, but we never liked hearing it. We thought the phrase was cold or callused. We often would say to ourselves, "but not for the person who just died." This was not any reflection of our belief in heaven, but rather the sadness that someone who was alive yesterday is not alive today and cannot experience earthly pleasures and pains. It is a striking reality that someone large in stature, generous, thoughtful, outgoing, strong, maybe even seemingly invincible could be silenced instantaneously.

During his treatment, Scott was among the living. The world seemed to slow down. The pain, discomfort, and uncertainty dragged on and on. For the first time in his life, he did not fall asleep when his head hit the pillow. Now he could understand what Charlene went through (she always was a light sleeper and often has difficulty going to sleep). Scott now understood what Frank Sinatra meant about "the wee small hours of the morning."

It is a strange feeling to be up when the rest of the world is sleeping. There is time to think. For a cancer patient, some of that time can be spent wondering whether there is a future. Pain and discomfort can prevent the mind from dwelling on these things too much. Scott hated the nights. To this day, he likes to keep the television set on all night. Maybe it reminds him that he is alive.

The world slowed down in other ways during those dog days of cancer treatment as well. Scott remembers Michael Jordon talking about how at crunch time during a basketball game things on the basketball court slowed down for him and enabled him to perform at such a high level. While the people around Scott were moving quickly, Scott and his world were not. He noticed and perceived things that he never took the time to notice before. Maybe this was because his work schedule was forcibly reduced a little or maybe he was just treating each day as if it were his last.

Having cancer did change Scott and actually made him a more complete person. He was more interested in public and community service—though he insists that Charlene dragged him in that direction. He emerged a deeper, more substantive person though he still prides himself on being a simple, superficial man.

Although cancer was a dominant part of our lives, we made it a point to recognize Scott was not a "cancer patient," he was the same person he was before the diagnosis, but with an important challenge that would require some time and attention. Scott mostly did his thing to the extent possible.

The hopes of cancer patients wax and wane from test to test. What are the results of the blood tests and the scans? Is the treatment working? Are the tumors bigger or smaller? Am I in remission? Your fate and future sometimes seems to hang on the test results. You are anxious before the tests, knowing that they are coming. You are anxious during the tests, knowing the importance of the results of the tests. Unlike college tests or law school examinations, you cannot improve the results by studying. Unlike taking a deposition, writing a brief, or trying a case, your experience, preparation, and expertise will not influence the result. Understandably, cancer patients are anxious about tests and test results. The term aptly coined to describe this is "scanxiety."

Time magazine described scanxiety as "one of those uniquely modern maladies, like carpal tunnel syndrome and BlackBerry thumb, that arise because we're experiencing something entirely new to human beings. For millennia, doctors and patients would have given almost anything to be able to look inside the human body. Now we have an ailment for the fear of what we might find when we do." For a cancer patient, you would almost have to be crazy not to have at least some level of scanxiety.

To make matters worse, doctors, hospitals, medical and non-medical staff often seem to contribute to the stress. We had many ways to try to beat the system and get Scott's test results more quickly. First, Scott always asked the technicians what the scans or x-rays show. There are two standard responses they gave—likely orchestrated by the lawyers representing the hospital or facility. "I'm sorry. I am not allowed to provide that information. You will have to get that information from the doctor." Alternatively, "I am not a doctor, I can determine whether the film is good, but cannot interpret the scans." As a lawyer, Scott fully understood these responses and the reasons for them. As a patient, however, he required immediate feedback and our job was to demand an answer. Many times, he would receive a response from a kind technician something along these lines: "I did not see any mass, but I am not a doctor and you will need to get the report from the radiologist." We always appreciated the kind technicians that took this approach. They knew what they were doing and provided information that afforded some level of relief to us with an appropriate disclaimer. It is important to realize that, when the technician will not give you a hint about the result, it does not necessarily mean you will be receiving bad news. Charlene would demand an instant preliminary reading from a radiologist if there was one around. Sometimes when the right doctor was there and we were willing to wait a few minutes, we got our quick preliminary answer.

We generally had to wait to get a call back with the results. The fellows were good about trying to push the radiologists to deliver at least a preliminary report. When the test results are not provided when expected, the natural fear is that the results are not good and the doctors are not in a hurry to tell you or that they are formulating a new treatment plan. Usually, it just means someone was busier than usual, on vacation, misplaced the results, failed to dictate or proof the report, or forgot to tell you earlier. We both worried, we would attempt to assure each other everything would be alright and provided the analysis for why that would be the case.

Once in remission, we tried to approach periodic scans as a positive thing. Many people have cancer in them for a long time. By getting periodic scans, Scott was assuring himself of catching any disease quickly when it can be most effectively treated. This approach did not eliminate the anxiety, but it did help us cope with it better. The longer in remission, the less anxiety you feel because you become more conditioned to hear good news, particularly if you are feeling well. You never truly lose all of the scanxiety, but you learn to deal with the stress and uncertainty because you have no choice.

Another phenomenon a lot of people experience once they are labeled a "cancer patient" is a new self-awareness with respect to health. Any pain or ache can be worrisome. Things Scott would not have noticed or given a second thought about before could keep us up nights and merited a report or a trip to the doctor.

Being a lymphoma patient, Scott naturally felt all sorts of phantom enlarged lymph nodes. He was shaving one morning and noticed what he thought was a swollen lymph node. Instantly, he felt the cancer had returned. Scott showed Charlene and she said she did not feel anything abnormal. She actually did not feel anything, but was concerned that Scott thought he felt something. She made an appointment with the oncologist. Scott was glad that Charlene did not feel anything because her sense of touch is excellent. But was she just saying that she did not feel a lump to keep him from worrying? Between working on cases, Scott was dreading the prospect of undergoing further treatment. But he had a worse fear: what if there is no treatment this time? Scott tried to resign himself to accept his fate, whatever it was, and returned his focus to his cases. The next couple of days, he checked the area multiple times. He thought he could feel it growing, yet objectively it seemed to be the same size.

Finally, we met with the oncologist. Everything turned out to be alright. The oncologist told us what Scott was feeling was his salivary gland. The doctor said, "it's alright, you were born with it." Maybe so, but Scott never noticed it before. Just a scare, but the cancer had not returned. This is the life of a cancer survivor. Every ache, pain, or lymph node (even if swollen from an infection) is taken seriously and is a cause for concern. It is not unreasonable because relapse always is possible. Developing a cancer secondary to many cancer treatments also is a possibility. You have to learn to live with this reality and control the fear. You have to be vigilant to catch any possible relapse quickly, but not be consumed with fear. It can be a delicate balance, but this is just one of the ways a cancer survivor's life is never the same. When you are not feeling right or are concerned about something, raise it with your doctor. If there is something wrong, it can be addressed. If not, you can relieve your concerns.

Cancer can leave emotional and mental scars, particularly where the treatments are prolonged, the prognosis is poor or uncertain, or the physical symptoms and resulting disabilities are significant. One complaint about the criminal justice system is that, once released, the ex-con is left to fend for himself or herself without the tools needed to be successful. Similarly, the healthcare system traditionally has not done an effective job of providing cancer survivors with the tools needed to function effectively after or outside of the cancer treatment.

Until recent years, very little attention was paid to long-term survivorship issues by the medical profession and non-profits. Once patients finished active treatment they often were left to their own devises, except for periodic follow-up testing. In recent years, cancer "survivorship" has become a cottage industry, with considerably more attention paid to the physical, emotional, psychological, social, vocational, and financial issues associated with cancer and its treatments. Part of it is the economics. With 17 million cancer survivors now in America, this is a pretty big market. However, it has been the efforts, demands, and awareness generated by survivors and advocates that has resulted in more attention and resources being devoted to issues of survivorship and needs of survivors.

Some effects, such as the loss of hair during treatment, can present body image issues, particularly for women. Cancer and its treatments can change a person's physical appearance and impact body functions, sometimes in a significant way. Examples include amputation of a limb, a mastectomy, a colostomy, infertility, or sexual incapacity.

Apart from the physical consequences, there can be emotional consequences associated with the experience of being a cancer survivor. They can be minor such as a temporary loss of confidence or they can present long-term issues regarding one's self-worth or even depression. First, you should realize that most cancer survivors experience one or more of the following: fear of recurrence; anxiety; profound sadness or unhappiness; isolation or loneliness; depression; grief; loss; guilt; uncertainty; and anger. Many have experienced these feelings or issues before cancer and the cancer experience rarely cures them. Even if you managed to avoid being overcome by these feelings before, the cancer experience can bring them out.

Also, cancer and the associated stresses can sometimes interfere with relationships, employment, and marriages. It is important to get help with the mental and physical consequences of cancer and its treatments. For many, talking with family, friends, and other cancer survivors can help. Depending upon the intensity and length of your feelings and the degree to which they are interfering with your life, professional help may be required.

When you have cancer, you need an angel. Where can you get an angel? Our friend, Jonny Imerman, will send you one. Jonny was diagnosed with testicular cancer as a young man (he still is a young man) and founded Imerman Angels to provide one-on-one cancer support to cancer patients and their family members. Imerman Angels matches cancer patients who they call "cancer fighters" with "cancer survivors" who had cancer of the same type. Having a friend that has made it through the same type of cancer or treatments is a tremendous resource. We had Jonny on the *Battling and Beating Cancer Radio Show*, you can listen to him discuss Imerman Angels and testicular cancer on demand at www.blogtalkradio.com/battling-and-beating-cancer. You can get hooked up with an angel at www. imermanangels.org.

Local medical and cancer centers may provide information about support groups as do many of the cancer organizations such as the

American Cancer Society, Gilda's Club, and Cancer Wellness Center. One organization that helps people in their 20s and 30s cope with cancer can be reached at www.imtooyoungforthis.org. There are other resources for cancer survivors. These include: The National Coalition for Cancer Survivorship (www.canceradvocacy.org) and Cancer Support Community (www.cancersupport.org). Additional resources include: www.cancer.net/patient/survivorship; www.survivorshipguidelines.org; www.journeyforward.org; www.oncolife.org/oncolife; www.nccn.org/patients/resources/life_after_cancer/default.aspx.

Cancer does not erase other problems, issues, or responsibilities. It only adds to them. Accordingly, once the treatment is completed, all of the tasks and problems you had before are still there with additional stresses. You still have the same bills and expenses and cancer only adds to your debts. The calls, letters, visits, and expressions of concern generally fade away, often leaving the patient to deal with survivorship in isolation. It is easy to understand that being a cancer survivor does carry its burdens. As they say, it is better than the alternative.

For some patients like Scott treatment ends within a discrete period of time (in his case within a year of diagnosis). Many patients go through long-term treatment or treatment over decades requiring them to hopefully be living well with cancer over an extended period of time. The take away point is that cancer and its treatments impact the mind, relationships, and the human spirit. Too often, cancer survivors fail to get the necessary help in dealing with these issues. Too often loved ones fail to recognize and help with these issues as compared to the physical symptoms. If you have not done so, get back to the business of living and doing what you like doing. If you need help, seek it out. Getting help does not make you less of a warrior. To the contrary, it is one of the cogent steps a sage warrior will take to survive and fight effectively.

CHAPTER 9

COUNTING OUR BLESSINGS (FORTUNATE TO BE ALIVE)

We get tired of hearing people talk about cancer being a blessing. Cancer is a monster that kills millions of people, ends lives prematurely, and makes wives widows, men widowers, and children orphans. From our experience, cancer seems to impact kind and good people in disproportionate numbers. Even survivors lose control of their lives for a period of time. The economic cost both in terms of expenses and opportunity costs is enormous. The human toll it exacts is immeasurable. We will not accept the notion that cancer is a blessing. As with many disasters, good people and the human spirit can make positive things happen. We do agree that people's reaction and what they do in response to cancer can result in good things and that cancer is a life-altering experience.

Being diagnosed with cancer in his mid-30s is not something Scott wanted, expected, or was prepared to handle. God gave him the strength to bear this burden and endure the treatment and for this we are grateful. But looking past the feelings of anger, self-pity, and loss of control, Scott realized as he was going through the treatment that he was blessed in many respects. Through all of those anxious, sleepless nights during the dark days of treatment, he did not do what Bing Crosby sang and Irving Berlin suggested: "count your blessings, instead of sheep." Scott will count his blessings now in writing for you. The next few paragraphs Scott penned himself.

According to Scott

I will start and end with my wife Charlene. Charlene was there for me every step of the way. She loved me, supported me when I needed it, kicked me when I needed it, cared for me, served as my inspiration, and provided the courage I needed to get through this ordeal. Charlene learned everything about lymphoma. She researched, read, talked to organizations, patients, and doctors, and was the best advocate any patient could hope to have. She convinced me to go through the treatments. She obtained the necessary information for us to make the proper decisions and, when that meant physically blocking the door to prevent a doctor from leaving before all of our questions were fully answered, that is exactly what she did. When it meant discovering errors and preventing medical personnel from making mistakes or demanding better care, she did that as well. I cannot say enough about the love of my life.

The concept for this book was derived from the keynote address that I was honored to deliver at the 2006 North American Educational Forum on Lymphoma in California. The address was entitled, "It Takes A Good Wife To Beat Lymphoma." We altered the title of this book, but the sentiment remains the same. Charlene tops my gratitude list.

I also am grateful for other supportive family members, partners, clients, and friends. Having reasons to live and people to support you make an important difference.

I was fortunate to have good insurance. Having cancer was bad enough, but not having insurance or the means to pay for the best doctors and treatments available or being unable to avail oneself of advantages of modern medicine, such as those shots that built up my immune system, would have been much worse. Having insurance or financial resources to get the best treatments by the best doctors is a blessing.

I am not sure that I was promptly diagnosed, but I was diagnosed in time. Although information now known would have resulted in a more precise diagnosis and a treatment course that would have been altered to prevent the heart attack that I subsequently sustained, I was diagnosed in accordance with the information known and standard of care at the time.

I had good doctors, not everyone is so fortunate. My cancer responded to surgery, chemotherapy, and radiation. Not all cancers do. Even with the proper treatment and good doctors, there were lots of glitches along the way. Never forget that God, family, friends, and good luck also are important parts of the survival equation.

The reality is that most people will beat cancer and that survival rates will continue to increase. Yet, sometimes I think that it is amazing that anyone beats the disease. There is a long list of things that could have gone wrong or decreased my chances of success: not seeking medical treatment when I did; the local convenient care facility not sending me to the hospital; the hospital not taking the appropriate tests or a misdiagnosis at the hospital; going to the wrong surgeon, oncologist, or radiologist-oncologist (either one less capable, one who was capable, but made a mistake or just did not pick up on something or do something as well on a given day); a mass that could not have been removed or removed completely; a mass in a fatal location; cancer that would not respond to chemotherapy or radiation; and sustaining any one of the number of possible severe complications from the treatment. One of the things we have learned is how to eliminate as many of the pitfalls along the way as possible. There are lots of things you can do to increase your chances of survival and we will discuss them in Part 2. Having an advocate and support group, being an active participant in your treatment, and having an appropriate state of mind all make an important difference.

Now I know you are thinking, "if being an active participant and having a positive state of mind is important, how did he survive?" I was not Mr. Optimist and I did not read everything out there on my disease and treatments—you've got me there. However, I did have a sense of humor, faked myself out to some extent by putting on a positive public face and, most important, I had Charlene to take care of the knowledge and participation elements. What I lacked in terms of the power of positive thinking, I made up for with a strong will to live and I was preparing to live.

As a man, I did not and probably still do not completely understand or acknowledge the psychological impact of cancer. Once again, in our family, that part of life falls under Charlene's job description. Fortunately and because of Charlene, I was able to cope with the mental and emotional aspects and was able to bounce back quickly after treatment. The cancer experience caused me to make some positive changes. Naturally, my love and appreciation for Charlene grew as a result of her love, loyalty, and advocacy during my illness. Also, I made a concerted effort to cut loose some people that I realized were vexations to the spirit. We are not guaranteed time on this planet and why waste more time than necessary on people you do not like or people with whom it is unhealthy to associate. You will learn about people as a result of the cancer experience. Some people you thought would be supportive may abandon you. Others who were not especially close to you before may prove to be supportive and become genuine friends.

I do not know how to be a good caregiver, but I do know how important it is to have one. I happen to know one of the best caregivers. Charlene is a cancer warrior's warrior and I will leave it to Charlene to cover this subject in the next chapter.

CHAPTER 10

CHARLENE TO THE RESCUE (THE CAREGIVER AND ADVOCATE)

According to Charlene

I have had the privilege of working with, counseling, and advocating on behalf of countless cancer patients and families. I have worked with men, woman, and children of all ages and from a variety of backgrounds. They have been referred to me through charitable organizations, websites, chat groups, patients and families, friends, doctors, and healthcare providers. Sometimes, the involvement is minimal such as a telephone call or e-mail where I provide some information or respond to a specific query. Other times, the involvement is substantial and personal, where I become very involved on behalf of a patient or family.

It is wonderful to help people and see them beat the disease. Some move on with their lives, others stay in touch, become friends, and even join our mission to cure cancer. But it is very hard and emotional when someone loses their battle. I can't give advice about not taking it personally because I do take it personally. Going to a funeral can take its toll even if the person extended their life beyond what the doctors had expected.

People need help—the diagnosis can be overwhelming and they need somewhere to turn. It is one thing to provide them with sources of information, such as those we have included in this book. But people often need more. Some need help learning their treatment options or evaluating their options, others need hand-holding, and still others require help making a doctor appointment or need someone to go with them to the doctor. Often patients need help identifying or getting into a clinical trial. All need hope and encouragement. Volunteers play such an important role and fill a huge vacuum. Some people have loving families, but need outside help. Others do not have friends or families that they can turn to for help. I still remember Scott asking me, as he was about to leave the hospital after his surgery, what someone would do if they did not have a loved one to take care of them.

The calls and e-mails can come at any time. I don't always have a good answer, but I always try to help. We have never said no to a patient or family and usually can find a way to help, even if only by providing encouragement. That is the role of a cancer champion and patient advocate. I am not going to spend much time on that role in this chapter because you have a sense of what I did from the prior chapters and will learn the substantive elements later in Part 2 of this book.

The roles of caregiver and patient advocate are different—though there can be some overlap and they may be filled by the same person in many instances. I have been a caregiver for people with cancer: my mother; my friends; and my husband. I am happy to help others as an advocate and continue to do a lot of this work. But I hope that I never have to play the role of caregiver again. I had a lot more information and tools than many other people who have to care for someone with cancer. But the emotional aspects of having someone you love go through cancer and the treatment can be difficult, and it can be physically demanding for the caregiver as well.

When Scott was diagnosed with lymphoma I knew I had to take control. I locked myself in survival mode and did everything I could to help Scott survive cancer. I could not go through the surgery, chemotherapy, and radiation treatments for him. But I tried to do everything else. I probably did more than the normal person, but I didn't care, I wanted him to live and I was going to do everything I could to make sure he had that chance. I was on top of all of the medical issues and double checked everything that was being contemplated and that was being done. This is important because medical facilities and hospitals miss things and mix up things because they are dealing with so many people. For example, they initially scheduled Scott's chemotherapy sessions four weeks apart. I knew this was wrong because I read the research studies and the protocols called for the chemotherapy to be administered three weeks apart. I asked the oncology nurse to double check with the oncologist and it turns out that I was correct. So they made the proper adjustment.

A woman we know was going though treatment the same time as Scott and she was not happy with her husband because he wasn't like me in terms of care-giving or involvement in her treatment. He seemed to her to be somewhat distant and detached. I told her that everyone is different and people handle things in their own way. Everyone has to find their comfort zone. Scott knows I am a take charge person when the going gets tough.

There were many times I went off and cried alone fearing Scott would die. We supported each other, but the biggest burden that I took on was keeping my fears from Scott because I thought I had to be strong for him and I was afraid that he would take on my fears. I knew that he had to be strong and felt it was my job to keep him as positive as possible. The other parts of being a caregiver were tough at times, but holding back my feelings from my partner in life was almost unbearable.

There are no rule books for being a caregiver because the needs of each patient, the role and tasks of each caregiver, and the circumstances differ based upon the needs of the patient and the relationship between the patient and caregiver. For our purposes, we are addressing family or volunteer caregivers as opposed to paid healthcare providers. Often the primary caregiver is a spouse, adult child, other family member, or close friend. But sometimes co-workers, neighbors, volunteers, or others undertake this role. Many times, people share the role or divide responsibilities by time, days, or functions. With the prevalence of outpatient treatments, insurance limitations, and more people getting and surviving cancer, today caregivers often do things that used to be done by trained healthcare professionals.

I have seen cancer bring families closer together, but sometimes it can create strains and even rifts. In our case, there was no question that I would take care of Scott. I would not have had it any other way. I had to make sure that he made it through. But I also appreciate the fact that others feel overwhelmed, unduly burdened, frustrated, angry, or even cheated by having to take on the responsibilities of being a caregiver.

The role of a caregiver: As a caregiver, you can have enormous influence on how the cancer patient deals with his or her disease. Your encouragement can help the patient stick with a demanding treatment plan and take other steps that are necessary to get well, like eating nutritious meals or getting enough sleep. You are the coordinator of care, the interface between the healthcare providers and the patient, the taskmaster making sure the patient does what he or she is supposed to do and refrains from things that the patient is not supposed to do. You are the patient's eyes and ears while he or she is in the hands of physicians and healthcare providers and the physician's eyes and ears while the patient is at home. Caregivers have to keep track of prescriptions, know which tests must be done, and communicate with the physicians and other family members. You have all of these things to do and still have to fulfill your other responsibilities. It really is quite a responsibility on the one hand and it can be quite rewarding on the other hand. In many ways, it is like being a parent when your child is sick. But when the patient is an adult it can make some things easier to the extent the patient is knowledgeable, appreciative, and cooperative. Sometimes, it can make things more challenging.

The tasks of a caregiver: Obviously the tasks vary depending upon the patient's needs, but they can run the spectrum from cooking, housecleaning, providing personal care and hygiene, shopping for food, medications, and health aids, making doctor appointments, transporting and accompanying patients on appointments and treatments, managing finances, solving problems, giving medications, shots, oxygen, and other treatments for which a medical professional is unnecessary or unavailable, keeping the patient company, taking phone calls, updating people on the patient's condition and needs, communicating with healthcare providers, dealing with insurance issues, explaining things to the patient and the physicians, monitoring and watching the patient's condition and health, bathing or bathroom monitor, fetching things, doing all sorts of things for, or on behalf of, the patient that the patient used to do for himself or herself. The tasks depend upon what the patient wants or needs and what you are willing and able to do.

Qualities of a caregiver: Being a good caregiver means being realistic, positive, resourceful, and creative. Knowing when the patient needs uplifting and optimism and knowing when the patient needs a kick in the rear end. It means identifying situations and symptoms that need immediate care and attention and being calm and collected when the patient is nervous or anxious. You have to be assertive in obtaining information and yet know when to respect the patient's privacy and know how to maintain the patient's dignity. You have to know when to lead and be assertive and when to defer to the patient. Medical knowledge and good judgment are always big pluses when you are taking care of someone with cancer or any major disease.

A few tips: Once again, there are no rules or static roles. But the greater the trust and better the communication between the patient and caregiver, the better the relationship will be.

- Keep organized. Maintain a running list of tasks and appointments and use Appendices "G" and "H" to maintain information regarding the patient's health issues. Help the patient prioritize and schedule.
- Involve the patient as much as possible because it is their health and life at stake.
- Step in and help the patient or protect his or her interests to the extent the patient is not able to do so and to the extent that you are able to do so.
- Keep in mind that the disease and treatments have emotional, mental, and financial as well as physical impacts on the patient. People confronting a disease may act differently than they do normally. They may be quiet, depressed, withdrawn, angry, or offensive. They may take their frustrations, fears, and pains out on you. Nobody wants to be sick and when you are not feeling well it is easy to be crabby. Try to realize the actions directed at you are not actually directed at anything that you did wrong. Sometimes you may let things roll off your back, but there are times when you have to set boundaries and rules.
- Everyone handles cancer differently. Some people don't want to talk about cancer at all. The patient may be afraid to talk about it or may be in denial. Let them know that you are there for them. Don't push the patient to talk about things, just let him or her lead the way. If the patient wants to talk about things in the past, just go with it. If he or she wants to talk about being scared or afraid of dying, provide encouragement and hope. Sometimes, people become more spiritual than they were in the past and that is good. Other patients want to talk about cancer and their condition as much as they can and become consumed with cancer. At some point, you have to try to get them to focus on living and on other topics.
- Apart from the physical sickness, the patient may feel he or she is a drain on the caregiver and may feel guilty, inadequate, or that things would be much easier for you if he or she were not around. Sometimes patients do need a little kick, reminding them that they are not just fighting for themselves, but also are fighting for us, our children, grandchildren, family, and friends. Sometimes that revives their fighting instincts because they do not want to leave their loved ones. Sometimes you have to help patients along

because they get discouraged and say they don't want to do this anymore. It is important that you let them know there is a light at the end of the treatment tunnel for them.
- Help the patient where he or she needs it, but encourage the patient to do things for themselves to the extent that they are able. Help the patient to lead as normal a life as possible.
- Give a hug and a smile.
- Develop a sense of when the patient needs to be alone and needs company.
- Don't put too much on the patient at one time. Many things can be done gradually. Sometimes a one-step-at-a-time approach is appropriate so that the patient does not feel overwhelmed and has time to adjust.
- Know your limitations. There are some things that you may not feel qualified or comfortable doing and you may have to rely upon others.
- Sometimes you cannot do or get to everything. Focus your efforts on the important things.
- Call upon support from family members if the patient is avoiding treatments, not doing what needs to be done, or doing things that are harmful.
- It is normal to feel frustrated, upset, and stressed sometimes when caring for someone with cancer. Use the resources and services of the healthcare team and other family members. There are support groups for caregivers and we have listed some in Appendix "C."
- Caregivers may feel isolated, depressed, stuck, or anxious. These feelings and the physical demands associated with care-giving can take a toll on the caregiver's health. Remember to take care of yourself and your health. Eat, sleep, and tend to your health issues.
- Make arrangements for others to step in and provide care so that you can take a break, relax, and enjoy life. You need a break and to take some time for yourself. A caregiver needs time to get away and recharge. Do something once a week that you like or ask someone to do something that will lessen the burden on you.
- Educate yourself about the disease. The more you know, the better you will know what to expect and how to care for the patient. Ask doctors and nurses about your loved one's condition and what you as a caregiver need to know. The internet is also a very good way

to learn more about your loved one's disease. Several resources are listed in Appendix "C."
- You must take all precautions against the patient contracting an infection, particularly if the patient is undergoing chemotherapy or a stem cell transplant. Limit the people they come into contact with and keep them clean. Monitor their blood counts closely and get immediate medical attention at the first sign of any cold or infection. We lost a friend who was undergoing a stem cell transplant due to infection.

Apart from spending time with your loved one, there is comfort and satisfaction knowing that you are there to care for them, comfort them, and make sure their needs are met with love and kindness.

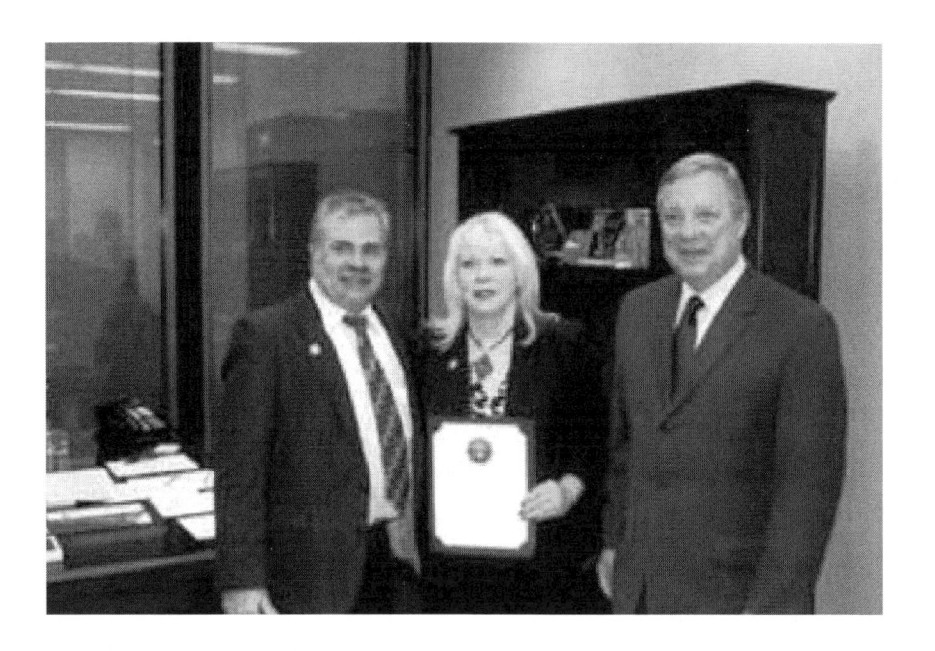

Charlene, Scott, and Illinois Senator Richard Durbin discussing legislation to keep an important cancer treatment on the market and the landmark Students in Action program.

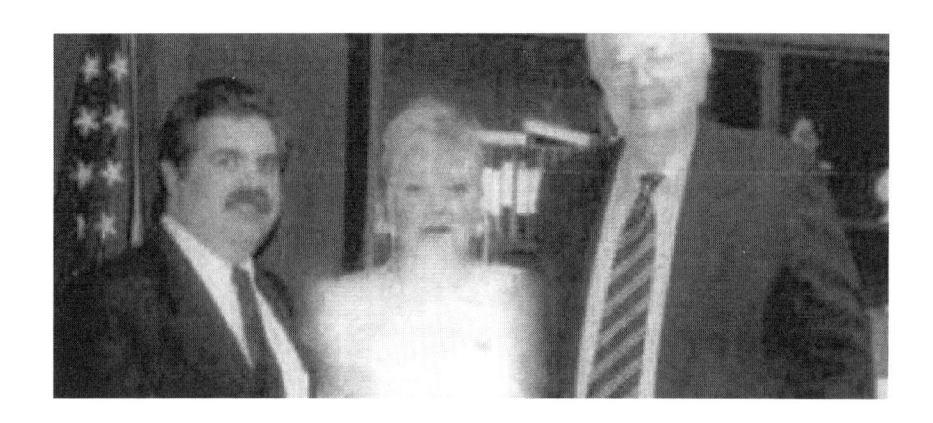

Charlene and Scott meeting with Congressman Henry Hyde to push the blood cancer agenda.

CHAPTER 11

PUTTING OUR NATION'S "LEADERS" TO WORK FOR US (OUR PUBLIC POLICY ADVOCACY EFFORTS)

With the active treatment behind Scott, he was anxious to get back to the business of living and litigating at a high level. He declared that "the word 'cancer' shall be stricken from all tablets and shall not be spoken in our house again." Charlene felt differently and said that we must do everything that we can do as laypeople to defeat cancer and to help others so that they did not have to go through what we went through. Scott's standard line is, "as a lawyer, the notion of helping other people never occurred to me. I am engaged in the battle against cancer because Charlene enlisted me."

Our mission to cure cancer during our lifetime has become a passion. We know we are not alone in this goal and many others are doing much more than us, but we have had an impact. Helping others was hardly new to Charlene, as she had helped cancer patients and been involved in charitable work long before cancer struck Scott.

Right after Scott's treatments, Charlene did some private fundraising through a letter writing campaign. Basically, Charlene wrote people saying her husband has lymphoma and asking people to donate money so we can find a cure. We donated the funds to a major medical center for cancer research. This was laudable and raised some money, but did not have the broad impact we were looking to achieve.

Charlene communicated frequently with senators and congressmen about a variety of health-related issues, including breast cancer. We now know what Charlene was doing was called public policy advocacy. Now she had a specific area of focus, although she has continued to champion various causes. Through what was then called the Cure for Lymphoma Foundation, she learned of the need to get lymphoma and blood cancer language in the appropriations bill for the National Institutes of Health and National Cancer Institute. There was specific language that was requested, and Charlene was determined to have that language included in the legislation.

Charlene set up a meeting with the late Congressman Henry Hyde, who was the representative for our congressional district in Illinois. Although we have made exceptions, we generally have decided not to spend our time with congressional aides or staff unless we have a prior relationship with them or have previously made contact with the senator or representative. We understand that is the opposite of how many people work, but for better or worse this is our methodology. We met with Congressman Hyde at his home office in Illinois. It saved us a trip to Washington D.C. and Charlene thought he would have more time for us at his local office.

Charlene did some background research and planned a presentation. Congressman Hyde's staff was very kind and accommodating. While waiting to meet with the Congressman, we spoke with representatives or lobbyists for HMOs that also were scheduled to meet with the Congressman after us. Congressman Hyde was ready to meet with us exactly on time, which impressed us. We went into his office and met with him alone for about 40 minutes and then his legislative aide joined us for a few minutes.

Charlene told him Scott's story in abbreviated fashion. She showed him the only picture of Scott from the dog days of chemotherapy. We gave Congressman Hyde an overview of lymphoma, its treatments, and advances on the horizon. The Congressman was supportive of our efforts, but said that he did not have a great deal of knowledge about lymphoma until meeting with us. He now understood something about lymphoma and its human toll. He said, "now I have a face and a story to put with the disease." We talked about cancer generally. He told us that his late wife had uterine cancer and he had bladder cancer.

We asked Congressman Hyde to support language in the appropriations bill directing the various agencies, including the National Cancer Institute, to dedicate additional efforts and funding for lymphoma research and treatment. Congressman Hyde said that he was very impressed with Charlene's presentation. He promised to support the language and also to express his support to Congressman Porter who sat on the appropriations sub-committee. While we were in this office, Congressman Hyde picked up his phone and called Congressman Porter. He told Congressman Porter what we requested, gave a couple of highlights from Charlene's presentation, said he supported including the language and asked for Congressman's Porter's support. Congressman Porter said he would support the language and asked that we provide him with the exact language that wanted in the bill. We left Congressman Hyde some written materials on lymphoma and the lymphoma organization. We thanked him for his time and support. At Congressman Hyde's suggestion, we followed up with Congressman Porter. Representatives Hyde and Porter were true to their word and the requested language appeared in the bill. Needless to say it was a productive meeting.

We maintained a relationship with Congressman Hyde on health issues. His office consulted with Charlene from time to time on cancer-related issues. Congressman Hyde asked Charlene to speak on stem cell transplantation as part of an effort to have Medicaid pay for stem cell transplantation. Charlene made a very compelling case for funding stem cell transplantation.

We realize that many of you are asking why get involved in public policy advocacy. After all, politicians are worse than lawyers. In fact, many of them are lawyers. The answer for Scott was simple. Charlene set up the appointment and made him go with her. The better answer is that, as cancer survivors and concerned citizens, we need to let our public officials know that more money must go to cancer research. We need to let them know what we expect on various issues relating to patient rights and other issues relating to health.

We have done a lot of public policy advocacy over the years and believe this is one of the important arrows in the cancer advocacy quiver. Mostly our focus has been on cancer, but we have been involved in other health issues (such as hospital infections and health insurance) and public and community service matters. The government can fund a whole lot of cancer research in one fell swoop. There is synergy in cancer research and research on one type of cancer may benefit other types as well. But there is competition among cancers and among diseases for a limited universe of funding. Believe it or not, most politicians listen to their constituents particularly when inundated with contacts and squeaky wheels do tend to get oiled. One of our complaints about cancer and lymphoma survivors is that, as a group, we are too stoic and quiet. We need to make more noise and have our voices heard. Lymphoma, leukemia, and myeloma are under-publicized diseases and that is one thing we aim to change.

There is some merit to simply contacting your senators, representative, governor, and the White House and demanding more money be appropriated for cancer research. Public policy advocacy, however, is much more effective when you are requesting a particular action. A "dear colleague" letter, a vote on a specific bill, or request for a hearing on a particular issue is much more likely to be effective.

Most major cancer-related organizations and medical institutions have people who monitor legislation and generate a legislative and public policy agenda. One way to keep informed of developments and to have an impact is by working with an appropriate non-profit cancer organization. They usually welcome volunteers and provide training and information. Before you invest too much time, make sure that the organization's agenda is something that you actually support and actually supports your mission. Although non-profit organizations are extremely competitive, they often join forces in support of legislation and in lobbying leaders.

There are courses, degrees, and careers in public policy advocacy. But as the Sammy Cahn song says, we will "give you the whole magilla in a one word speech: reach." Effective public policy advocacy boils down to: (1) having a specific request or agenda; (2) contacting the correct officials (those capable of supporting or advancing your request); (3) having the best person contact the public official (the contact hierarchy is someone with a personal relationship with the public official or aide, a constituent, an invested advocate such as a patient, survivor, or family member, and a non-profit staff person); (4) providing the appropriate information (the specific bill, letter, bill language, background, and research information regarding the cause and request) and appropriate background; (5) determining the best manner and time to communicate (letter, e-mail, call, or appointment); (6) "making the ask" and properly communicating the request (streamline and organize the presentation); (7) following up; and (8) enlisting as much support as possible—the more calls, letters, and emails, the better.

These folks are very busy and have competing demands for their time and attention. Respect their time. Be respectful to them and be professional. Be clear, direct, and organized in your presentations and communications. Unless you are a "one legislation Charlie," develop relationships with the public official and staff. This makes it more likely your communications will be received and acted upon. Charlene has made an effort to develop relationships. From time to time, officials reach out to Charlene to get her views on health-related issues and to alert her to activities.

Non-profit organizations can provide important insights, background, and materials. Employees of non-profits have an important role to play. But people relate to "real" people and those impacted by cancer usually have much more impact in meetings and hearings than people just advocating for a living. Many people feel intimated by the prospect of communicating with public officials or by the process. As long as you are willing to share your story and are passionate about your mission, you can be an effective public policy advocate.

Actually, public policy advocacy on health-related issues, particularly cancer, in some respects is easier than in some other areas because cancer is something that impacts so many people and it is a subject that generally is more non-partisan in nature than many subjects. We have found widespread support from Democrats, Republicans, and Independents alike. The main limitation we confront is that "there is only so much money to go around." Our job is to make funding for cancer research a greater priority and to fight to make this a reality. This is part of the national call to action to cure cancer.

The landscape has changed somewhat over the years. In particular, the internet and social media have empowered patients and provided great platforms for raising issues and becoming aware of issues, engaging and activating others on issues, and getting out the "word" directly.

Increasingly, more and more decisions impacting patients are made by non-elected government bureaucrats. Getting the attention and proper response from these folks can be a frustrating, time-consuming, and challenging process.

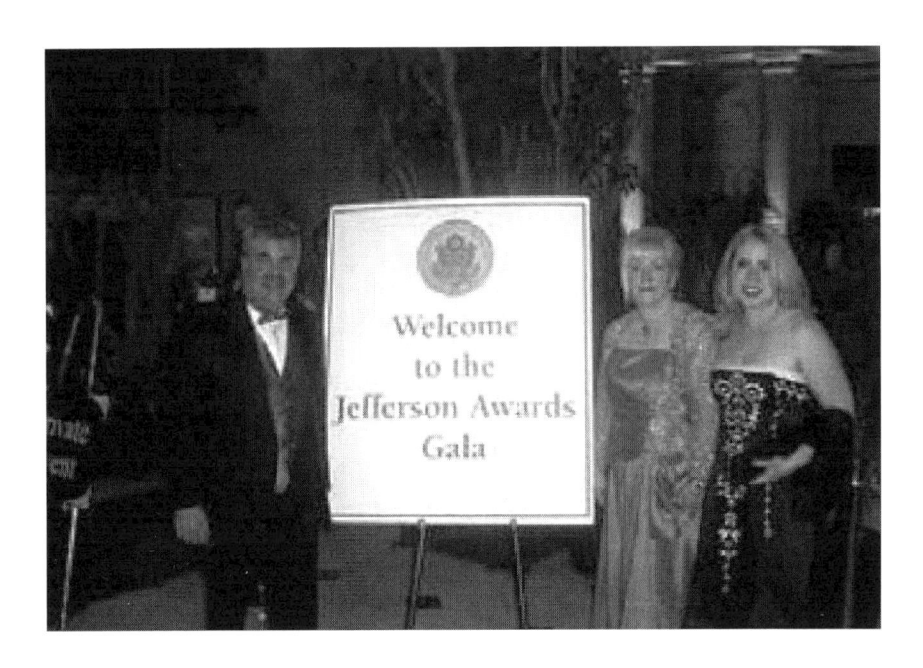

Charlene and Scott at the National Jefferson Awards Ceremonies in Washington, D.C., where Charlene received her Jefferson Award.

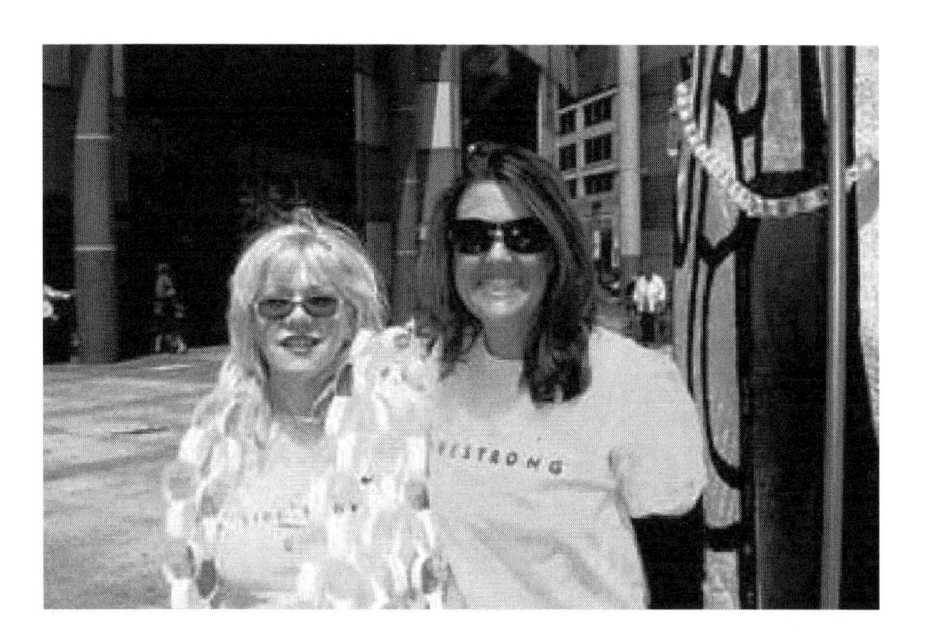

Charlene helped organize the first Livestrong Day in Chicago.

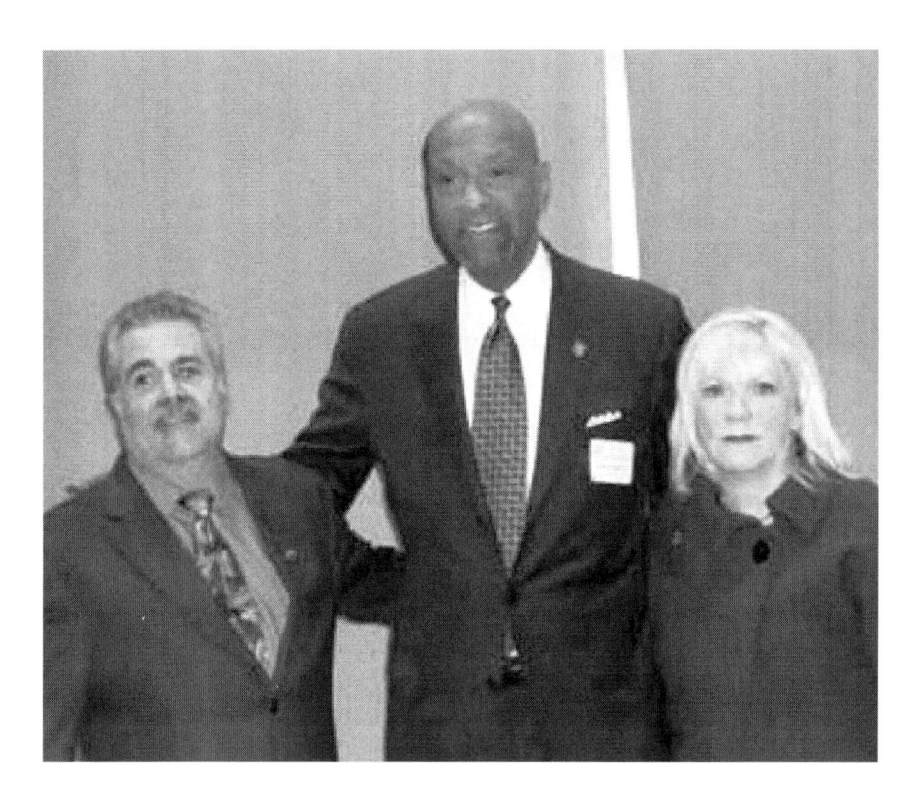

Charlene and Scott with NBC 5 Chicago's news anchor Warner Saunders co-chairing "Celebrate Chicago."

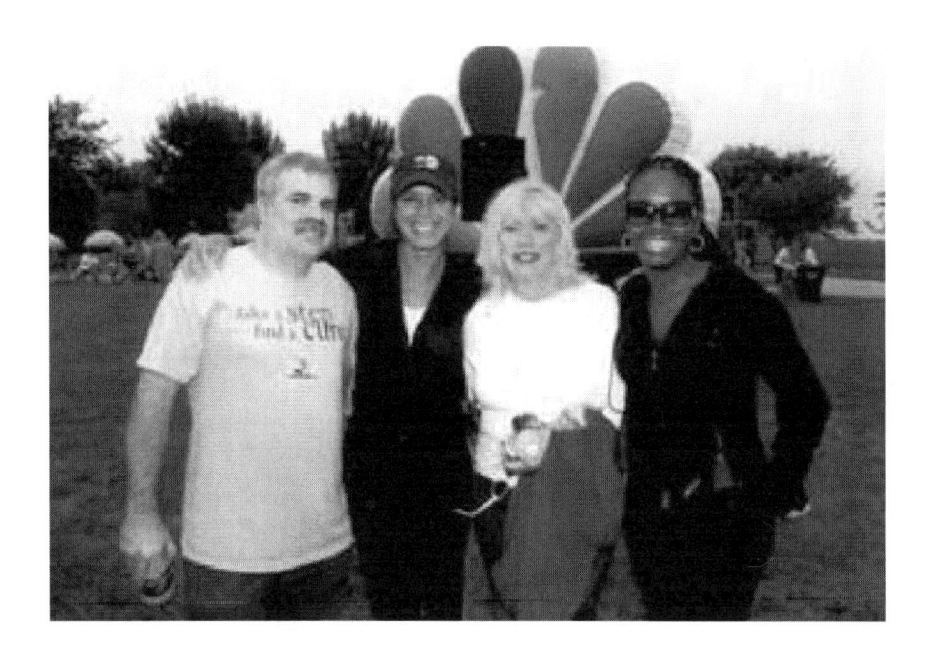

Charlene and Scott with Zoraida Sambolin, NBC 5 Chicago and Telemundo Chicago news anchor and reporter, and Deborah Brown, NBC 5 Chicago's Director of Station Relations.

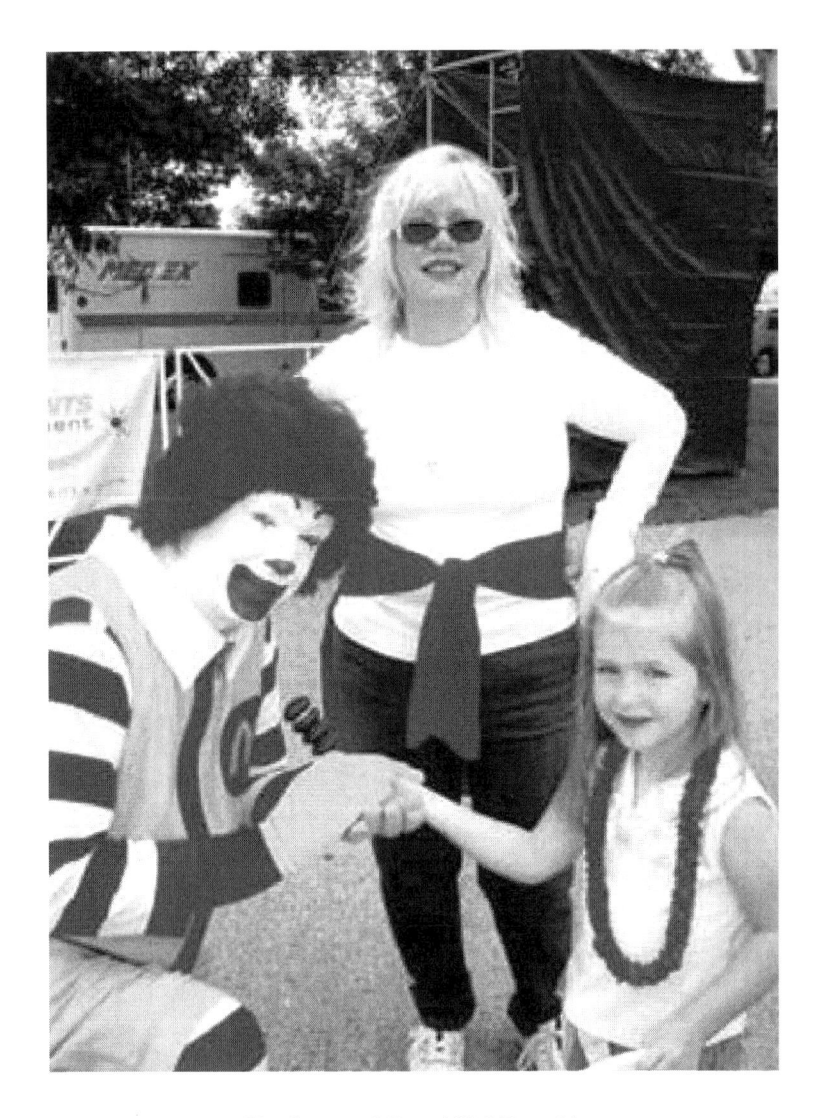

Charlene and Ronald McDonald.

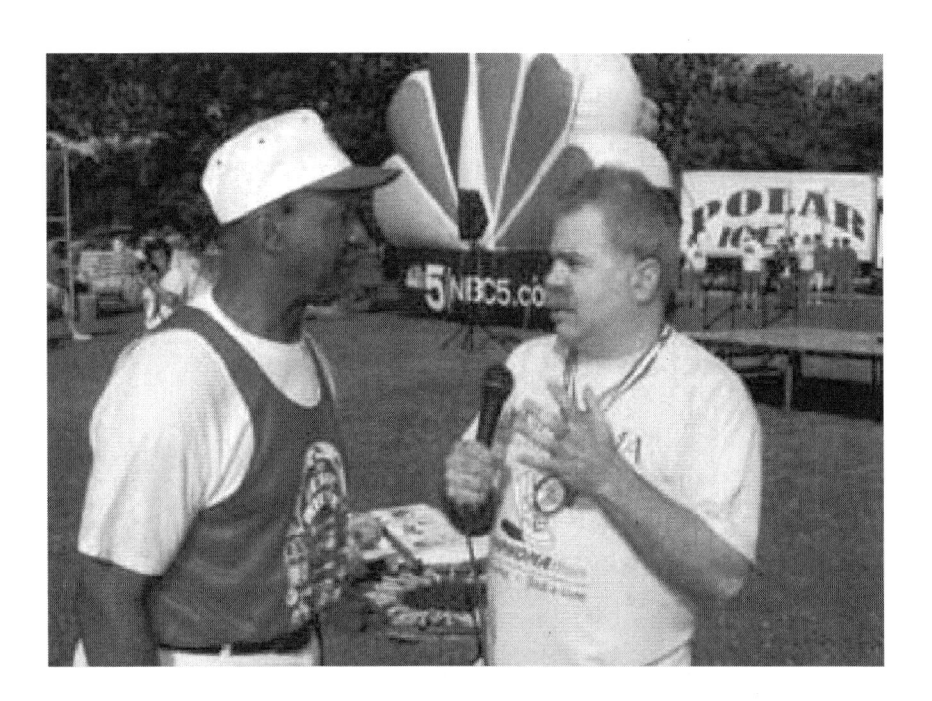

Scott and Illinois Secretary of State Jesse White, discussing the fabulous Jesse White Tumblers and the importance of "giving back."

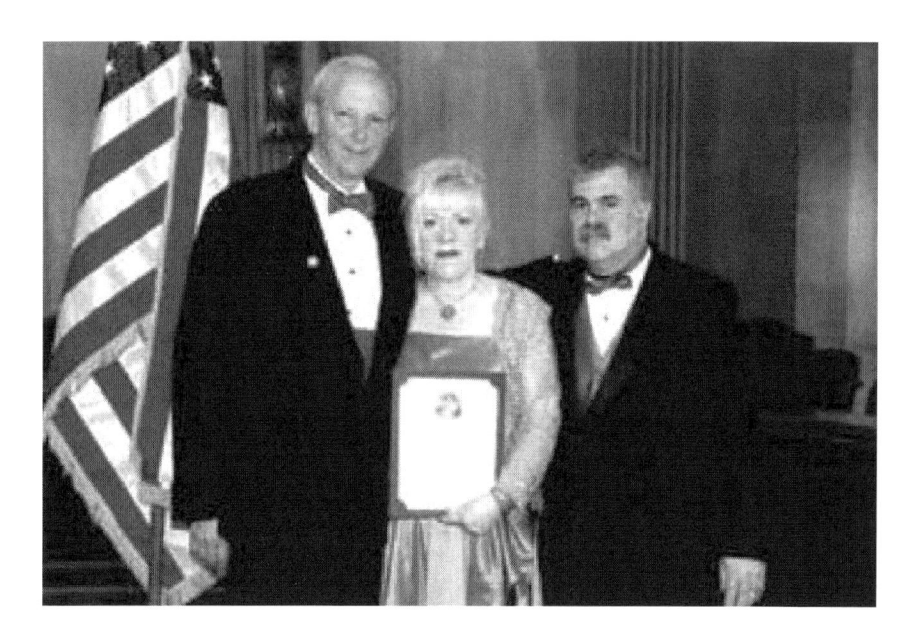

Charlene and Scott with Sam Beard, co-founder of the Jefferson Awards for Public Service and Chairman of the National Development Council, at the United States Senate Office Building.

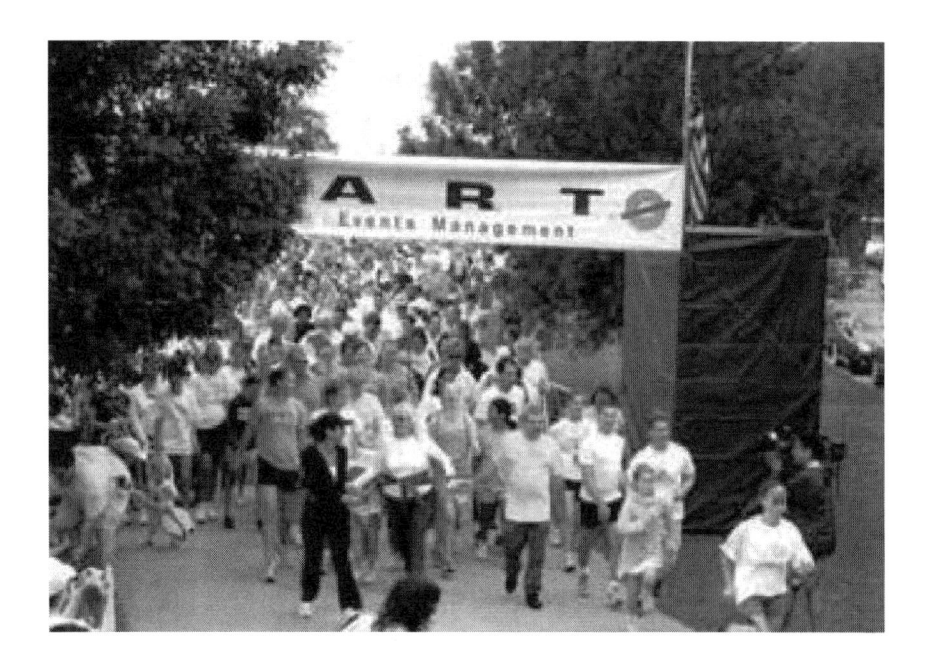

Zoraida, Charlene, and Scott are getting overtaken after starting off the Lymphomathon one year.

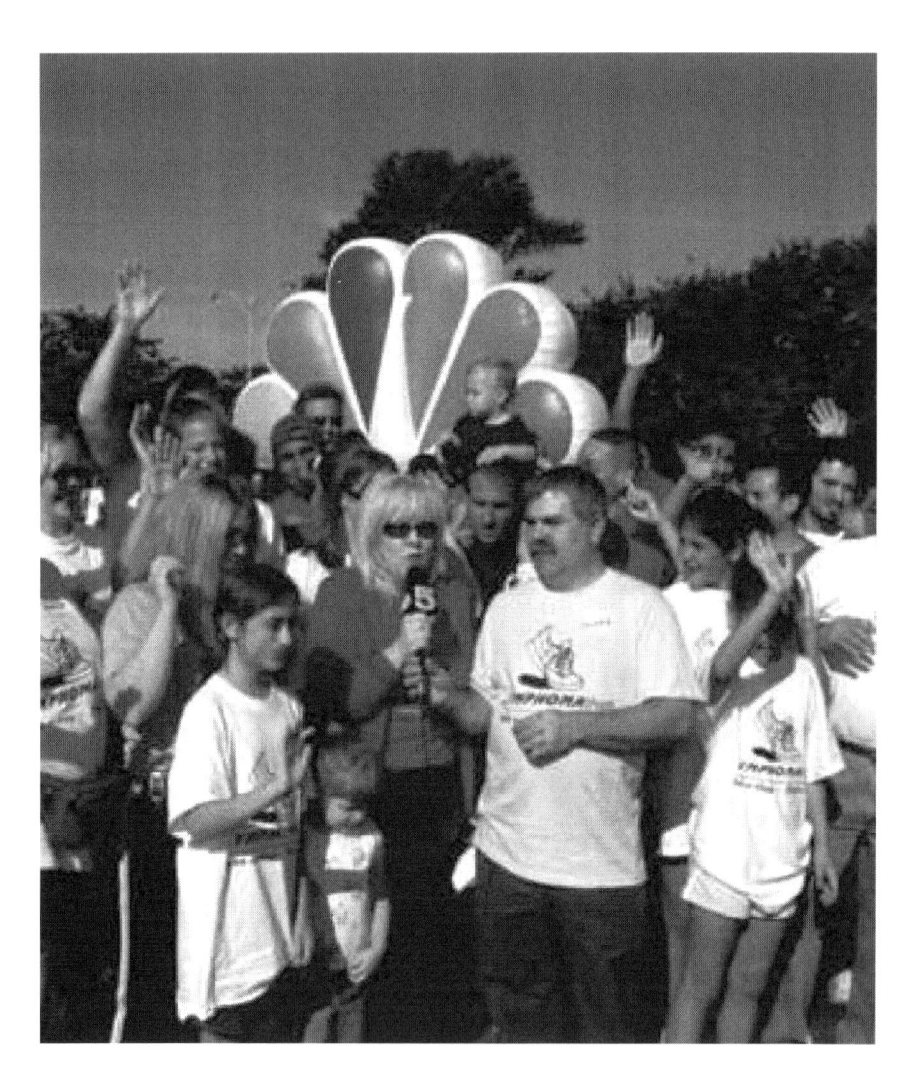

Charlene, Scott, and the gang live "on-air."

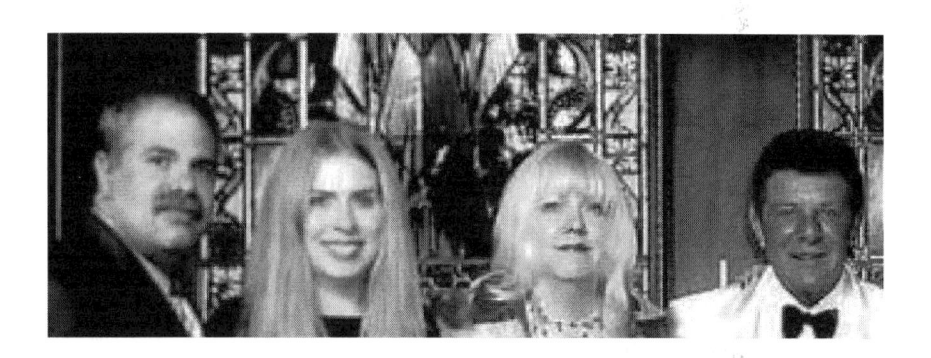

Charlene and Scott with Frankie Avalon at a cancer fundraising event.

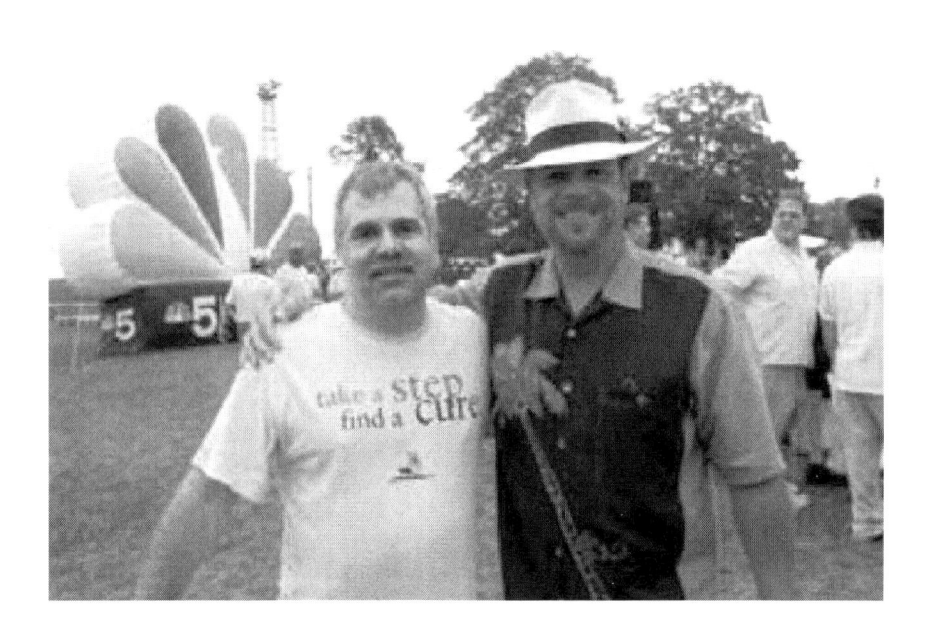

A couple of friends and fellow cancer survivors Scott and Chicago's Entertainer, Ron Hawking.

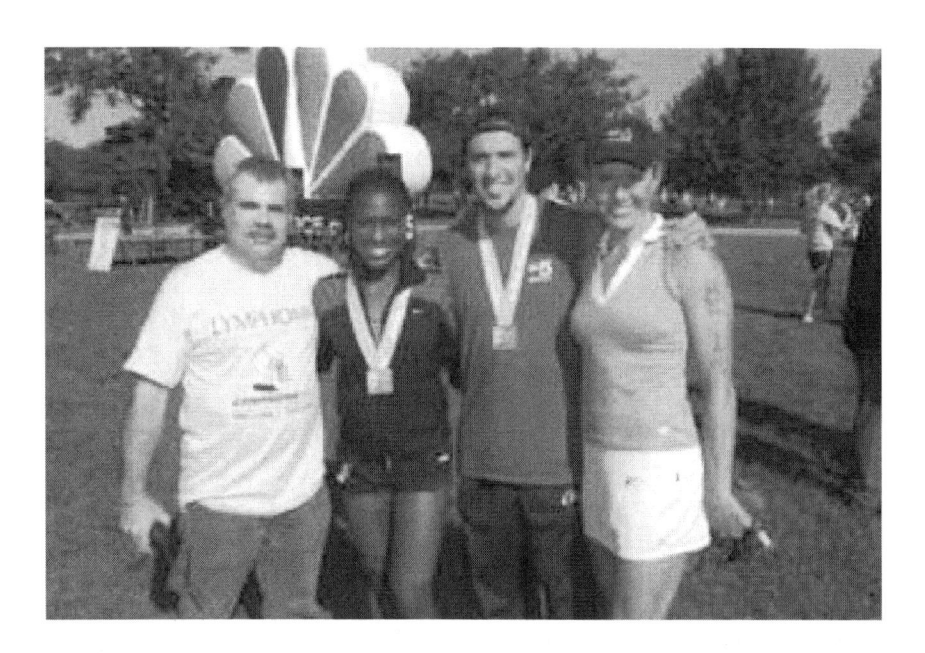

Sergio Rojas, Saran Dunmore, and Andrea Metcalf "The NBC 5 Fitness Team" urging Scott to get in shape.

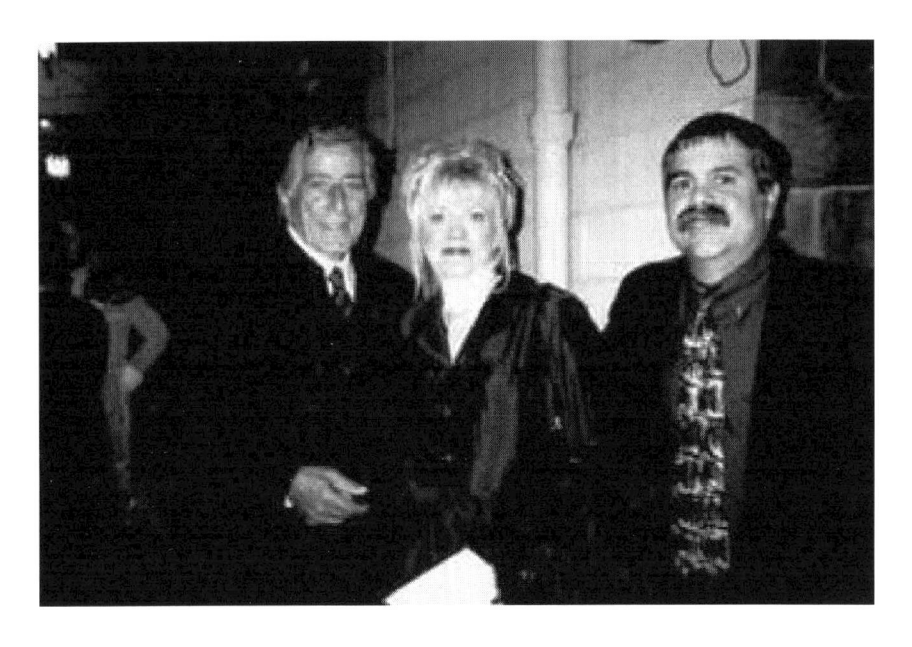

Charlene and Scott with the legendary Tony Bennett.

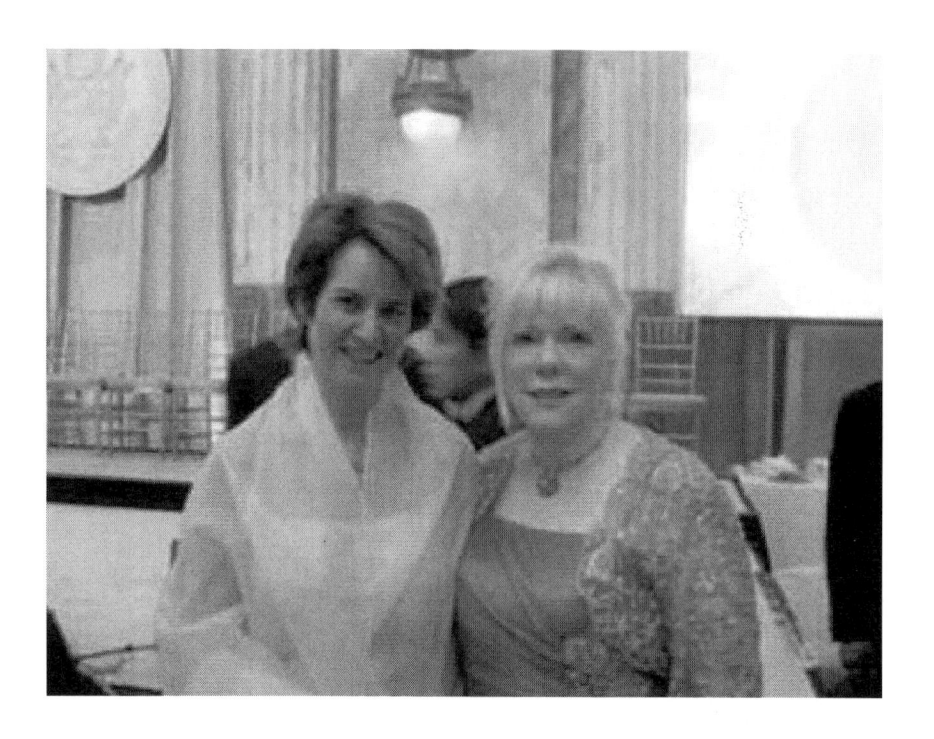

Charlene and Kathleen Kennedy Townsend discussing dresses and public service.

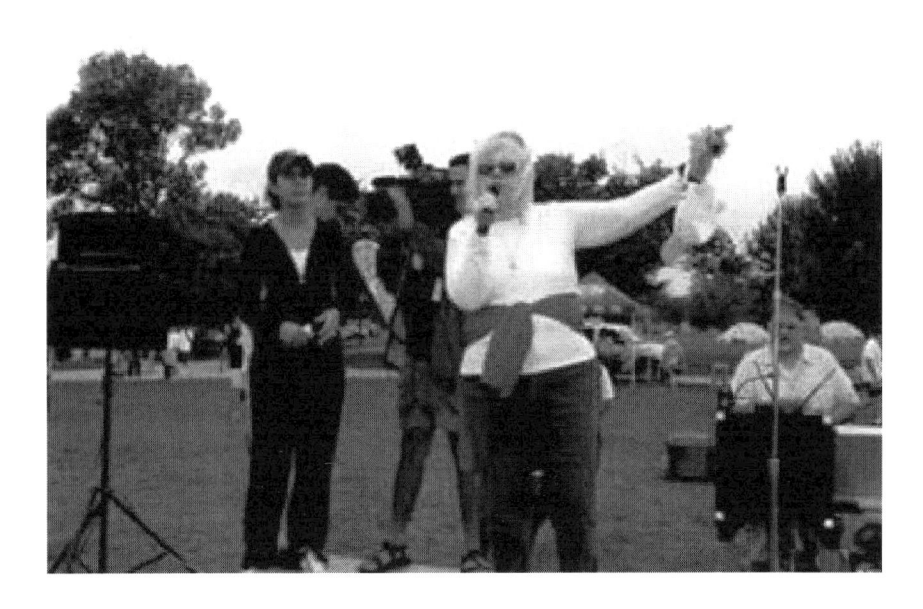

Charlene and Zoraida inspiring participants.

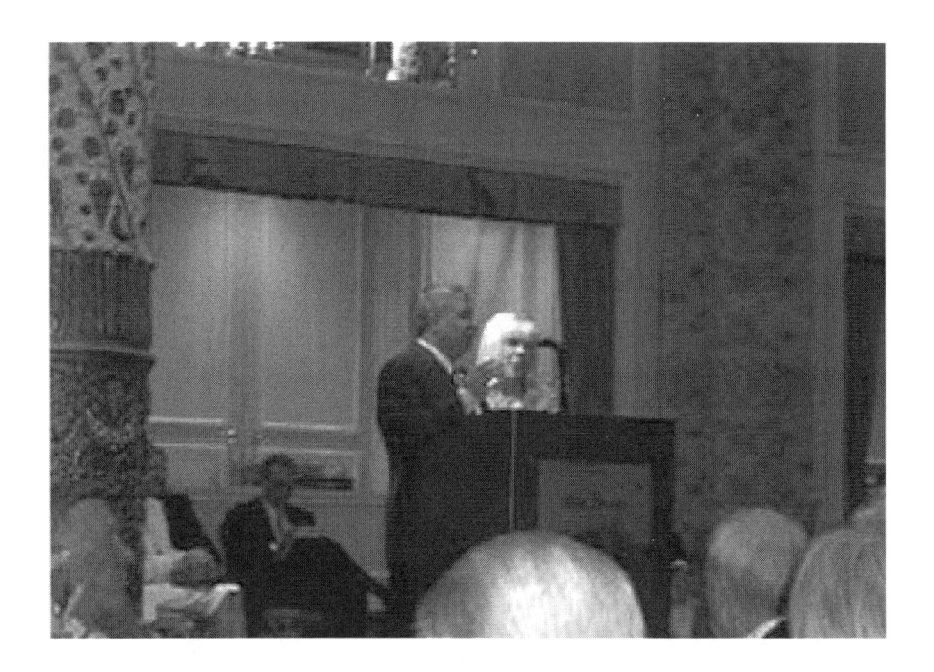

Charlene and Scott speaking at the First Annual Lymphoma
Dinner after receiving the LRF Tribute Award

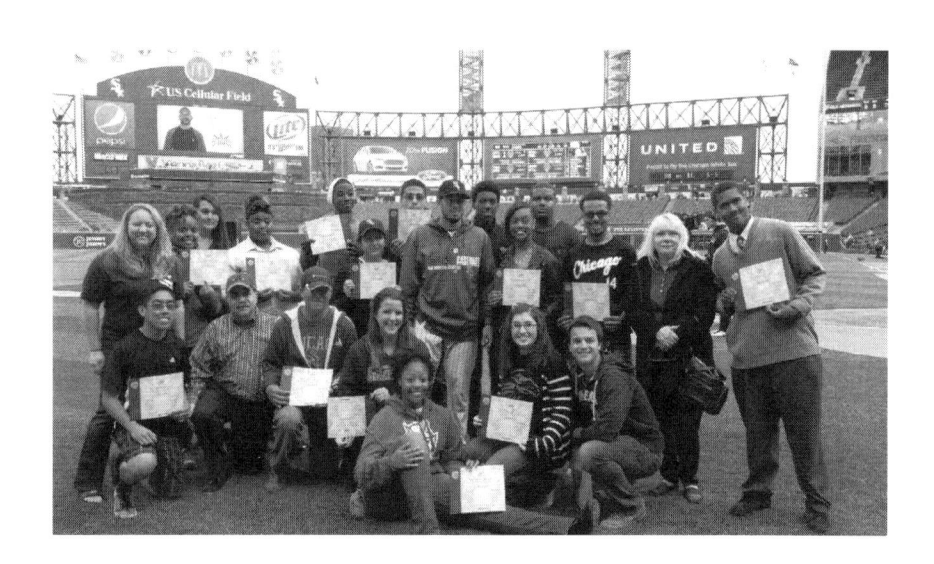

Charlene and Scott on the field with high school student leaders who were being recognized for their community leadership and philanthropic efforts.

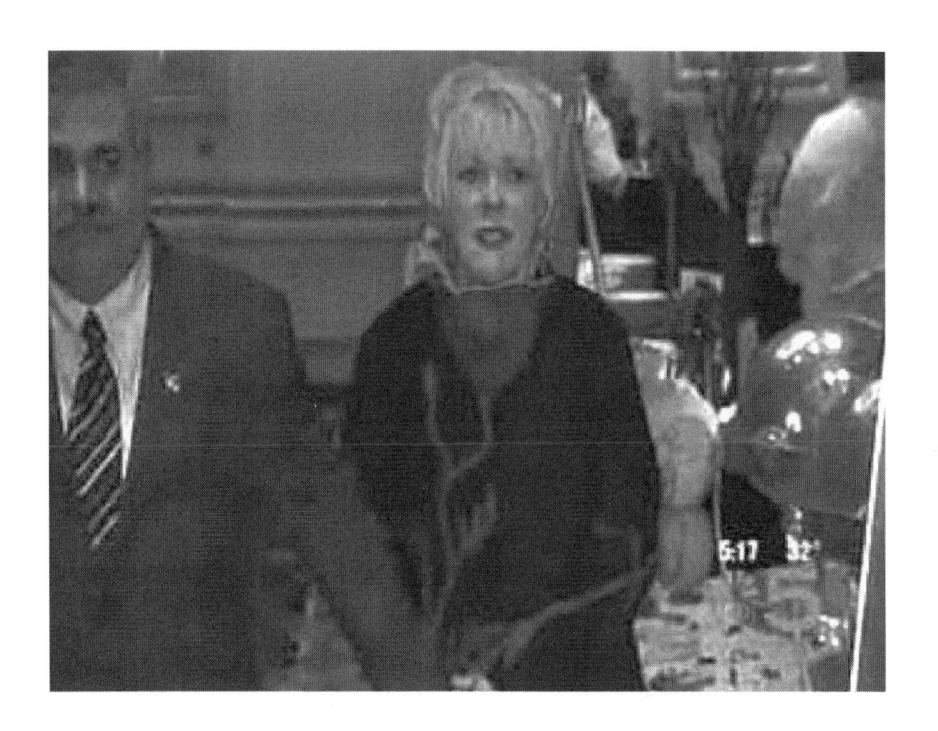

Charlene and Scott at the Second Annual Lymphoma Dinner.

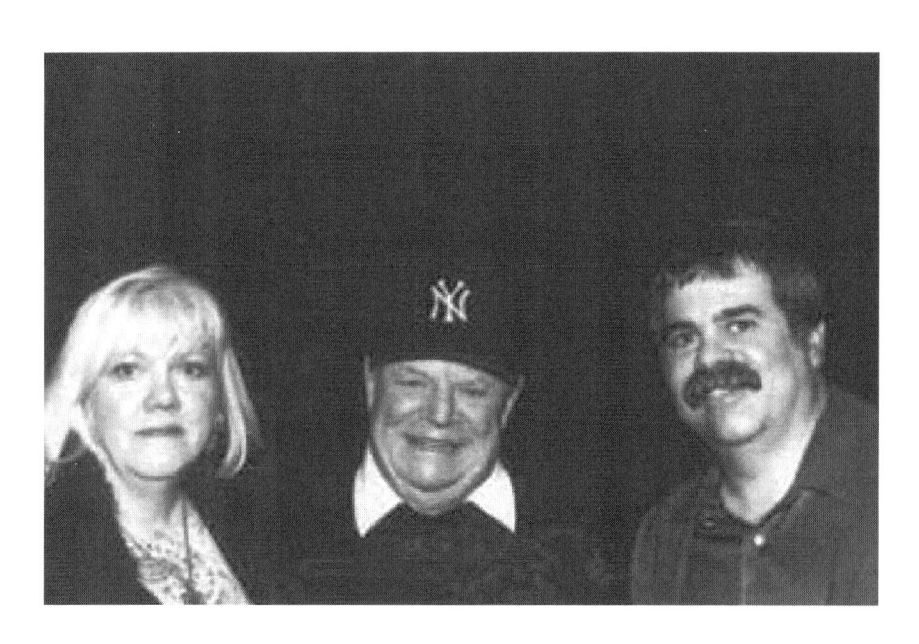

Charlene and Scott with the legendary Don Rickles.

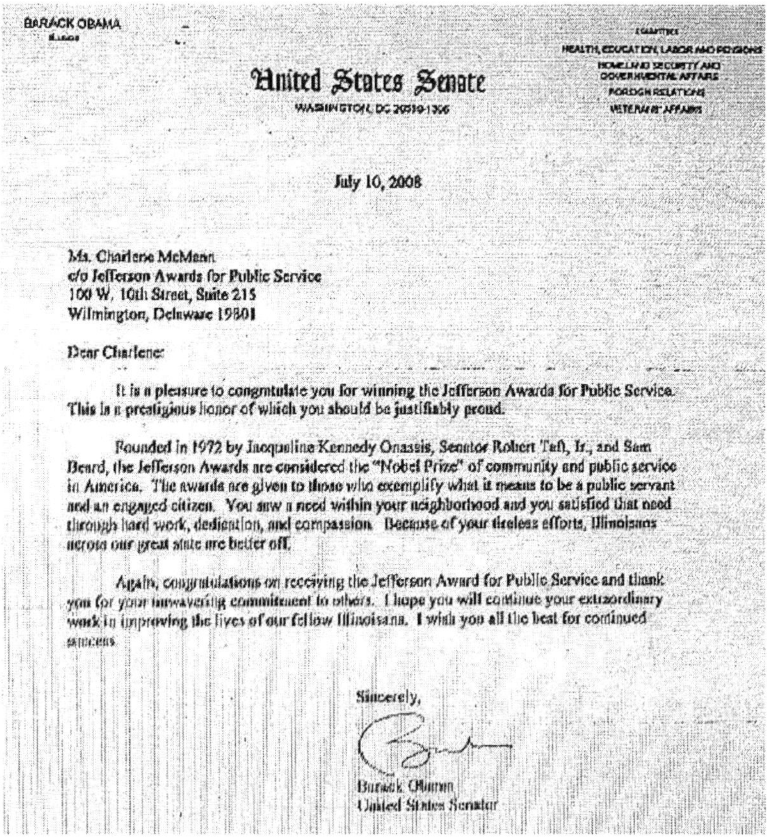

BARACK OBAMA
ILLINOIS

United States Senate
WASHINGTON, DC 20510-1306

COMMITTEES:
HEALTH, EDUCATION, LABOR AND PENSIONS
HOMELAND SECURITY AND GOVERNMENTAL AFFAIRS
FOREIGN RELATIONS
VETERANS' AFFAIRS

July 10, 2008

Ms. Charlene McMann
c/o Jefferson Awards for Public Service
100 W. 10th Street, Suite 215
Wilmington, Delaware 19801

Dear Charlene:

It is a pleasure to congratulate you for winning the Jefferson Awards for Public Service. This is a prestigious honor of which you should be justifiably proud.

Founded in 1972 by Jacqueline Kennedy Onassis, Senator Robert Taft, Jr., and Sam Beard, the Jefferson Awards are considered the "Nobel Prize" of community and public service in America. The awards are given to those who exemplify what it means to be a public servant and an engaged citizen. You saw a need within your neighborhood and you satisfied that need through hard work, dedication, and compassion. Because of your tireless efforts, Illinoisans across our great state are better off.

Again, congratulations on receiving the Jefferson Award for Public Service and thank you for your unwavering commitment to others. I hope you will continue your extraordinary work in improving the lives of our fellow Illinoisans. I wish you all the best for continued success.

Sincerely,

Barack Obama
United States Senator

Letter to Charlene from President Obama (then Senator) Congratulating Her on Winning the Jefferson Award for Public Service.

CHAPTER 12

CHARLENE'S IDEA BECAME A MISSION (FIGHTING BACK THROUGH CANCER FUNDRAISING, AWARENESS, AND ORGANIZING EFFORTS)

Back at the time that our cancer nightmare began, there was nowhere near as much information available on the internet as there is today. In fact, the internet was in its infancy. Charlene worked hard to get useful information about lymphoma. She was reading and calling doctors and organizations. During her information earthworm activities, she called a blood cancer organization. She spoke to a wonderful lady who provided her with information about lymphoma, feedback on oncologists, and she also provided Charlene with hope. It turns out that her husband had the same type of lymphoma that Scott had and it originated in the same approximate area. She told Charlene that her husband was doing really well and that he had been diagnosed about five years earlier. He still is doing well and they have done tremendous things for people impacted by cancer. They used his diagnosis and the lack of information then available about lymphoma as the impetus to start an organization. At some point, Charlene told her that, if they ever wanted to start a chapter in Chicago, to let her know and she would help.

Learning someone else had the same type of cancer and survived lifted Charlene's spirits and gave her hope. Charlene stayed in contact with the organization and occasionally did things with or through it. A couple of years later, this organization merged with another and became interested in forming chapters. With national offices in New York and Los Angeles, Chicago was the natural place for the organization's first chapter.

Subsequent to Charlene's initial dialogue, others expressed interest in participating as a result of an educational event.

We had both done charity work through other organizations, but this mission was personal. The co-founder and executive director of the organization came to Chicago in the summer of 2002 for an initial meeting to see whether the time was right to form the organization's first chapter. They felt if we could raise $50,000 during the first full year we would be self-sustaining and contributing to the mission. Naturally, Scott declared that the figure was too low and we should easily double that figure. Many of the faces that appeared at that meeting were never to be seen again in the organization. A few continued on and made valuable contributions. New faces would appear over time. We wound up with three core families that drove the effort and another four or five that were reasonably active. Over the years, numerous generous people contributed as volunteers, board members, sponsors, donors of goods, services, and money. As the line from Kevin Costner's movie *Field of Dreams* goes, "build it and they will come." This is may be true, but it does not happen automatically.

It was difficult getting the chapter off the ground. We were a small, but capable core group of people. We had no budget, no local staff, and the national organization was just underway as a combined entity and had growing pains and things to learn. There were no rules or blueprints. No officers or board members. We had a meeting or two with a lot of talk and no action. Charlene quickly became impatient and wanted action, not talk. Scott realized that we needed to appoint officers and a board to get things moving. There was some resistance to making appointments out of the concern that others may want to join and we did not want to leave anyone out. Charlene wanted there to be something to join and we all agreed we could always add officers and board members. So Scott went around the table and appointed the initial officers and board. Charlene and another lady were the only ones not to duck down, so they became our initial executive vice president and president. We left positions open for a couple of people who expressed interest, but were not at the meeting. The other 3 or 4 of us became board members. The Chicago chapter was born.

One of the families was formulating plans for an initial fundraising event. There were a couple of ideas that fell through. The small board knew the importance of having the initial event be successful and was concerned there was not enough time to put the event together. The board voted against the event. Charlene and the lady who was putting the event together were outraged. Afterwards, she convinced us that the space and entertainment were lined up and ready to go. Charlene got angry and declared, "we cannot just sit around and talk about curing cancer, we have to do something about it." She added, "if we aren't going to do anything, then I will quit. I am not wasting my time." She asked Scott to call the board members the next day and get them to change their vote so this event could get off the ground. Scott made the calls and easily convinced the others to allow the event to proceed. People simply had doubts about whether there was enough time to put the event together and thought we might be biting off more than we could chew. They were happy to allow us to go forward, which we did. The event was beautiful and raised about $90,000. One of our cherished members said if the event was successful given the tight time frame he would eat his hat. In the middle of the event, he approached us with a big smile on his face and his hat in his hand.

Now the fun really began. The organization wanted to have a 5K walk and, naturally, Chicago was the place to start. We needed to find someone to chair the event and no one was willing to step up. Enter Charlene. She said, "I will chair the walk—it is a great idea." The event was scheduled for September 13, 2003 and that marked the birthday of the Lymphomathon. Scott was not pleased Charlene volunteered because he knew she would drag him into it.

Scott had mixed feelings about us taking on the walk. We faced several challenges. First, we had never organized an event like this before. Second, the Chicagoland calendar already was loaded with walks, runs, and similar events throughout the spring and fall. Third, the organization was completely unknown in Chicago. So neither the organization nor the event had any name recognition whatsoever in Chicago. Fourth, the timing was difficult because the gala was held just a couple of months earlier so we just had our hands out to people we knew. But Charlene had committed to do the walk and that was the end of that discussion.

An event planner was hired to handle the logistics (permits, site selection, set-up, and equipment). We developed a good relationship with her and she went beyond her contractual requirements in helping us to get the event off the ground. Although we started out knowing nothing about organizing an event like this, we spoke with other event organizers and over the years have become as knowledgeable as anyone. We were motivated by the strong desire to raise money and awareness about lymphoma. We were equally motivated by the fear of failure and embarrassment.

Once we got started, we both realized that this would not only be a successful event in its own right, but also would be a springboard to promote awareness about lymphoma, the organization, and our chapter. We thought we could use the publicity to put the organization on the map in the Chicagoland area, to develop recognition, credibility, and a positive track record that would serve to pave the way for other events and other chapters. We felt we needed to create an identity or personality for the walk so that it did not get lost in the already overcrowded calendar of fundraisers in the Chicagoland area. We did. Regardless of how many people came or how much we raised the first year, it was important that people had an enjoyable, meaningful, and rewarding experience so that they would return in future years. To grow the event, we wanted to bring back a core of key people year after year. People are battling a sickness and have other things going on in their lives. It is common for people to participate for a year or two and move on. Fortunately, we have enjoyed a strong rate of return in our event over the years.

We put on a full court press involving many friends and people we knew and encouraged other chapter members to do the same. After all, people walking, running, and donating are the main revenue sources along with corporate sponsorships. Scott's firm and partners were very supportive. Scott went to the leading grocery store chain in the Chicagoland area, which he had represented years early in major litigation involving what was then the largest food borne outbreak of disease in the United States. Having them serve as a sponsor provided name recognition and credibility to the event and organization. They did not provide money, but provided food and beverages. They also provided a source for us to display posters and brochures at a couple hundred store locations. It was an instant chain of promotion. Their community relations director, a friend of Scott's, was a wonderful source of information and a great sounding board for ideas, having been involved in so many fundraising events over the years.

We needed press and had absolutely no advertising budget. We formulated a media and publicity plan. One of our dear friends is a wonderful, talented, community-minded, caring person who also happens to be one of the best news anchors and reporters in the business. The station did not sponsor first-year events, but she got us on a newscast and paved the way for the station to serve as our television media partner in future years. The next year she would serve as our emcee, but a couple of wonderful radio talk show hosts emceed the first year. We had many media friends and talked a couple of radio stations into interviewing us about lymphoma and the Lymphomathon. Another station agreed to air some public service announcements. Charlene recorded a 60-second public service announcement and her voice was the first to hit the airwaves in Chicago for the organization and the event. An on-line fundraising website, facilitated team-building and fundraising.

In Chicago on September 13, 2003, the world's first Lymphomathon took place. Our fundraising goal was $50,000, but we wound up raising about $137,000. Each year, we increased the media exposure with the same non-existent budget and added some entertainment so there always was something new. We have grown steadily from the 300 to 400 participants in the first year to well over 2,000 in the sixth year. We raised nearly $3 million at our first few events. It has been rewarding to see that what started out as a simple walk in Chicago has turned into more than 20 walks across the country raising money and awareness for lymphoma annually. It was not until the fifth year that we had any staff members in Chicago—it was volunteers that organized and ran the events. Every year, we were touched by the stories and support of so many lymphoma survivors.

Over the years, we built important partnerships with many media members, two television stations, multiple radio stations, a newspaper, and various other outlets. This provided important publicity about the Lymphomathon, the Chicago chapter, and the national organization. It also promoted public awareness about the disease. The event and the related publicity is a vehicle to get more people involved in various ways. The atmosphere has always been supercharged with wonderful people gathering to support each other. It is a giant support group and an opportunity to network with doctors and about treatments and beating the disease. Every year, we would see many people buoyed by the event and their spirits lifted by friends and families coming out to support them. During the first walk, for example, a very nice, articulate, elderly lady approached Scott praising the event and all of the associated publicity regarding the signs and symptoms of lymphoma. She handed him a check and returned every year. It turns out that she was the widow of a famous, ground-breaking lymphoma doctor who himself ultimately died of lymphoma.

We would appear often on radio and television to promote events and educate the public about blood cancer. The educational component was as important as the fundraising. Many people have come to the

Lymphomathon (now called the lymphoma walk) or contacted us and we have been able to help them.

Chicago drove the organization's chapter network, being the first chapter formed, the first to hold a Lymphomathon, and the first to have staff and an office. We led the way in terms of fundraising, educational events, public awareness, and advocacy. We served as a blueprint for other chapters. We had the opportunity to meet and speak with many of the talented volunteers across the country and marvel at the amazing things they have done. Charlene served as president for a couple of years and we co-chaired the Lymphomathon for each of the first six years. We made outreach efforts into all communities and developing relationships with doctors, media, and strategic partners a priority. We hosted numerous free educational events for patients and their families. Most of the people involved with us are alive and doing well and that is the main thing. But we have lost friends along the way, which serves as a sharp reminder that we still have a lot of work to do. Charlene put it aptly in an article she wrote a few years ago:

> We have met so many wonderful people, each with his or her own needs, values, and ways to contribute. But the thread of continuity that binds us together is the noble goal of eradicating lymphoma. You may start out invested in finding a cure for yourself or a family member, but your investment is increased dramatically as you meet new friends battling blood cancer. We have accomplished much, but have a lot more work to do.

The lymphoma walk has continued as an annual event in Chicago and at numerous locations across the country. We have since undertaken many other efforts to fund cutting edge, impactful research at leading institutions; promote awareness about cancer; educate patients, families, and health care providers about cancer and treatments; and foster patient access to information and health care.

We subsequently produced and hosted a radio show called *the Battling and Beating Cancer Radio Show* on which we interviewed doctors, survivors, caregivers, and others and talked about issues of importance to people impacted by cancer. The show aired live worldwide on the Blog Talk Radio Network and people can still listen on demand at www.blogtalkradio.com/battling-and-beating-cancer, and on other outlets. Our

Battling and Beating Cancer television series originated from the CAN TV studios in Chicago. We served as the National Cancer Examiner and the Chicago Cancer Examiner.

You do not have to form an organization or a chapter. You do not have to give away your wealth to find a cure. Naturally, you do have to take care of your health first and foremost. However, when and to the extent you are able to do so, we strongly encourage you to make some significant contribution to help others battling cancer. Whether it is assisting in the advancement of public awareness or knowledge, funding the search for better treatments, or talking to or mentoring people suffering from cancer, in some way, make a difference! Do not do it because it is noble or the right thing to do—although that certainly is the case. Do it for selfish reasons. Do it because if your cancer returns or someone you love gets diagnosed down the road there will be more effective or less toxic treatments available or even a cure. Do it because it is a way to be empowered and to lose the feeling of being victimized by cancer. Do it because you will meet so many wonderful people and you will be given so many meaningful gifts that money cannot buy.

We realize that people react differently to cancer. Some wish to avoid remembering or thinking about cancer, in some ways we all do and who could blame us. We will not attempt psychoanalysis, but it seems to us that even those who completely "move on" and distance themselves from cancer or people afflicted with the disease actually are stuck. Rise above focusing upon your own circumstances, condition, and pain. Notwithstanding the truism that no good deed goes unpunished, helping others will help you.

There have been several people who befriended our mission although they were cancer-free, but who would later turn to us for help when a loved one was diagnosed with cancer. It is remarkable how small the world can be at times. It is unfortunate that the reach of cancer is so broad.

You do not just want to feel like you are doing something positive, you want to make sure that you actually are doing something positive. For those who are afraid or hesitant to ask others to contribute to the cause, remember you are not asking them to give money to you, you are asking them to do something that will benefit society. You would be surprised by the generosity of people. Still, be reasonable and remember that people have financial constraints and other causes to support.

The last thing we set out to do was fundraising. We were more interested in patient advocacy, education, and public policy advocacy than in fundraising. Working with people is a more direct and tangible way of helping people. It also can be very draining, demanding, and, at times, depressing because there is no way not to become involved or invested in the people you are working with and not all outcomes are what we want. Mostly through Charlene's insistence, we have never stopped these activities.

The more involved we became in this mission to eradicate cancer, the more we realized the most important long-term impact we can have as laypeople is helping to raise money for cancer research. Research is the key to defeating cancer and the ticket to all of our long-term survival. So we believe that it is important to include fundraising in the mix.

It is private philanthropy that drives cancer research. It provides seed funding to explore new frontiers in cancer research. The reality of the competitive pursuit of limited governmental funding of research is that the pace of research can be incremental – taking a project previously funded and vary it or advance it slightly. Private fundraising is more flexible and leads to more breakthroughs.

There is no magic to fundraising, advocacy, and fighting cancer. From our experience, cancer survivors and their families are much more effective than professional fundraisers and organizational staff. To professionals, it is often just a job. To survivors and family members, it is a passion and a mission. Our experience has taught us that, in most instances, volunteers impacted by cancer have to lead the efforts and make sure the organizations do not lose their way. Keep in mind that you can always contribute directly to medical researchers and institutions. Fundraising, organizing, and participating are critical components of the national call to action to cure cancer and help those impacted by cancer.

Our current efforts include being a modest part of the great scientific and wonderful philanthropic teams supporting the Hippocratic Cancer Resource Foundation ("HCRF"). HCRF supports the world class research of Leonidas C. Platanias MD, PhD, Director of the Robert H. Lurie Comprehensive Cancer Center of Northwestern University and his renowned team of scientists.

More specifically, the mission of the Hippocratic Cancer Research Foundation is to eliminate cancer and save lives by funding the discovery, development, and implementation of effective new therapies and groundbreaking research at the Robert H. Lurie Comprehensive Cancer Center of Northwestern University. We empower Dr. Platanias and his interdisciplinary research teams to address the most urgent questions in the fields of cancer biology and oncology in daring and innovative ways. By investing in cutting edge, "out of the box," impactful research, with an emphasis on translational cancer research, HCRF seeks to accelerate and heighten the impact of scientific discoveries. HCRF has supported impressive research impacting various forms of cancer including research identifying cellular pathways that affect all cancers, promising new drug targets for brain cancer, pancreatic cancer pathways opening doors for new treatment options, developing novel treatments for blood cancer, strategies to help curb the spread of the pandemic, and identifying potential antiviral therapy.

HCRF's signature event is the annual Wings to Cure Gala held in Chicago in November. Each year, this event brings together people from across the globe – raising a lot of money for cancer research, featuring touching stories of survivorship, and reporting remarkable research developments. HCRF also hosts fashion shows and other events.

Since the outset of the pandemic, HCRF has hosted *Cancer & COVID Talks with Dr. Platanias* to update and inform the cancer community on pertinent issues. Numerous leading physicians and investigators on the forefront of COVID and cancer from around the globe have joined Dr. Platanias, Dr. Liadis, and HCRF Board Members for these sessions. So many fine people are involved and contribute to HCRF. Our friend, Eleni Bousis, is the driving force and the leader of HCRF. Her passion for curing cancer is inspiring. The advances funded to date by HCRF have been impressive and our work continues. We invite you to join us at: https://hcrfwingstocure.org.

Whatever efforts or organizations you support, as people impacted by cancer, it is incumbent upon us to lead the way to better treatments and to cures for the various types of cancer. Simply stated, more committed cancer warriors are needed! We hope you are or will be a cancer warrior!

PART 2

WHAT YOU NEED TO KNOW AND DO TO CONQUER CANCER (YOUR STORY OF SURVIVORSHIP)

CHAPTER 13

THE WORLD'S WORST TERRORISTS LIVE WITHIN US (DEVELOPING A WARRIOR'S MENTALITY AND COGENT BATTLE PLAN TO DEFEAT CANCER)

Cancer can suck the enjoyment right out of life if you let it and sometimes even though you resist mightily. It has sucked the life out of a lot of people. Some say cancer is something that you "live with," but we believe that cancer is something that you need to destroy so that it does not destroy you. Some do not like analogies between cancer and war, but we think it can be a useful framework. Indeed, there are some striking similarities between the war on terrorism and the war against cancer.

For those who do not like the analogy, we will not carry it forward beyond this chapter. For younger readers the analogy may not resonate as strongly. If you are about to undergo treatment or are in the middle of treatment, you may want to skip this chapter for now and return to it after reading the rest of the book.

You remember where you were and how you felt: September 11, 2001 is a day that changed our country forever. We will never forget where we were when we learned that the two planes struck the World Trade Center or the sick feeling in our stomachs when we learned that America was under attack. Scott was in the Sears Tower (now called Willis Tower) where his offices were at the time and there were reports that Sears Tower was the next target for attack. It is difficult for citizens to enjoy their freedom when national security is in doubt.

Similarly, no one diagnosed with cancer will ever forget the day that he or she heard the three dreaded words "you have cancer." Without your health, it is difficult to enjoy the freedoms associated with the American way of life. Scott was diagnosed with cancer and endured major surgery, chemotherapy, and radiation therapy prior to September 11, 2001. We felt no less afraid, vulnerable, insecure, sick, and not in control during that "cancer period" of time than we did in the wake of September 11, 2001. In fact, the cancer was worse. It is hardly surprising that being diagnosed with cancer traditionally tops the list of worst fears of Americans.

Forces that aim to destroy your life and way of life: Terrorists aim not only to kill people, but to destroy freedom and our way of life. Cancer is a brutal, merciless, vile, life-threatening disease. To us, it is a terrorist that lives within us—nothing less. It is an indiscriminate killer, politically correct only in that it seeks to destroy people regardless of their race, creed, color, age, socio-economic status, or gender. We are all at risk for cancer. It actually is the worst form of terrorism because there are cancer terrorist cells already living inside our bodies and capable of destroying us. In order to defeat this enemy, you have to know what you are dealing with and you need a plan.

A war is a war no matter what you call it: There was no official "declaration of war" in response to the attacks of September 11, 2001. Nonetheless, to the brave men and women engaged in combat in Afghanistan and Iraq they were at war. Similarly there has never been an official "declaration of war" on cancer. President Nixon's so-called war on cancer took place in 1971. He did not actually use the phrase "war on cancer." In his January 1971 State of the Union address, he said "I will also ask for an appropriation of an extra $100 million to launch an intensive campaign to find a cure for cancer, and I will ask later for whatever additional funds can effectively be used. The time has come in America when the same kind of concentrated effort that split the atom and took man to the moon should be turned toward conquering this dreaded disease. Let us make a total national commitment to achieve this goal." As part of this national effort, the Army's Fort Detrick, Maryland, biological warfare facility was converted to a cancer research center and, in December of 1971, the National Cancer Act was signed into law. Whether officially declared or not, a war is a war.

Heroes to help us: The war on terror and the war against cancer both feature ordinary citizens being transformed into heroes. Every September 11, we pay tribute to all Americas who lost their lives as well as to those heroes who keep us safe and fight to preserve our freedoms. Special gratitude must be expressed to the first responders, the plane passengers aboard flight 93, and the wonderful young men and woman in the armed forces.

Every day in America, thousands of people mourn the loss of loved ones to cancer. There is an important difference between cancer patients and members of our armed forces. Our brave men and woman in the armed forces voluntarily place themselves in harm's way. Cancer patients do not raise their hands to get cancer. Yet, cancer patents and military members alike are properly referred to as "fighters." The commonality is that they all are fighting for their lives and to preserve their way of life for themselves and their families. As people impacted by cancer, we believe that those dedicated researchers, physicians, nurses, caregivers, and advocates are heroes and they save lives.

Deployment of effective weapons: America has deployed the mightiest fighting machine on the planet in the war against terror. To defeat the terrorist living within them, many cancer patients are forced to endure the potent and sometimes toxic components in the cancer treatment armamentarium such as surgery, chemotherapy, and radiation therapy. In both wars, you attempt to deploy the most effective weapons that cause the least amount of collateral damage. Investment in cogent cancer research is key. Once the terrorist has moved inside, you need potent ammunition to kill it before it kills you. We know there are cancers that people can "live with" for years, but the analogy generally holds true.

Awareness and education are important: To fight the war on terror, it was necessary to get a critical mass of public support and will. Awareness and education are important to prevail in the long-term war against terrorism and to beat cancer. We lack perfect information and have to base decisions on available information. Public awareness and education have been important in the war against cancer, for example, in reducing smoking and, therefore, some forms of cancer. Screenings, such as colonoscopies and pap tests, have had an impact as well. But most progress has been made because of investment in cancer research, education, and awareness.

Too many lives lost: The terrorist attacks of September 11, 2001 resulted in approximately 2,977 deaths (we exclude the hijackers who sought to die in the process of killing innocent people). It breaks down as follows: 246 died on the four planes, 2,606 died in New York City in the towers and on the ground, and 125 died at the Pentagon. When you add the thousands of people in our armed forces whose lives have been lost, there is no question that terrorism has exacted a tremendous toll on American lives. By any measure, the lives lost to the attacks of September 11 and the resulting military engagements are far too large.

Yet, this death toll pales by comparison to the number of American lives lost to cancer. Over 1.9 million new cases of cancer are expected to be diagnosed in the United States in 2021 according to the American Cancer Society, This figure does not even include people with basal and squamous cell skin cancers or people with carcinoma in situ (non-invasive cancers). According to the American Cancer Society, approximately 608,570 Americans are expected to die of cancer in 2021 (1,670 deaths per day). Cancer is the second most common cause of death in the United States exceeded only by heart disease. These estimates do not take into account the impact of COVID-19.

The economic cost of the war: The National Cancer Institute estimates that cancer-related direct medical costs in the US were $183 billion in 2015 and were projected to increase to $246 billion by 2030, a 34% increase based only on population growth and aging. This does not include the indirect costs such as lost earnings. The economics and humanomics compel the same conclusion – we must invest more to eradicate cancer and help those impacted by the disease. The statistics will change and vary somewhat from source to source, but the foregoing provides a very good order of magnitude of the problem.

Too little invested in cancer research: It has been reported that, from 1971 to about 2009, the federal government, private foundations, and drug companies collectively have spent less than $300 billion to find a cure for cancer. About one-third of this amount was government funded research. To be sure, there are many individuals, organizations, advocates, medical professionals, researchers, and drug companies fighting on the front lines of this war every day. By any reasonable account, however, the investment in cancer research is a pittance considering that cancer actually is a couple hundred diseases, many of which have numerous forms and sub-types. Appendix "B" contains a listing of some of the types of cancer. Whatever you think about the amount spent on the war on terror, the amount spent on the war against cancer has been utterly insufficient.

Progress has been made, but much more remains to be done: Regardless of whether you believe that many elements of the war against terror were necessary and appropriate, the record does demonstrate some degree of success. Supporter's properly point out that there has not been a major, foreign-led terrorist attack on the United States in decades, Saddam

Hussein and Osama Bin Laden and other terrorist leaders are dead, and—although still woefully lacking and many Americans may be becoming more complacent—America's state of alert and preparedness has improved at least to some extent. Unlike a conventional war, the war on terror is not limited in time or space.

How about progress in the war against cancer? There has been an extensive debate as the 50th Anniversary of the National Cancer Act approached concerning whether the war against cancer has been a success or a failure. The reality is that progress has been made, progress has been too slow, and that the pace of development has increased dramatically in the last few years.

According to the National Cancer Institute, there were more than 16.9 million Americans with a history of invasive cancer alive on January 1, 2019. Some still have cancer, but most were diagnosed many years ago and have no current evidence of the disease. The overall age-adjusted cancer death rate rose during the 20th century, peaking in 1991 at 215 cancer deaths per 100,000 people. As of 2018, the rate dropped to 149 per 100,000 (a 31% decline), in large part, because of reductions in smoking and improvements in early detection and treatment for some cancers. This decline translates into about 3.2 million fewer cancer deaths from 1991 to 2018. The 5-year relative survival rate for all cancers combined has increased substantially since the early 1960s, from 39% to 68% among white people and from 27% to 63% among black people. Improvements in survival reflect advances in treatment, as well as earlier diagnosis for some cancers. Survival varies greatly by cancer type and stage and more progress has been made for some types of cancer than for others.

Progress has been dramatic for some forms of cancer, but virtually non-existent for other forms. From 1975 to 2005, death rates for melanoma, liver, bile-duct cancer, and pancreatic cancer have all increased. Overall, the death rate from cancer fell 7.5% during that 30-year period. Yet, during this same period, the death rate from cardiovascular disease has fallen approximately 70% according to one report. All of this demonstrates that we should have invested more money and done much more to eradicate cancer in the past and we must invest more now. Like the war on terror, the war against cancer is not limited in time or space.

The enemy is not static: Terrorist organizations use new techniques to recruit members and to impose terror on the world. Similarly, the fight against cancer is complicated by the fact that the enemy is not static.

Cancer cells are capable of changing and seeking to avoid attack. Just as bacteria and infectious agents find ways to evolve and develop resistance to antibiotics, cancer cells develop resistance to drugs. This is one of the reasons that individualized treatments likely will be emphasized more in the future. Sometimes when a staff member spoke of taking a day off or going on vacation, we would jokingly question their commitment. We would point out that cancer does not sleep or take vacations. It is in constant formation, on the attack 24-7-365.

Understanding what we are fighting: You have to understand some things about the enemy in order to defeat it, especially where the geographic dispersion and temporal duration of the war is great. The more you know, the better. The intelligence gathering on terrorist organizations has contributed to success in the war on terror. Just as terrorists fall into different factions, with different motivations and *modus operandi*, so do cancers.

With a better understanding of cancer at the molecular level, more forms and sub-forms have been identified. Microarray technology has given scientists the ability to detect and quantify small molecules, such as proteins and antibodies, as well as DNA variations and expression levels. With the ability to identify these unique disease characteristics, scientists can develop sophisticated diagnostic tools and provide insight into the mechanisms behind the clinical course observed by physicians.

American resolve, economic commitment, and cogent regulations: American politicians impressed upon the public that, to win the war on terror, we must have long-term resolve and we must devote sufficient resources. Americans were told that government and intelligence agencies must have the flexibility and tools needed to protect American's from the threat of terrorism and that existing regulations were barriers to fighting terrorism. Unfortunately, some of the tools have been abused.

Similarly, to defeat cancer, Americans must impress upon politicians the importance of having the resolve to win the war against cancer. America must invest substantially more money in cogent cancer research. We also must change the regulatory *status quo* so that regulation and regulatory agencies do not harm cancer patients and hinder their recoveries under the guise of protecting them. Fast track approval of treatments shown to be effective, fast track funding for elite researchers with proven records and cogent protocols, and proper funding and reimbursement policies for treatments demonstrated to be effective are sensible ways to help win the war against cancer. Cancer survivors and those advocating for them must be vocal, relentless, and organized to impose their will upon elected officials especially in these times in which our country is burdened with debt.

Prevention and early diagnosis: A substantial proportion of cancers could be prevented, including all cancers caused by tobacco use and other unhealthy behaviors. According to the American Cancer Society Cancer Facts & Figures 2021: "Excluding non-melanoma skin cancer, at least 42% of newly diagnosed cancers in the US – about 797,000 cases in 2021 – are potentially avoidable, including the 19% of cancers caused by smoking and at least 18% caused by a combination of excess body weight, alcohol consumption, poor nutrition, and physical inactivity. Certain cancers caused by infectious agents, such as human papillomavirus (HPV), hepatitis B virus (HBV), hepatitis C virus (HCV), and Helicobacter pylori (H. pylori), could be prevented through behavioral changes or vaccination to avoid the infection, or by treating the infection. Many of the more than 5 million skin cancers diagnosed annually could be prevented by protecting skin from excessive sun exposure and not using indoor tanning devices. In addition, screening can help prevent colorectal and cervical cancers by detecting and removing precancers in the colon, rectum, and uterine cervix. Screening can also detect these and some other cancers early, when treatment is often less intensive and more successful. Screening is known to reduce mortality for cancers of the breast, colon, rectum, cervix, lung (among people who smoke, or used to smoke), and probably prostate." Almost 1 in 5 cancers is caused by excess body weight, alcohol consumption, poor diet, and a sedentary lifestyle according to the American Cancer Society. These are key components to direct education and awareness campaigns.

Cancer warrior mentality: To defeat cancer, you need to develop the mentality of a cancer warrior. This means that you must get past the initial shock, panic, fear, denial, and take the offensive. You must understand the enemy at your gate and respond with a cogent battle plan. You need to get the most capable, experienced, and compassionate soldiers, marines, and sailors to formulate and implement the plan—so draft your doctors, medical professionals, advisors, and advocates wisely. Select the proper hospital or cancer center as your theatre of operations. Make sure proper training and safety rules are in place and implemented. Assemble the best weapons and assets for the battle—the precise treatments, drugs, and procedures to beat this enemy. Pray to your god. Live life and stay among the living to the maximum extent possible. Laugh and enjoy life as much as possible. A good sense of humor will serve you well as you go through your treatments. A positive attitude is very helpful, but a strong will to live and warrior mentality are indispensable to surviving.

A cogent battle plan: In this age of personalized or precision medicine it remains helpful to know about treatment options in general. However, with an increasing ability to identify genetic and molecular components of an individual's cancer and to select treatments that will be most effective to eradicate the individual's cancer, it is increasingly crucial for patients and their physicians to develop individualized treatment plans where possible. It also is important to continue to review the plan and revise it based upon changes in the individual's cancer as emerging treatment options, studies, and technologies become available.

We discuss these subjects in the chapters to follow. For a cancer patient going through treatment and fighting for his or her life, the discussion in portions of this chapter may be too academic. You can return to it later, once you have conquered or contained the cancer that is terrorizing you. We will drop the war on terror analogy from this point forward, but not the fighting spirit.

CHAPTER 14

THE CANCER LANDSCAPE (SOME BASIC INFORMATION ABOUT CANCER IN GENERAL AND BLOOD CANCER IN PARTICULAR)

What is cancer? Cancer is a term used for diseases in which abnormal cells divide without control and are able to spread and invade other tissues. Cancer cells can spread to other parts of the body through the blood and lymph systems. If uncontrolled, cancer can result in death. All cancers begin in cells, the body's basic unit of life. The body is made up of many types of cells. These cells generally grow and divide in a controlled way to produce more cells as they are needed to keep the body healthy. When cells become old or damaged, they die and are replaced with new cells. However, sometimes this orderly process goes astray. The genetic material of a cell can become damaged or changed, producing mutations that affect normal cell growth and division. When this happens, cells do not die when they should and new cells form when the body does not need them. The extra cells may form a mass of tissue called a tumor. Not all tumors are cancerous; tumors can be benign (non-cancerous) or malignant (cancerous). Some cancers do not form tumors. For example, leukemia is a cancer of the bone marrow and blood.

Most cancers are named for the organ or type of cell in which they start. Cancers fall into various categories, including: sarcoma (cancer beginning in bone, cartilage, fat, muscle, blood vessels, or other connective or supportive tissue); carcinoma (cancer beginning in the skin or in tissues that line or cover internal organs); and blood cancers.

More is known about the cause of some forms of cancer than others. In general, cancer may be caused by both external factors (*e.g.*, tobacco, infectious organisms, chemicals, and radiation) and internal factors (*e.g.*, inherited mutations, hormones, immune conditions, and mutations that occur from metabolism). These causal factors may act together or in sequence to initiate or promote the development of cancer. Often the amount or dosage of exposure is an important determinant and sometimes there can be a long latency period of years or even decades between exposure to external factors and detectable cancer. Asbestos exposure and mesothelioma is a good example of a cancer that can take decades to produce discernable symptoms. The immune system response is fundamentally important as well.

Pervasive impact: *Cancer Facts & Figures 2021* from the American Cancer Society provides some good insights into the scope and magnitude of these diseases collectively referred to as cancer. As previously stated, one in two men in America will get cancer during their lifetime and more than one in three women will get cancer during their lifetime. More than 16.9 million Americans with a history of invasive cancer were alive on January 1, 2019. The National Cancer Institute projects the number of cancer survivors is projected to increase to 22.2 million by 2030. Almost 1.9 million new cancer cases are expected to be diagnosed in the United States in 2021. This estimate excludes basal cell and squamous cell skin cancers (which are not required to be reported to cancer registries) and carcinoma in situ (noninvasive cancer). Approximately 608,570 Americans are expected to die of cancer in 2021 (1,670 deaths per day). Cancer is the second most common cause of death in the United States. Heart disease remains the most common cause of death.

The risk of developing cancer increases with advancing age. In fact, approximately 75 to 80% of all cancers in the United States are diagnosed in people 55 years of age or older. The 5-year relative survival rate for all cancers combined has increased substantially since the early 1960s – from 39% to 68% among white people and from 27% to 63% among black people. Survival rates do not distinguish between patients who have no evidence of cancer and those who have relapsed or are still in treatment, nor do they represent the proportion of people who are cured as cancer death can occur beyond 5 years after diagnosis. Survival rates are a lagging indicator because they do not reflect the most recent advances in detection and treatment as they are based on people who were diagnosed several years in the past. In 2021, new cancer cases will be diagnosed in an estimated 10,500 children in the United States (ages 0 to 14 years) and

5,090 adolescents (ages 15-19 years). Cancer is the second-leading cause of death among children ages 1-14 years, after accidents. It is estimated that approximately 1,190 children and 590 adolescents will die from cancer in 2021. It is important to keep in mind these estimates do not reflect adjustments for the COVID-19 pandemic.

Worldwide, cancer accounts for about 1 in every 6 deaths. In 2018, there were an estimated 17 million new cancer cases and 9.5 million cancer deaths globally. According to the National Cancer Institute, by 2040, the number of new cancer cases per year is expected to rise to 29.5 million and the number of cancer-related deaths to 16.4 million.

According to the National Cancer Institute the most common cancers are breast cancer, lung and bronchus cancer, prostate cancer, colon and rectum cancer, melanoma of the skin, bladder cancer, non-Hodgkin lymphoma, kidney and renal pelvis cancer, endometrial cancer, leukemia, pancreatic cancer, thyroid cancer, and liver cancer. Prostate, lung, and colorectal cancers account for an estimated 43% of all cancers diagnosed in men in 2020. For women, the three most common cancers are breast, lung, and colorectal, and they accounted for approximately 50% of all new cancer diagnoses in women in 2020.

We are about to embark upon a fairly detailed discussion about the blood and lymph systems and blood cancer – lymphoma, leukemia, and myeloma. Unless you are impacted by blood cancer, you may wish to skip the balance of this chapter. Even if you are impacted by blood cancer, you may want to only review the portions pertaining to the type of blood cancer that impacts you or a family member. Keep in mind, the information about treatments is general and offered for illustrative purposes. The treatments discussed may be inapplicable to your cancer and/or outdated by the time you read this. Of course, whether dealing with blood cancer or a solid tumor, you will want to consult with your health care team and obtain the latest, most applicable information. Nonetheless, we have become fairly knowledgeable about blood cancer and wanted to include this information for those interested in obtaining a more detailed overview.

Some basic information about blood and the lymph system: There are three major classes of blood cells. The first type is red blood cells (or erythrocytes), which carry oxygen from the lungs to tissues throughout the body and remove carbon dioxide waste produced by cells and bring it to the lungs for exhalation. People with a low number of red blood cells are called anemic and often feel week, tired, and sometimes short of breath.

The second type is white blood cells. These cells are part of the immune system, helping the body fight infections. There are several categories of white blood cells. Lymphocytes are discussed in greater detail in Chapter 21. B lymphocytes (B cells) make antibodies to fight infections. T lymphocytes (T cells) quarterback the immune system and help direct immune responses. There are many kinds of T cells. Some T cells help B cells make antibodies, some attack and kill infected cells, some make chemicals called cytokines that help target the immune response so that it eliminates viruses and cancer cells. Others help control or regulate the way that other parts of the immune system function. Natural killer (NK) cells attack and kill cancer cells and virus-infected cells. They also make cytokines. Granulocytes come in three forms neutrophils, basophils, and eosinophils. Neutrophils fight bacterial infections. A low number of neutrophils in the blood is called neutropenia. People with neutropenia are more likely to get infections (mostly bacterial infections). Basophils are cells that take part in inflammatory reactions. Eosinophils help fight parasites. Monocytes and macrophages also help the immune system fight infections.

Finally, platelets are tiny cells that clump into blood clots to stop bleeding from broken blood vessels. A low number of platelets is called thrombocytopenia. People with thrombocytopenia are more susceptible to bleeding and bruising from minor trauma and to suffer from recurring nosebleeds and gums bleeds.

All blood cells have a limited lifespan requiring the body to continuously replenish its supply of these cells. Red blood cells live for about 120 days. White blood cells live for a few hours up to a few weeks. New blood cells are made by hematopoietic (blood-forming) stem cells, which are immature cells that can develop into any kind of blood cell. Hematopoietic stem cells are found mainly in the bone marrow.

The lymph or lymphatic system is a network of tissues, vessels, and organs that work together to move a colorless, watery fluid called lymph back into your circulatory system. Approximately 20 liters of plasma flow through your body's arteries, blood vessels, and capillaries every day. After delivering nutrients to the body's cells and tissues and receiving their waste products, about 17 liters are returned to the circulation by way of veins. The remaining three liters seep through the capillaries and into your body's tissues. The lymphatic system collects this excess fluid, now called lymph, from tissues in your body and moves it along until it ultimately returns it to your bloodstream. The lymph system maintains fluid levels in the body, absorbs fats from the digestive tract, transports and removes wastes and abnormal cells from the lymph, and protects the body against foreign invaders.

The body has groups of small, bean-shaped organs called lymph nodes. They filter the lymph fluid, removing bacteria, viruses, and other foreign substances from the body. Hundreds of lymph nodes are found throughout the body, most notably in the neck, underarms, chest, abdomen, and groin. Lymphocytes can mostly be found in lymph nodes, where they patrol for signs of infection. The lymph nodes can change in size, becoming bigger or smaller depending on the number of lymphocytes inside them. Lymph nodes are often tender when they react to an infection, but they may or may not be tender or painful when they are enlarged due to lymphoma. The thymus gland, tonsils, and the spleen also are part of the lymph system.

Blood cancers: As contrasted with "solid tumors," blood cancers are cancers of the blood and lymph systems. There are three major categories of blood cancer: lymphoma, leukemia, and myeloma. Blood cancers are prevalent. Every three minutes someone is America is diagnosed with blood cancer and someone dies from the disease every 9 minutes. Over 178,000 Americans were diagnosed with blood cancer in 2020, and approximately 56,840 died in 2020 from blood cancer accounting for approximately 9.9 percent of new cancer cases diagnosed in the United States and 9.4% of the cancer deaths. Blood cancer is the most common form of cancer in children, with leukemia causing more deaths in children and young adults under the age of twenty than any other cancer. Leukemia, lymphoma, and myeloma cause more than 54,000 deaths per year in the United States. It is estimated that more than 1,297,000 Americans are living with or in remission from blood cancer. www.seer.cancer.gov.

Lymphoma basics: Lymphoma is the most common blood cancer. It is cancer of the lymph system and white blood cells known as lymphocytes, which fight infection and disease. There are two major types: Hodgkin's disease and non-Hodgkin's lymphoma (NHL) and dozens of subtypes that range from indolent or slow growing to aggressive subtypes.

With a better understanding of cancer at the molecular level, more forms have been identified. If we were writing this book before the fall of 2008, we would have written that there are more than thirty-five types of lymphoma, five forms of Hodgkin and more than thirty types of non-Hodgkin. The Fourth Edition of the World Health Organization Classification of Tumours of Haematopoietic and Lymphoid Tissues described sixty-one subtypes of non-Hodgkin lymphoma and six forms of Hodgkin lymphoma. Now there are approximately nighty forms of Non-Hodgkin lymphoma identified. Microarray technology has given scientists the ability to detect and quantify small molecules, such as proteins and antibodies, as well as DNA variations and expression levels. With the ability to identify these unique disease characteristics, scientists can develop sophisticated diagnostic tools and provide insight into the mechanisms behind the clinical course observed by physicians. This emphasizes the need to seek the best treatment for the specific subtype that each individual has and not settle for getting treated with a "one size fits all" approach. In this respect, science has come a long way since lymphoma was first described in 1832 by pathologist Thomas Hodgkin. Although many forms of cancer have been declining, the rate of incidence of non-Hodgkin lymphoma has nearly doubled since the 1970s. These figures may be outdated by the time you read them, but they at least gives you an idea about the prevalence of blood cancer.

The treatments, prognoses, and survival rates can vary significantly depending upon the type and stage. Accordingly, it is not enough to know someone has lymphoma or even non-Hodgkin lymphoma—you need to know the subtype. There are over 791,000 lymphoma survivors in the United States (over 644,000 of which are non-Hodgkin), over 85,000 new cases (over 8,400 Hodgkin and 77,000 non-Hodgkin), and more than 20,000 deaths from lymphoma (1190 Hodgkin and nearly 20,000 non-Hodgkin) annually.

There are many signs and symptoms potentially suggestive of blood cancer. It is important to note, however, that many of these symptoms are general and do not necessarily mean the individual has blood cancer or any serious illness for that matter. Also, many people with blood cancer do not experience any of these symptoms. Accordingly, it is important to seek medical attention when you are not feeling well, to avoid self-diagnosis or jumping to conclusions, to get regular physical examinations and routine blood work, and to be on the lookout for symptoms that persist.

The classic sign of lymphoma is enlarged lymph nodes. Lymph nodes are located throughout the body, but generally the ones patients can identify are located in the head, neck, under the arms, or in the groin area. The swollen lymph nodes are usually painless. Keep in mind that it is common for lymph nodes to be enlarged while fighting a cold or infection. If the lymph node persists or remains enlarged, seek medical attention. Other lymphoma symptoms may include: fever; night sweats; unexplained itching; unexplained weight loss; weakness; fatigue; and chronic infections or infections that do not seem to resolve. The overall 5 year survival rate of Hodgkin's is about 86% and NHL is about 70% (but there is considerable variance among subtypes). This represents significant progress over the past couple of decades. Let's take a closer look at some of the types of lymphoma, starting with Hodgkin lymphoma.

Hodgkin's Lymphoma: Classical Hodgkin lymphoma accounts for most of the cases of Hodgkin lymphoma and is recognized as one of the most treatable cancers. The classical types are nodular sclerosis (accounting for between 60 percent and 80 percent of all cases of Hodgkin lymphoma) in which the Reid-Sternberg cells (which are visible under a microscope and named after the researchers who identified them) mix with normal white blood cells. The lymph nodes often contain prominent scar tissue, hence the name nodular sclerosis (scarring). The disease is more common in women than men, and it usually affects adolescents and adults under 50. The great majority of patients are cured with current treatments.

Mixed Cellularity Hodgkin accounts for more than 15 percent of all cases of Hodgkin lymphoma and is found more commonly in men than women. This subtype primarily affects older adults and may be associated with HIV and the Epstein-Barr virus. More extensive disease is usually present by the time this subtype is diagnosed. Lymphocyte Depletion accounts for fewer than 5 percent of all Hodgkin cases. It is characterized by few normal lymphocytes, but abundant Reid-Sternberg cells. Lymphocyte Depletion is aggressive and usually not diagnosed until the disease is widespread. Lymphocyte-Rich accounts for less than 5 percent of all Hodgkin cases. The disease may be diffuse (spread out) or nodular (knot-like) in form and is characterized by the presence of numerous normal lymphocytes and very few abnormal cells and classical Reid-Sternberg cells. This subtype of Hodgkin lymphoma is usually diagnosed at an early stage in adults and has a low relapse rate.

Lymphocyte Predominant Hodgkin Lymphomas account for 5 percent to 10 percent of all Hodgkin cases. It affects more men than women and is usually diagnosed in people under 35. Most of the lymphocytes found in the lymph nodes are not cancerous. Typical Reid-Sternberg cells are usually not found in this subtype, but large, abnormal B-cells can be seen as well as reactive small b-cells. This subtype is usually diagnosed at an early stage and is not aggressive. In many ways, this form of Hodgkin lymphoma resembles indolent b-cell non-Hodgkin lymphoma. Diffuse Lymphocyte Predominant is very rare and disease recurrence is common in this final subtype of Hodgkin lymphoma.

Classical Hodgkin disease generally is treated with multi-agent chemotherapy often along with radiation therapy. A stem cell transplant may also be recommended for some patients. Brentuximab vedotin (Adcetris) has been approved to treat Hodgkin disease in certain patients who failed to respond to previous therapies. For those diagnosed with nodular lymphocyte predominant Hodgkin lymphoma, radiation alone may be appropriate for patients with early stage disease. For those with later-stage disease, chemotherapy plus radiation, as well as the monoclonal antibody rituximab may be recommended. Until recently, the relative high survival rates for most forms of Hodgkin disease resulted in less research focus and development of treatments for Hodgkin disease.

Non-Hodgkin Lymphoma: Some of the subtypes of non-Hodgkin lymphoma include: anaplastic large-cell lymphoma; angioimmunoblastic lymphoma; blastic NK-cell lymphoma; Burkitt's lymphoma; small lymphocytic lymphoma (SLL); cutaneous t-cell lymphoma; diffuse large b-cell lymphoma; follicular lymphoma; hepatosplenic Gamma-Delta t-cell lymphoma; mantle cell lymphoma; marginal zone lymphoma; pediatric lymphoma; peripheral t-cell lymphomas; transformed lymphomas; central nervous system lymphoma; and Waldenstrom Macroglobulinemia. There are many other subtypes. Some lymphomas are aggressive—such as diffuse large b-cell, which is the most prevalent type of lymphoma. Others—such as follicular lymphoma—are slow growing or indolent. Sometimes indolent lymphomas can "transform" and become aggressive.

Follicular, chronic lymphocytic leukemia (CLL)/small lymphocytic lymphoma (SLL), Walderstrom Macroglobulinemia, and marginal zone lymphomas generally are considered indolent. DLBCL, anaplastic large cell, angioimmunoblastic T-cell, Burkitt's, mantle cell are among the aggressive lymphomas.

Diffuse Large B-Cell Lymphoma: DLBCL is the most common form of non-Hodgkin lymphoma, accounting for up to 30 percent of newly diagnosed cases. DLBCL is an aggressive lymphoma. It can arise in lymph nodes or outside of the lymphatic system, in the gastrointestinal tract, testes, thyroid, thymus gland, skin, breast, bone, or brain. Certain factors can predict risk of relapse of DLBCL, including age at diagnosis, blood levels of specific proteins, a person's ability to function without help, the disease stage, and whether the lymphoma cells appear in organs outside of the lymphatic system. Because DLBCL advances very quickly, it usually requires immediate treatment. A combination of chemotherapies and the monoclonal antibody rituximab (Rituxan) can lead to a cure in a large number of people with this form of lymphoma. The most widely used treatment for DLBCL is R-CHOP, which is a mixture of rituximab (Rituxan) and several chemotherapy drugs (cyclophosphamide, doxorubicin, vincristine, and prednisone). Etoposide sometimes is added to R-CHOP, resulting in a drug combination called R-EPOCH. This is the type of lymphoma Scott had. For patients with refractory disease (disease that does not respond to treatment) or relapsed disease (disease that returns after treatment), secondary therapies such as a stem cell transplant may be used and in many cases can be curative.

When Scott was diagnosed and treated, DLBCL was a single category. More recently, he would have been diagnosed with a specific type called primary mediastinal B-cell lymphoma (PMBCL). It is a form of DLBCL that arises in the thymus gland and is usually limited to the mediastinum (a compartment in the central part of the chest that includes the heart, thymus, esophagus, and trachea). Most patients are 30 to 40 years of age at diagnosis though teenagers may also develop PMBCL. Symptoms may include cough, chest pain, fever, weight loss, night sweats, shortness of breath, and swelling of the face and arms from compression of the major vein delivering blood to the heart. Patients with PMBCL usually have a better prognosis than those with other subtypes of DLBCL. The treatment now is considerably different than the CHOP and radiation Scott received or the R-CHOP and radiation subsequently used. More recently, the preferred treatment usually is R-EPOCH as opposed to R-CHOP. One of the CHOP components contains too much potential heart toxicity. Importantly, the treatment no longer includes radiation therapy. It turns out that our hesitation to undergo the radiation therapy was well-taken due to the development of heart disease secondary to the treatment. Once again, we are able to differentiate cancer subtypes much better now and this favorably impacts treatment and survival rates and avoids side-effects.

Follicular Lymphoma: This is the most common indolent or slow-growing form of NHL that arises from b-lymphocytes. Follicular lymphomas account for roughly 15 percent of all non-Hodgkin lymphomas and usually take several years to develop. Although follicular lymphoma may impact people at any age, the average age at diagnosis is 60. Follicular lymphoma is graded from 1 to 3 depending on the number and pattern of certain large cells called centroblasts seen in biopsy samples. Patients with grades 1 and 2 follicular lymphoma have no or only a few centroblasts are considered to be low grade. Grade 3a is considered to be low grade and similar to grades 1 and 2. Grade 3b has more large cells, behaves more aggressively, and are typically treated the same as transformed lymphoma/diffuse large B-cell lymphoma (DLBCL).

Traditionally, "watch and wait" has been a common strategy. Importantly, this is only applicable to some indolent lymphomas and generally is a dangerous strategy for most cancers. Often a single agent, immunotherapy rituximab (Rituxan) or rituximab together with chemotherapy is used to treat the disease. There are many drugs and combinations of drugs that can be used to manage this disease, including: bendamustine (Treanda); CHOP (cyclophosphamide, doxorubicin, vincristine, prednisone); CVP (cyclophosphamide, vincristine, prednisone); and Fludarabine. For patients with relapsed follicular lymphoma, high dose chemotherapy and stem cell transplant may provide a prolonged disease-free interval in some patients. Some patients with follicular lymphoma will eventually transform into an aggressive lymphoma, which are usually treated with combination chemotherapy. Many treatments are being tested in clinical trials for relapsed or refractory follicular lymphoma patients, including: bortezomib (Velcade); ofatumumab (Arzerra or HuMax-CD20); lenalidomide (Revlimid); and mTOR inhibitors. As we detail elsewhere, though in the past it was commonly said to be treatable but not curable, we believe that with treatments like radioimmunotherapy (RIT), follicular lymphomas are curable in some patients.

Mantle Cell Lymphoma: MCL is a rare form of NHL, constituting only about 4 percent of all NHL cases in the United States. Although traditionally it has been considered to be an aggressive b-cell lymphoma, many physicians believe it is more appropriately classified as an indolent lymphoma. In any event, it most often affects men over the age of 60. Frequently, MCL is diagnosed at a later stage of disease and in most cases involves the gastrointestinal tract and bone marrow. The disease gets its name because mantle cell tumors are composed of cells that come from the "mantle zone" of the lymph node.

Treatments include watch and wait, chemotherapy regimens such as R-CHOP, HyperCVAD-MTX/AraC (hyper-fractionated cyclophosphamide, vincristine, doxorubicin, dexamethasone, methotrexate and cytarabine) combined with rituximab (Rituxan). Stem cell transplantation has also shown promising results. Proteosome inhibitors, drugs that disrupt a molecular pathway that is critical for the elimination of proteins in both normal and cancer cells such as bortezomib (Velcade), may be used. Bendamustine (Treanda) in combination with other drugs such as rituximab (Rituxan) also may be used. Gemcitabine (Gemzar), a drug that interferes with cell growth, is being tested in MCL patients. It is also being studied in combination with bortezomib (Velcade). Other treatments under investigation include Bcl-2 directed therapies; rituximab (Rituxan); RIT; lenalidomide (Revlimid); thalidomide (Thalomid), and mTOR (mammalian target of rapamycin) pathway inhibitors.

Marginal Zone Lymphoma: Marginal zone lymphomas are indolent b-cell lymphomas that account for approximately 12 percent of all b-cell lymphomas. The median age for diagnosis is 60. There are at least three types of marginal zone lymphoma. The first, extranodal marginal zone lymphoma of mucosa-associated lymphatic tissue (MALT) occurs outside the lymph nodes, such as in the stomach, small intestine, salivary gland, thyroid, eyes, and lungs. MALT is divided into two categories: gastric MALT, which develops in the stomach, and non-gastric MALT, which develops outside of the stomach. Nodal marginal zone lymphoma (sometimes called monocytoid b-cell lymphoma) occurs within the lymph nodes. Splenic marginal zone lymphoma occurs mostly in the spleen and blood.

For gastric MALT lymphoma, the initial treatment generally has been antibiotic therapy, which is typically given for two weeks. Approximately 70 percent to 90 percent of patients respond to antibiotic therapy and approximately half of the patients require no further treatment. If patients relapse after antibiotic therapy, there are additional treatment options available, including: bendamustine (Treanda), bortezomib (Velcade), various chemotherapies, low dose radiation, rituximab (Rituxan), and surgical excision. Non-gastric MALT treatment typically includes surgery or radiation therapy with or without a system-wide approach, such as chemotherapy. Nodal marginal zone lymphoma is usually a slow-growing disease and often a patient is on watch and wait. When treatment is necessary, options include radiation therapy and/or chemotherapy. Several treatment options exist for splenic marginal zone lymphoma. Some patients have the spleen removed or are given low-dose radiation of the spleen. Other patients may receive rituximab (Rituxan) with or without chemotherapy such as fludarabine, cladribine, or cyclophosphamide. Several other treatments are under investigation.

Waldenstrom Macroglobulinemia: Waldenstrom, also called lymphoplasmacytic lymphoma or immunocytoma, is a rare, slow-growing b-cell lymphoma that occurs in about 3 percent of people with NHL. The disease usually affects older adults and is found primarily in the bone marrow, although lymph nodes and the spleen may be involved. Waldenstrom is characterized by a high level of a protein called immunoglobulin in the blood, which can cause a thickening of the blood and result in nosebleeds, headaches, dizziness, and blurring or loss of vision. Other symptoms may include tiredness, night sweats, pain or numbness in the extremities and increased size of the liver, spleen, and lymph nodes. Waldenstrom is diagnosed with blood and urine tests as well as with a bone marrow biopsy.

For patients without symptoms, a watch and wait approach may be appropriate. Some patients receive a procedure called plasmapheresis to reverse or prevent the symptoms associated with the thickening of the blood. This procedure involves removing the patient's blood, passing it through a machine that removes the part of the blood containing the IgM antibody, and returning the blood to the patient. Doctors often combine plasmapheresis with other treatments, such as chemotherapy. There are many drugs or combinations of drugs that can be used to manage this disease, including: single-agents such as chlorambucil (Leukeran); cCladribine or fludarabine; rituximab (Rituxan) or a combination such as R CHOP; R cyclophosphamide dexamethasone; R fludarabine; R bendamustine (Treanda); or R bortezomib (Velcade).

The choice of treatment is based on individual patient needs, as well as considerations for short and long-term side effects. In patients with high IgM levels, it has been suggested that rituximab should be used with caution due to a potential flare phenomenon leading to abrupt increases in IgM levels and aggravation of serum viscosity. In patients, with an IgM level of 5000 mg/dL or higher or who have hyper viscosity symptoms (such as headaches, blurry vision, nosebleeds), plasmapheresis may be performed before rituximab is used, and IgM levels should then be closely followed. In younger, stem cell transplant eligible patients the use of chlorambucil and nucleoside analogue agents such as fludarabine or cladribine generally should be avoided due to possible toxicity to stem cells. An increased risk of secondary cancers has also been reported with chlorambucil and nucleoside analogues. An increased risk of neuropathy is associated with vincristine and bortezomib based therapy.

T-Cell Lymphomas: T-cell lymphomas are much less common than b-cell lymphomas, particularly in the United States. They develop from abnormal t-lymphocytes and account for approximately 15 percent of all non-Hodgkin lymphoma cases in the United States. There are many different types of t-cell lymphomas, some of which are very rare. Among the more common t-cell lymphomas are peripheral t-cell lymphoma not otherwise specified (PTCL-NOS), which accounts for about a quarter of all t-cell lymphomas. These lymphomas are often aggressive and may show up in lymph nodes, skin, or other organs of the body. Anaplastic large cell lymphoma describes several types of t-cell lymphoma and accounts for approximately 15 percent of all t-cell lymphomas in adults. It is subdivided into three subtypes: ALK positive, ALK negative, or a skin only type called primary cutaneous anaplastic large cell lymphoma. The systemic types are usually fast-growing while the skin only type is usually more slow-growing, Angioimmunoblastic lymphoma is a fast-growing t-cell lymphoma accounting for more than 15 percent of all t-cell lymphomas in the United States. It often presents with swollen lymph nodes and systemic symptoms such as fever and rash. It is generally treated like other fast-growing t-cell lymphomas, but can be managed sometimes with milder therapies. Cutaneous t-cell lymphoma accounts for 2 percent to 3 percent of all NHL cases and mostly affects adults. These are slow-growing cancers that start, and are most often confined, to the skin. Mycosis fungoides is the most common type of cutaneous t-cell lymphoma. It appears as skin patches or plaques, and is often controlled over many years. Less common forms include Sezary syndrome, primary cutaneous anaplastic large cell lymphoma and lymphomatoid papulosis among others. Even rarer t-cell lymphomas include adult t-cell leukemia/lymphoma, which is caused by the HTLV virus. This virus is more commonly found in people from the Caribbean, southern Japan, and central Africa. The virus often is acquired from breast feeding, but only about 2 percent who carry the virus will develop lymphoma. The great majority will remain asymptomatic carriers throughout their life.

Blastic NK-cell lymphoma is a very rare cancer that only impacts a small number of people each year. This lymphoma is fast-growing and can be difficult to treat. It can arise anywhere in the body. Dark red or purple skin lesions are a common feature. Enteropathy-type t-cell lymphoma is an extremely rare subtype of t-cell lymphoma that appears in the intestines and is strongly associated with celiac disease. Hematosplenic gamma-delta t-cell lymphoma is an extremely rare and aggressive disease that starts in the liver or spleen. It may occur in those with inflammatory bowel disease who are immunosuppressed. Lymphoblastic lymphoma can appear in both b-cells and t-cells, but is much more common in t-cells, comprising 80 percent of all lymphoblastic lymphomas. This lymphoma is most often diagnosed in children. With intensive chemotherapy, the complete remission rate can be very high. Nasal NK/t-cell lymphomas are relatively rare in the United States, but are fast-growing and typically originate in the lining of the nose or upper airway. They are treated with radiation and various combinations of chemotherapy. Treatment-related t-cell lymphomas sometimes appear after solid organ or bone marrow transplantation. The immune system suppression that is required to transplant patients can put them at risk for developing post-transplant lymphoproliferative disorders, certain unusual forms of peripheral t-cell lymphoma and other types of NHL.

Treatments depend upon the type and other factors. Due to the rarity of t-cell lymphomas, most treatments have been borrowed from other types of lymphoma. Treatments include chemotherapy, radiation, stem cell transplantation and surgery. Treatments aimed at the skin, such as ultraviolet light therapy or electron beam therapy are effective for many slow-growing t-cell lymphomas that appear in the skin. For most subtypes of PTCL, the frontline treatment regimen is typically a combination chemotherapy, such as CHOP (cyclophosphamide, doxorubicin, vincristine, prednisone) or EPOCH (etoposide, vincristine, doxorubicin, cyclophosphamide, prednisone) or other multi-drug regimens. Drugs that have been approved specifically for t-cell lymphomas of the skin include: bexarotene (Targretin); denileukin diftitox (Ontak); romidepsin (Isotodax); and vorinostat (Zolinza). A procedure called extracorporeal photopheresis, which involves removing a patient's blood and treating it with ultraviolet light and drugs that become active when exposed to light is approved to treat the blood of people with mycosis fungoides or Sezary syndrome. Pralatrexate (Folotyn) has been approved for relapsed and refractory peripheral T-cell lymphoma. Relapsed PTCL patients may also be treated with combination chemotherapy programs such as ICE (ifosfamide, carboplatin, etoposide), followed by an autologous or allogeneic stem cell transplant. Gemcitabine (Gemzar) appears effective against some forms of relapsed PTCL and is often given in combination with other chemotherapies, including vinorelbine (Navelbine) and doxorubicin (Doxil) in a regimen called GND. Other chemotherapy regimens include DHAP (dexamethasone, cytarabine, cisplatin) and ESHAP (etoposide, methylprednisolone, cytarabine and cisplatin). In June 2011, the U.S. Food and Drug Administration (FDA) granted accelerated approval of romidepsin (Istodax) for injection for the treatment of peripheral t-cell lymphoma (PTCL) in patients who have received at least one prior therapy. In 2011, the U.S. Food and Drug Administration (FDA) granted accelerated approval of brentuximab vedotin (Adcetris), an antibody-drug conjugate which targets CD30, for the treatment of patients with relapsed or refractory systemic anaplastic large cell lymphoma (ALCL). Many drugs are being studied for the treatment of PTCL, including: ABT-262; AT-101; bortezomib (Velcade); decapeptide; obatoclax; (GX15-070); panobinostat (Faridak); PXD101 (Belinostat); romidepsin (Istodax); vorinostat (Zolinza); lenalidomide (Revlimid); zanolimumab; and brentuximab vedotin (Adcetris).

ALCL appearing in multiple sites on the body may require systemic treatment such as mild chemotherapy (single agents or mild combinations); bexarotene (Targretin) pills; CVP (cyclophosphamide, vincristine, prednisone) chemotherapy; or methotrexate (Trexall). There are several drugs in clinical trials that are showing promising results, including pralatrexate (Folotyn). Novel combination chemotherapy regimens are also being studied in ongoing trials for patients with systemic t-cell lymphomas such as CHOP plus bevacizumab (Avastin) and PEGS (cisplatin, etoposide, gemcitabine and solumedrol).

Angioimmunoblastic t-cell lymphoma is usually first treated with chemotherapy regimens such as CHOP (cyclophosphamide, doxorubicin, vincristine, prednisone), dose intense regimens such as Hyper-CVAD (cyclophosphamide, vincristine, doxorubicin, dexamethasone), or non-adriamycin based chemotherapy, radiation or high-dose chemotherapy followed by an autologous stem cell transplant (stem cell transplant in which a patient receives their own stem cells). Once a patient has disease that has relapsed, alternative therapies are indicated such as pralatrexate (Folotyn). Other salvage chemotherapies such as a gemcitabine (Gemzar) containing regimen, or an allogeneic stem cell transplant (stem cell transplant in which a patient receives stem cells from a donor). Several drugs currently being tested in clinical trials are showing promise. For example, a new class of drugs, known as histone deacetylase inhibitors, which include the drugs suberoylanilide hydroxamic acid (SAHA) and vorinostat (Zolinza), have been effective in the treatment of a variety of t-cell lymphomas.

For mycosis fungoides, treatment is either directed at the skin or the entire body (systemic). Because Sezary syndrome is chronic and systemic (affecting the entire body), it is usually not treated with skin-directed therapies alone. Treatments may be prescribed alone or in combination to achieve the best long-term benefit.

Other treatments include: ultraviolet light (PUVA, UVB); denileukin diftitox (Ontak); narrow-band UVB); extracorporeal photopheresis; topical steroids; gemcitabine (Gemzar); nitrogen mustard; interferon; liposomal doxorubicin (Doxil); retinoids (bexarotene gel); mMethotrexate (Trexall); local radiation; oral retinoids (bexarotene capsules); total skin electron beam therapy; romidepsin (Istodax); vorinostat (Zolinza). Some second-line therapies include the above or bortezomib (Velcade), chlorambucil (Leukeran), cyclophosphamide (Cytoxan), etoposide (Toposar), pentostatin (Nipent), and temozolomide (Temodar). There are several treatments being tested in clinical trials for cutanious t-cell, including allogeneic stem cell transplant; lenalidomide (Revlimid); autologous dendritic cell vaccine; mogamulizumab (KW-0761); bortezomib (Velcade); pralatrexate (Folotyn); enzastaurin; vorinostat (Zolinza); forodesine (BCX-1777); and zanolimumab (HuMax-CD4).

T-cell leukemias are a poorly defined group of diseases that show up in the blood. These include slow-growing diseases such as t-cell granular lymphocytic leukemia, or faster-growing diseases such as aggressive NK-cell leukemia. There are other rare cancers of the immune system that are neither b-cell nor t-cell lymphomas, but involve other types of white blood cells such as histiocytic and dendritic cell neoplasms.

Leukemia fundamentals: The next most common category of blood cancer is leukemia. Leukemia is cancer of the blood and bone marrow, the spongy center of bones where our blood cells are formed. The disease develops when blood cells produced in the bone marrow grow out of control. The cell undergoes a change and becomes a type of leukemia cell. Once the marrow cell undergoes a leukemic change, the leukemia cells may grow and survive better than normal cells. Over time, the leukemia cells crowd out the development of normal cells. The rate at which leukemia progresses and how the cells replace the normal blood and marrow cells are different with each type of leukemia.

The most common types of leukemia are: acute myeloid leukemia (AML); chronic myeloid leukemia (CML); acute lymphocytic leukemia (ALL); and chronic lymphocytic leukemia (CLL). These types account for approximately 90% of leukemias. There also is hairy cell leukemia, chronic myelomonocytic leukemia, and juvenile myelomonocytic leukemia. Once again, the stage and type often are important determinants of treatment and prognosis.

In 2020, 60,530 people in the United States were expected to be diagnosed with leukemia. There are an estimated 376,000 people living with or in remission from leukemia in the United States. The overall 5-year survival rate for leukemia has more than quadrupled, from about 14 percent from 1960 to 1963 to 65.8 percent for all races from 2009 to 2015. From 2009 to 2015, the five-year survival rates overall were: ALL 71.7 percent overall (91.9 percent for children and adolescents); AML 29.4 percent overall (68.7 percent for children and adolescents); and CLL 88.2 percent. In 2020, 23,100 people ware expected to die from leukemia (13,420 males and 9,680 females). From 2012 to 2016, leukemia was the sixth most common cause of cancer deaths in both men and women in the United States.

There is a wide range of potential symptoms of leukemia, including: easy bruising or blood with no clear cause (due to low platelet count); pinhead size red spots under the skin; cuts that take a long time to heal; fatigue or chronic lack of energy and paleness (due to enema); shortness of breath during normal physical activity; mild fever; night sweats; swollen gums; frequent minor infections (due to low white blood cell count); unexplained weight loss; chronic aches or discomfort in bones or joints; and pain or discomfort in the upper left part of the stomach (caused by an enlarged spleen).

Leukemia developing in the lymphocytes (lymphoid cells) is called lymphocytic leukemia. Leukemia developing in the granulocytes or monocytes or myeloid cells is called myelogenous leukemia. Acute leukemias (either lymphocytic or myelogenous) involve new or immature cells (or blasts) that remain immature and incapable of performing their functions. The blasts increase in number rapidly, and the disease progresses quickly. Chronic leukemias involve some blast cells, but they are more mature and are able to perform some of their functions. The cells tend to grow more slowly and the number increases less quickly, so the disease progresses gradually.

Acute Lymphocytic Leukemia: ALL is a rapidly progressing disease in which too many immature lymphocytes (type of white blood cell) are produced in the bone marrow. It is the most common cancer diagnosed in children. ALL generally is diagnosed by a Complete Blood Count (CBC) with differential, a bone marrow biopsy, and flow cytometry examined by a hematopathologist.

The first phase of treatment is induction therapy. The goal of induction therapy is to destroy as many cancer cells as possible in order to achieve (induce) a remission. Typically, initial therapy requires a hospital stay of 4 to 6 weeks. Induction regimens for ALL generally use a combination of drugs that include Vincristine (Oncovin), Anthracyclines (daunorubicin), Corticosteroids (prednisone, dexamethasone) and may include asparaginase (Elspar, Rylaze) and/or cyclophosphamide (Cytoxan). At the conclusion of induction therapy, doctors will check to see whether the patient has achieved a complete remission. A complete remission is achieved when no more than 5 percent of cells in the bone marrow are blast cells, blood cell counts return to normal, and the signs and symptoms of ALL have resolved.

Approximately, 25 percent of adults have an ALL subtype called "Ph-positive ALL" (also known as either "Ph+" or "Philadelphia chromosome-positive ALL"). In Ph+ ALL the Philadelphia chromosome contains the abnormal BCR-ABL fusion gene that makes an abnormal protein that helps leukemia cells to grow. Tyrosine kinase inhibitors (TKIs) are used to treat Ph+ ALL by blocking (inhibiting) the BCR-ABL protein from sending signals that cause leukemia cells to form. TKIs are a type of targeted therapy. Targeted therapy uses drugs or other substances that target and attack specific cancer cells but are less likely to harm normal cells. TKIs generally are added to a chemotherapy regimen and are taken in pill form. Imatinib (Gleevec) is approved for adult patients with relapsed or refractory Ph+ ALL and pediatric patients with newly diagnosed Ph+ ALL in combination with chemotherapy. Dasatinib (Sprycel), taken by mouth, is approved for adults with Ph+ ALL with resistance or intolerance to prior therapy, d older with newly diagnosed Ph+ ALL in combination with chemotherapy Ponatinib (Iclusig), is approved for the treatment of adult patients with *T315I*-positive Ph+ ALL. Sometimes stem cell transplantation is used for ALL. One of the most serious potential long-term side effects of ALL therapy is the development of AML. This occurs in about 5% of patients after they have received chemotherapy drugs called epipodophyllotoxins (*e.g.*, etoposide or teniposide) or alkylating agents (*e.g.*, cyclophosphamide or chlorambucil). Less often, children cured of leukemia may later develop non-Hodgkin lymphomas or other cancers. Among children with ALL, more than 95% attain remission and 75%-85% are free of recurrence for at least 5 years after diagnosis.

Acute Myeloid Leukemia: AML usually is diagnoses through a complete blood count (usually patients with AML have lower than average red blood cells and platelets), a peripheral blood smear (usually patients with AML have too many immature white blood cells or blasts and too few mature white blood cells) and bone marrow biopsy. Genetic tests may help identify changes (mutations) in the genes or chromosomes of a cell. Identifying these specific changes can help determine the patient's treatment options and prognosis. The following tests may be done to examine the genes of a patient's leukemia cells: cytogenetic analysis (karyotyping); Fluorescence In Situ Hybridization (FISH); and molecular testing. Blast cells normally comprise 1 to 5 percent of marrow cells. Having at least 20 percent blasts is generally required for a diagnosis of AML. But AML can also be diagnosed if the blasts have a chromosome change that occurs in a specific type of AML, even if the blast percentage is less than 20 percent. Characteristic markers (antigens) on the surface of blast cells, such as CD13 or CD33 may be identified through flow cytometry.

AML treatment is generally done in two phases (cycles) induction therapy and post-remission or consolidation therapy. Different subtypes may be treated differently. Most AML patients are treated with a combination of an anthracycline (such as daunorubicin, doxorubicin, idarubicin, or cytarabine), Gemtuzumab, Midostaurin, Daunorubicin and cytarabine (Vyxeos), Venetoclax (Venclexta), Glasdegib (Daurismo^M), Ivosidenib (Tibsovo). Other drugs may be added or substituted for higher-risk, refractory or relapsed patients. Some patients may also receive radiation therapy or a bone-marrow transplant using their own or a closely related sibling's cells.

Chronic Myeloid (or Myelogenous) Leukemia: CML typically is diagnosed by the same tests discussed above. We discuss CML and the revolutionary treatment made possible through the work of Dr. Janet Rowley elsewhere. In recent years, the standard of care for CML is to treat with a type of targeted drug called a tyrosine kinase inhibitor (such as imatinib or Gleevec). These drugs are very effective at inducing remission and decreasing progression to the accelerated phase. These drugs have had a major impact for patients with this disease.

Chronic Lymphocytic Leukemia: One person's CLL may be another's small lymphocytic lymphoma (SLL). Leukemia and lymphoma are sister diseases. When the cancer cells are located mostly in the lymph nodes, the disease is called SLL. When most of the cancer cells are located in the bloodstream and the bone marrow, the disease is referred to as CLL, although the lymph nodes and spleen are often involved. CLL tends to be an indolent (slow-growing) cancer, but it can progress to a more aggressive disease. About one-third of CLL patients will live for years or decades without symptoms. Another one-third will require therapy immediately or will be symptomatic within three to five years and require treatment. The final one-third will experience intermediate disease progression with waxing and waning disease that responds to treatment.

The chemotherapy regimens most commonly used for treatment of CLL are R-CHOP (rituximab, cyclophosphamide, doxorubicin, vincristine, prednisone); FR (fludarabine, rituximab); FCR (fludarabine, cyclophosphamide, rituximab); BR (bendamustine, rituximab); BCR (bendamustine, cyclophosphamide, rituximab); and PCR (pentostatin, cyclophosphamide, rituximab). Monoclonal antibodies used include alemtuzumab (Campath) approved for use in patients with advanced CLL who are no longer responding to other treatments; ofatumumab (Arzerra) approved for patients with CLL refractory to fludarabine (Fludara) and alemtuzumab (Campath); and rituximab (Rituxan) approved in combination with fludarabine and cyclophosphamide for patients with untreated or previously treated CD20-positive CLL. Stem cell transplantation is a treatment option typically reserved for patients whose CLL does not respond to other therapies. Patients whose disease has transformed into a more aggressive form potentially could benefit from a reduced intensity allogeneic transplant.

There have been several promising developments for CLL patients in recent years. For example, PCI-32765 is one of several drugs in clinical trials with the common theme that they all interfere with b-cell receptor signaling. When you ligate the b-cell receptor, you provide a very strong signal for survival and proliferation to the cell. There are a number of different downstream kinases in that pathway, and the drugs that have been in clinical trials inhibit the message that tells the cell to survive and proliferate, but those drugs target totally different kinases. CAL-101 is a PI3

Kinase inhibitor; PCI-32765 is a Bruton's Tyrosine Kinase (BTK) inhibitor; and fostamatinib is a Spleen Tyrosine Kinase Inhibitor (SYK). One study showed a 67% response rate of patients with relapsed CLL. Also the drugs are oral, so they are easy to administer. PCI-32765 appears to have very minimal side effects. The most common side effect is diarrhea, which often tends to be self-limited. Also, the drugs are not myelosuppressive, which is particularly important to leukemic patients who, even when they are not myelosuppressed, do not have a normally functioning immune system, and, therefore, are prone to infections. Many including Dr. Andre Goy believe that the b-cell inhibitors will be a game-changer in CLL and b-cell lymphomas. A study using Bendamustine combined with rituximab (BR) in patients with relapsed and/or refractory CLL shows it to be effective and safe in patients with relapsed CLL and to have notable activity in fludarabine-refractory disease. Major but tolerable toxicities were myelosuppression and infections. Lenalidomide may be an option for elderly patients with chronic lymphocytic leukemia who may be unable to tolerate traditional chemoimmunotherapy such as FCR. Bendamustine (Treanda) is both more effective and less toxic than the standard CHOP regimen when both are combined with rituximab (Rituxan). According to Dr. Mathias Rummel of University Hospital in Germany, it should be "preferred as first-line therapy" in patients with follicular lymphoma and similar slow-moving diseases.

It is important to have multiple agents and alternatives—choices of monoclonal antibodies, kinases inhibitors, etc. One study, for example, concluded that, patients with fludarabine-refractory chronic lymphocytic leukemia that was resistance to rituximab, responded to ofatumumab. The Leukemia and Lymphoma Society is a good source of information about leukemia.

Other forms of leukemia: We have discussed the four most common types of leukemia above. More rare forms of leukemia include: hairy cell, chronic myelomonocytic, juvenile myelomonocytic, large granular lymphocytic, blastic plasmacytoid dendritic cell neoplasm, B-Cell prolymphocytic, and T-Cell prolymphocytic leukemias.

Myeloma overview: Myeloma is the final major category of blood cancer. Myeloma begins in the bone marrow and impacts certain white blood cells called plasma cells. Plasma cells produce antibodies, which are proteins that assist the body in ridding itself of harmful substances. Each plasma cell responds to one specific substance by producing one kind of antibody. The body has many types of plasma cells and, therefore, can respond to many types of substances. When cancer occurs, the body overproduces abnormal plasma cells, known as myeloma cells. Myeloma cells collect in the bone marrow and the outer layer of the bone.

An estimated 32,270 new cases of myeloma (17,530 males and 14,740 females) were expected to be diagnosed in the United States in 2020. An estimated 129,000 people in the US are living with or in remission from myeloma. The five-year survival rate has increased from 12 percent from 1960 to 1963 to 53.7 percent from 2009 to 2015. The 5-year survival rate is 76.2 percent for people with myeloma who were younger than 45 years at diagnosis. Approximately 12,830 deaths from myeloma were expected in 2020 (7,190 males and 5,640 females). Myeloma survivors in the United States are estimated to total more than 69,000, with over 21,700 new cases and 10,700 deaths a year.

There are several forms of myeloma identified by the areas of the body impacted and the rate of progression. Most patients, about 90%, have multiple myeloma, meaning the disease is in multiple areas of the body by the time of diagnosis. The disease is most common in older individuals—the medium age at diagnosis is 70 years—but younger people can have myeloma too. Many times, it is a broken bone that leads a patient to seek treatment and that results in the diagnosis. The most common signs of myeloma are bone fractures and bone pain without an apparent reason. Pain is most common in the back or ribs, but it can occur in other bones. The pain is usually made worse by movement. Other symptoms may include: weakness; fatigue; pale skin; recurring infections; neuropathy (numbness, tingling, burning or pain) in the hands or feet; increased thirst or urination; constipation; and kidney failure. Hyperviscosity syndrome is associated with myeloma. This may cause blurry vision, headaches, chest pain, abnormal bleeding, or shortness of breath.

There are various treatments for myeloma. Drugs include bortezomib (Velcade), thalidomide (Thalomid), dexamethasone (Decadron), lenalidomide (revlimid), Melphalan (Alkeran) which sometimes are used as single agents, but more often in various combinations. In addition, autologous stem cell transplants (sometimes tandem transplants) often are a component of treatment. There appears to be a role for maintenance therapy. There is no standard maintenance therapy at present, but research is ongoing and promising. Radiation therapy is used sometimes as a first-line treatment for patients whose myeloma is localized, in preparation for a stem cell transplant, or in carefully selected patients whose bone pain does not respond to chemotherapy. Carfilzomib (kyprolis) has been approved to treat refractory patients with multiple myeloma who have received at least two prior therapies. The number of immunotherapies and drugs has increased significantly as have promising clinical trials providing additional help and hope to patients with myeloma.

The "etiology" or cause of blood cancers: Cancer patients, after coming to grips with the diagnosis and forming a battle plan, often wonder "how did I get cancer" or "what caused my cancer?" We are learning more about what causes cancer. More is known about the cause of some forms of cancer than others. For example, everyone now knows that cigarette smoking (and second-hand exposure to smoke) causes lung cancer. We are past mere associations and can say definitively that there is cause and effect between cigarette smoking and lung cancer.

Similarly, the virus causing cervical cancer has been identified and should be tested for regularly in woman. There are associations between many cancers and inflammatory conditions: lung cancer and cigarette smoke; liver cancer and hepatitis; Malt lymphoma and stomach cancer and Helicobacter pylori; colon and rectal cancer and inflammatory bowel disease; cervical cancer and Papillomavirus; and mesothelioma and asbestos are some examples.

With respect to most blood cancers, the answer often is less clear. It is difficult to say what caused lymphoma in any individual person. There is evidence suggesting associations between some lymphomas and environmental and occupational exposures to some chemicals, including: benzene; petrochemicals and combustion by-products (such as polycyclic aromatic hydrocarbons and soot); some pesticides, fungicides, insecticides, and herbicides (such as Agent Orange used in Vietnam); hair dyes, polychlorinated biphenyls, and solvents (such as styrene, trichloroethylene, and tetrachloroethylene). The associations are stronger in some instances than in others. Benzene appears to be a significant culprit. People who suffer from some auto-immune disorders (such as Sorgen's Syndrome, rheumatoid arthritis, and Lupus) may be at a higher risk of developing some lymphomas than people who do not suffer from these disorders. Recipients of organ transplants also are more likely to develop lymphoma as are people with AIDS.

Even items intended to heal people may cause lymphoma. For example, there are associations between some prescription medicines—such as TNF

Blockers—and lymphoma. Cancer treatments—such as chemotherapy and radiation—may cause some lymphomas as well. We know that some leukemias are the result of prior cancer treatments. Hardly a week goes without a news report about possible links between diet and cancer.

Lymphomas are not contagious. But exposure to some bacteria and viruses causes some lymphomas. Epstein-Barr virus, for example, is linked to the endemic type of Burkitt's lymphoma in Africa. In Western Countries, a very high percentage of patients with Hodgkin lymphoma have or had Epstein-Barr virus. Helicobacter pylori and Hepatitis C are also associated with some lymphomas. Simply stated, there are associations between exposures to toxins, viruses, and other substances and some lymphomas.

We know that there is more to the equation than exposures to toxins and viruses. After all, many people exposed to these agents do not get lymphoma and many people with lymphoma do not have known exposures to these agents. Our immune system plays a critical role in defeating cancer and lymphoma actually is cancer of the immune system. This is why understanding what causes lymphoma is critically important not only for lymphoma, but also for unlocking the mysteries to other cancers and other diseases. This is one of the many reasons why we say that blood cancer research is the super highway to curing cancer.

Usually, when we discuss cancer research, the focus is on developing new and more efficacious treatments. But another critical aspect of cancer research involves the epidemiology of cancer—or the investigation into the causes of cancer. Understanding what causes cancer provides important insights into how to prevent cancer. It also fosters the development of better treatments. Fortunately, there are dedicated researchers around the globe investigating the causes of lymphoma. More importantly, they are working collaboratively—sharing their discoveries, statistics, and insights. Such collaborative efforts benefit all of us by hastening the pace of medical advancement. The International Lymphoma Epidemiology Consortium (InterLymph) is an international group of leading medical investigators engaged in research on the epidemiology of non-Hodgkin lymphoma. We interviewed three such dedicated researchers on the *Battling and Beating Cancer Radio Show* and you can listen to that interview on demand at www.blogtalkradio.com/battling-and-beating-cancer.

Many more treatments options available to patients: Through the investment in research, the treatment armamentarium for all blood cancers—as with solid tumors—has grown, with more effective and less toxic treatments available for many subtypes.

We also discuss generally some treatments for cancer in Chapter 19, but research of your particular type of cancer, consideration of factors unique to you and your cancer, your general health, prognostic indictors and tumor markers and consultation with your physician are required. In view of the individual factors and the pace of research and developments, websites and timely information from reliable sources should be consulted. By the time you read this, there will be more treatment options available and more information about the efficacy and safety of various treatments.

Now, we will focus on some of the important things that you can do to conquer cancer.

CHAPTER 15

PICKING THE BEST DOCTORS AND ASSEMBLING YOUR HEALTH CARE TEAM (CHOOSE YOUR DOCTORS WISELY)

Generally, the two most important medical decisions that a cancer patient will make are selecting the medical doctors and treatment facilities to entrust with their care and selecting the treatments to undergo and to forego. Usually, the doctor you select will play a major role in the treatment you undergo since you are relying upon his or her medical judgment. Sometimes, however, the medical treatment that you decide to undergo is a major determinant of the doctor you select. The completion of the Human Genome Project, the advent of targeted therapies, and recent developments in platform technologies to comprehensively diagnose and prognose a patient's cancer have paved the way for personalized or precision medicine as we now it. It is important to have doctors who are well-versed in the treatment options available and conversant with the latest technologies. Patients must be open to having more doctors on their team and be flexible if they need to change the composition of their medical team over time. You need to embrace personalized medicine, but not be overwhelmed by it.

Most people expend more time and effort in choosing a house painter or car mechanic than in selecting an oncologist or other medical specialist. People will get multiple estimates from a painter, speak with friends and neighbors, call the Better Business Bureau, and get additional references before letting someone work on their house or car. Yet, most people know very little about their oncologist, radiologist, or surgeon. It is uncanny how many times people put their lives and well-being in the hands of someone that they know so little about. Often they are in the hands of a specialist because their internist sent them to him or her, or they happen to be in the geographic area where the patient lives or have staff privileges at the hospital where the patient is located. Sometimes the circumstances are such that emergency treatment is required and you get who you get. But more often, the patient has the opportunity to have input in the doctor, be it a surgeon, oncologist, or radiologist-oncologist. Simply stated, getting the best physician possible is extremely important, particularly when you are dealing with a life-threatening condition such as cancer.

Getting the best doctor available does not guarantee a good result, but it is an extremely important factor in getting a good result. Good doctors make mistakes, have bad days, and some conditions are beyond any doctor's ability to treat effectively. Mediocre and bad doctors get lucky, have good days, and sometimes help patients in spite of their lack of skill. Our experience in dealing with cancer and Scott's experience as a lawyer (who years ago defended doctors in medical malpractice cases) informs us that there is a very broad variance among doctors in the same field. Skill, training, education, general experience, experience with particular disease types, treatments, and procedures as well as effort, energy, compassion, knowledge, ability to communicate, instinct, judgment, and pride run the gambit with doctors just as with people in the general population. The lack of medical experience on the part of the patient and caregiver may excuse selection of sub-par doctors, but this is no consolation whatsoever to the patient that does not receive the best available care. Hopefully, you already appreciate the importance of selecting the best doctor available. Admittedly, there is not a single touchstone. All of the factors listed above enter into the equation, as do such factors as the patient's comfort level and trust in the physician and the location of the physician.

According to Scott, the threshold test for selecting a doctor involves how the doctor refers to himself or herself. He found that most of the best doctors will introduce themselves to patients by saying their name without referring to themselves as "doctor." They know that you know that they are doctors – that is why you are there to see them. He is saying this somewhat tongue in cheek and we have allowed ourselves to be treated by physicians who introduce themselves as "doctor." Our main point is you want a doctor who respects and values you as a person and patient and understands that you intend to be an active partner in your treatment and recovery. So let's move to the substance of selecting doctors.

Proactive selection of a physician involves two basic elements: names and investigation. There are many good sources for recruiting your physicians. There are traditional sources and those available in these days of the worldwide web. They all have advantages and limitations.

Referrals from other doctors: Obtaining a referral from your internist or family doctor is a starting point. Many people obtain their oncologists and specialists this way and it often works out well. The value of a referral is a function of the level of trust and respect that you repose in the referring physician and the basis upon which the referring physician makes the referral. Many referrals are made on the basis that the oncologist works out of the same office, group, or hospital as the referring doctor. The referral may be made because the oncologist is one of the two oncologists that the referring doctor knows. Maybe there are cross-referrals between the doctors or other economic incentives for the doctor to make the referral. It does not necessarily make the referral bad, but it does not necessarily make the referral good either.

Referrals are more valuable where the referring doctor is knowledgeable about the specialist recommended and the specialty itself. The doctor may have referred multiple patients with the same condition to that doctor and knows the details of the treatments and of favorable outcomes. At a minimum, when dealing with cancer, you will not only want the doctor's name, but an explanation concerning the basis for the referral, the credentials and factors leading to the recommendation, and the experience the referring doctor has had with the doctor. Asking the referring doctor why he recommends the doctor and whether he knows of any other specialists with more experience or better credentials are fair questions.

Referrals from friends and relatives: This is another common source of doctor selection. Once again, it depends not only upon the trust and level of confidence you have in the person making the referral, but also their knowledge and ability to make a proper referral. They are not shrouded with medical knowledge, but may have an undue emotional or familial influence on your decision. Again, you must get behind the name and learn about the basis for the recommendation.

Referrals from cancer patients and survivors: Now these folks have had actual experience with cancer and presumably are at least alive to make the referral. They frequently are excellent referral sources, but you have to consider the type of cancer and treatment they experienced, any bias they may have, and any limitations on their ability to evaluate. Ask them for the basis for their recommendation. You are likely to get important details about the physician from cancer patients.

Referrals from organizations: Cancer and health-related non-profit organizations are not in the business of rendering medical advice. They are not qualified to do so and do not want to assume any liability for purporting to do so. Many of them do have staff members or volunteers who will identify doctors in various geographic areas and will share some collective experiences. They can identify doctors who have spoken at seminars, are involved in clinical trials, are leaders in the field, and have treated patients affiliated with their organization. Many times, these organizations have phone lines dedicated to speaking to people about doctors, treatments, and clinical trials. They may provide insights on technical skills, bedside manner, and they sometimes can assist in obtaining prompt appointments.

We have helped patients obtain prompt appointments and avoid protracted delays in being seen seeing by doctors many times when traditional channels failed. With cancer, time usually is of the essence. Some good sources of referrals, include: the American Society of Clinical Oncology (ASCO) www.cancer.net and search their oncologist database; the American Society of Hematology (ASH) at www.hematology.org/patients; and the American Board of Medical Specialties (ABMS) Certification Matters website at www.certificationmatters.org. Others are identified in Appendix "C."

Referrals from medical centers and institutions: There are several preeminent cancer diagnostic and treatment centers in the United States, such as Sloan Kettering, Northwestern University, Rush University Medical Center, Dana Farber, Stanford, Mayo Clinic, and M.D. Anderson. Speaking with doctors from such institutions or looking at their websites will provide information. In fact, most institutions identify doctors and have their credentials and biographies online. If there is an institution or doctor that you are particularly impressed with, you may select that doctor or ask the doctor to refer you to a specialist in your area.

Medical articles, periodicals, and online searches: In these days of computers, search engines, and various websites, it is relatively easy to conduct online searches to obtain important information about the type of cancer you have, treatments, studies, and results. This will help you to learn about doctors who are writing, speaking, and researching areas of interest and those who are quoted or cited in the area. It also will provide you with information about the disease and arm you with substantive questions to ask your doctors. Often videos of doctors are available online and they provide insight into the doctors personality, approach, communication skills, and knowledge.

Chat groups: Sometimes patients and caregivers participating in chat groups are a tremendous source of referrals as well as information on the disease. You have to remember that participants can range from flakes and phonies to serious people who are extremely knowledgeable, sophisticated, and attuned. The web can be a source of misinformation or incomplete information. Make sure you consider the reliability of the source and verify. One of the books we recommend in Appendix "J" is *The Web-Savvy Patient* by Andrew Schorr, a leukemia survivor and medical journalist.

Insurance provider lists: If your insurer, HMO, or PPO limits your choice of doctors and hospitals, the listing of available doctors or network providers may be the starting point for your review. There may be very qualified doctors and institutions within the network. We are not suggesting that it is an endpoint, as you may be able to obtain approval for another doctor under a variety of circumstances or may be willing and able to pay for the doctor of your choice. You should know the insurance and financial consequences associated with selection of a physician.

There is no magic answer, but there are a variety of sources of information. Once you get a few names, conduct some research and investigation and run the names by some of these sources. Often, the process of selecting physicians and obtaining information on the disease and available treatments goes hand-in-hand.

Listen to your spouse or your own instincts: The ability of the patient to connect with and have confidence in the doctor is a valid and important variable. Yet, we know many instances where people are not being given the optimal treatment because they are seeing doctors that they trust or believe in to a higher degree than objectively warranted.

There are some instances where immediate attention and treatment is required. However, there are many more instances where the patient at least has some time to select the doctor and treating institution. When being pressured by the doctor on the scene to undergo the procedure immediately, the patient and caregiver are placed in a difficult situation. Absent exigent circumstances, do not be rushed into making a decision. There are instances when patients are pushed into immediate action when it is not required so that the doctor or hospital secures the business and does not lose it to another health center or when the sense of urgency conveyed at the scene is overstated for whatever reason, including genuine interest in the patient and a genuine belief that this is the proper place for treatment. Whenever possible and without significant threat to the patient's life or well-being, the patient and advocate should attempt to secure some time to consider the treatment, doctor, and hospital. The patient is at a distinct informational disadvantage to be sure, but by thinking about the symptoms experienced, by asking detailed and probing questions, by following one's own sense of well-being and instincts, and by having knowledgeable people around you, better decisions can be made. There are no guarantees, but you want to be in the hands of the best, most capable, most experienced doctor available.

Several years ago, one of our friends saw a doctor who told her that she had cervical cancer and needed a hysterectomy. The doctor tried to rush her into having the surgery. She called us and faxed the pathology report to us. Although we are not doctors, it did not appear to us that she even had cancer. We had her see one of the leading oncologists in the area. She did not have cervical cancer and did not need a hysterectomy. There is a broad range of potential explanations for the first doctor's actions that include incompetence or an attempt to perform an unnecessary surgery for financial gain. The incident illustrates the importance of being in the hands of a good doctor, the wisdom of not being unduly rushed into a procedure, and the need for a second opinion.

Regardless of the sources of your referrals, the next step is to obtain information and evaluate your potential doctors.

Do your research: There are many ways to check out the doctor's credentials and to do your due diligence. Below are some things for you to consider in conducting your research.

Online resources: There are numerous helpful online resources. For example, the American Board of Medical Specialties website allows you to learn the board certification status and specialty of any physician certified by one or more of the 24 Member Boards of the American Board of Medical Specialties (www.abms.org). DocFinder is the health professional licensing database provided by Administrators in Medicine and its participating boards. (www.docboard.org). The American Society of Clinical Oncology website allows people to search by doctor's name, practice location, and medical specialty certification (www.asco.org). Surgeons accredited by the American College of Surgeons are listed at www.web.facs.org. The American Medical Association's Physician Select Service website contains information on physicians (www.ama-assn.org). These are just some examples of investigatory resources.

There are several websites that purport to rate doctors based on patient reviews. The quality of the sites and the information they base their ratings on vary considerably. Some may be based only upon one or more online reviews and the utility of such information may be suspect. Again, evaluate the source carefully.

The questions to ask: Let's talk about some of the things you will want to know about the doctor. The more you know before seeing the doctor, the better. Many patients do not feel comfortable asking the doctor questions about his or her experience or background. We do not have any qualms about doing so and have even requested a copy of the doctor's curriculum vitae if we did not already have the necessary information. Still, we recommend having as much information about the doctor as possible in advance of the appointment for three reasons. First, it will inform your decision as to whether even to meet with the doctor at all. Second, many doctors are put off by lengthy (or any) inquiries regarding their capabilities, and you want to avoid creating any unnecessary animosity at the outset that may interfere with a pleasant relationship with the doctor. Third, in view of the limited time available, you would be better served by using the time to focus on the treatment and medical issues pertaining to you during a consultation or appointment.

The areas of inquiry depend upon the situation and the patient. Here are some of the things that may inform or impact your evaluation of the physician.

The physician's background, education, and licensure: Standard areas of interest regarding the doctor's background include: medical school (school, degree, and year of graduation); residency, internships, and fellowships (institution, year, and focus); medical licensure (states, dates, and confirmation of good status); hospital affiliations and staff privileges (hospitals and dates); positions and jobs; professorships and teaching positions (schools and dates); board certifications (type and dates); professional associations (organization, committees, and dates); other credentials; and honors and awards. In short, you are looking to see that the doctor is qualified and experienced in the type of cancer that afflicts you and the treatments you may receive. If you are at a stage where the diagnosis is not yet clear or known, you need to assess the doctor's skills as a diagnostician.

Generally, you want a doctor that is board certified in the relevant specialty. Specialty boards are private, nonprofit organizations that conduct examinations and certify doctors that have taken and passed rigorous oral and written examinations given by other doctors who specialize in the practice area. Board certification is not an assurance of the care a doctor will provide, but it demonstrates that the doctor has met standards higher than those required to obtain a medical license. If a doctor is not board certified (or is only board eligible), in some instances you may want to find out why.

As a general rule, we prefer doctors with hospital-based practices or who practice as part of a specialty group rather than those who practice alone or with only another doctor or two. We prefer doctors that practice at a National Cancer Institute designated cancer center, a respected university hospital, or a hospital affiliated with a medical school.

Research, writings, and presentations: This will provide information as to how knowledgeable and invested the doctor is in the areas relevant to your treatment and whether he or she has any particular biases or interests.

Disciplinary actions and malpractice lawsuits against the doctor: This probably is not a good area to question the doctor about directly, but this information often is available online through such sources as the Public Citizen Research Group's site (www.questionabledoctors.org), Health Grades (www. healthgrades.com), or through the state licensing body. You can contact the state licensing body to ensure the doctor is duly licensed with no disciplinary proceedings. You can even check courthouse records or online sources to determine the nature of any malpractice actions. Keep in mind, many suits are not meritorious or may merely involve bad outcomes or indiscriminate naming of defendants who did not have any significant involvement in treating the patient or rendering the treatment that is at issue.

Experience and success rate in the relevant area and procedures: You want to know how many patients the physician has treated with your type of cancer, how many times he or she has performed the procedure or rendered the treatment that is being contemplated for you, over what period of time, and what their record is regarding the outcomes and complications. This is a *key* area (often the most important area of inquiry) and is worthy of specific inquiry and probing questions put directly to the doctor. The doctor's answers will inform your decision about what treatment to undergo and the realistic outcome. The substance of the answers and the doctor's demeanor will tell you something about the doctor's method of practicing and something about the doctor as a person. It should shed light on the doctor's command of the subject, ability to communicate, and commitment to patients.

An inquiry also should be made regarding the experience of the hospital in which treatment or procedures are rendered. The doctor may be the captain of the treatment ship, but the experience and quality of the hospital personnel are extremely important. There is a lot of information suggesting success rates are higher with physicians and institutions that have extensive experience in the procedure or treatments being performed. Practice may not make perfect, but it increases the skill set and provides a broader basis to avoid complications, refine procedures and protocols, spot complications, and treat patients with a higher level of expertise. It is not only important to know the historical record, but to know about any recent changes (such as key doctors leaving) which may impact the institutional experience. The questions are simple: how many patients with this cancer have you treated, how many of these treatments have you performed, what is the success rate, and what are the factors the doctor believes are important to the outcomes? At least one site, www.medicalconsumers.org, has data on the number of times some doctors have performed a particular procedure.

Interaction: Notice the way the doctor interacts with you, other patients, staff, and other doctors and how they, in turn, interact with the doctor. This can be very informative. Responses to phone calls and conditions of other patients foretell how the doctor will respond to your phone call.

Billing practices and insurance accepted: Unless you have ample resources, you need to know the financial consequences and realities that impact selection of the treating physician. Most notably, does the doctor accept your insurance? If you do not think about payment at the outset, the doctor's office will be sure to raise this issue.

Location and convenience: We firmly believe that obtaining the best available care and doctors is more important than selecting the closest doctor or hospital. This is particularly true when it comes to obtaining the correct diagnosis and selecting the best treatment. Nonetheless, many cancer treatments such as surgery, chemotherapy, and radiation involve a lengthy stay or multiple, long-term treatments. Travel can be difficult on a patient, particularly one who has work and family obligations that require attention and given the side effects of many treatments. Travel also can take its toll on the family. Sometimes there is a way to balance obtaining the benefit of a top doctor that is inconveniently located and minimizing the inconvenience. For example, sometimes the best option may be to go to a renowned doctor at a leading institution for your work-up, diagnosis, treatment plan, and for periodic visits and have the treatments or testing done at a nearby facility, particularly if the treatment selected is relatively common. Such an approach has benefits and drawbacks.

Doctor's compassion, bedside manner, accessibility, and character: First and foremost, you want a skilled physician that will correctly diagnose, properly treat, effectively steer you away from side effects and complications, and lead you to victory over cancer. Skill and competence come first. You also should have a doctor that genuinely cares about you, takes your outcome personally, answers your questions, provides you with authentic confidence and hope, and a doctor that you trust. Sometimes it seems that the young, relatively inexperienced doctors score high on some of the later categories, but are still developing their skill set. The prestigious doctors sometimes seem too busy, self-absorbed, and intolerant of questions.

We are here to tell you that we have had the privilege of meeting world-renowned doctors who are effective communicators, extremely caring and protective of their patients, and genuinely committed to curing cancer. The point is most times you can get an outstanding doctor that you like and trust. Some wonderful examples are the doctors we mentioned in the acknowledgements. Obtaining such a treasure is possible and worthwhile. If you have to choose between competence and bedside manner, however, choose competence every time. You can usually obtain the other elements from their fellows, nurses, your other doctors, family, and patients that have gone through this before you.

Your health care team: We have discussed selecting a doctor in the singular. The reality is that most cancer patients have multiple doctors. This often is the result of specialization. You may have a general internist or cardiologist, an oncologist, a radiologist, and other specialists depending upon the type and site of the cancer, side effects from the disease or treatments, and other health conditions. You may have multiple oncologists over time depending upon the cancer type and treatments. Another reality is that you may have multiple doctors because the senior doctor—the one you actually selected to treat you—uses junior attending doctors, residents, or fellows. You expect to be under the care of a leading doctor at the cancer center, but he or she may do an initial workup and treatment plan and leave it in the hands of juniors to implement it under his or her guidance (which varies greatly). This is something treating physicians in community hospitals often cite as an advantage of being under their care as opposed to being cared for in a major research university (or teaching hospital as they like to call them). One advantage—maybe the only significant plus—in having junior doctors participate in your care is that they tend to have more time and a better disposition for handholding and answering questions, although the degree to which they have the answers varies. Make sure you know the doctors who actually will be treating you. Ask this question upfront before making your doctor selection.

The presence of multiple doctors treating you means you have to make sure that nothing is falling through the cracks and avoid the movie line "what we have here is a failure to communicate." Effective communication is needed to avoid breakdowns in treatment, adverse drug reactions, repetitive testing, and other problems. Sure, it is the doctors' responsibility, but they may fail to do so or improperly rely upon staff. There are so many potential pitfalls associated with miscommunications and non-communications that the patient and advocate must be alert to these potential issues. Better to ask questions and confirm than to assume the doctors are effectively communicating. Have a packet of key medical records that you can share with the doctors so that you are providing an accurate history.

The doctor's philosophy and biases: Doctors have different approaches. In some instances, virtually all competent doctors may come up with the same treatment plan. But there are many instances where the course is not clear cut or where multiple reasonable treatment options are available. Some doctors are more aggressive, others more conservative. Some are more attune to complementary approaches. So you need to consider the doctor's philosophy and how it can impact your treatment. High caliber doctors recognize their own biases and philosophies and inform the patient so that the patient can make an informed decision.

There are some other important qualities to consider in a doctor. As the doctor is the captain of your treatment ship, you want a doctor with sufficient authority, seniority, and command to take responsibility for your care and ensure that you get the necessary priority in treatment, and to instill sufficient fear or respect on the part of hospital or medical center staff so that everyone is on their toes and operating at the top of their game in providing for your care. The next chapter will underscore the importance of these traits.

CHAPTER 16

HOSPITALS STAYS CAN BE SCARY, BUT HOSPITALS ARE PLACES OF HEALING (SURVIVING YOUR HOSPITAL STAY)

Another important decision—and one that often is related to your selection of doctors—is the hospital or facility in which you will be treated. Most doctors work out of a single hospital or have staff privileges at only a hospital or two. Doctors may be able to obtain special privileges or associate with doctors that have staff privileges at a hospital where necessary.

Your doctor or doctors will not be with you around the clock and your care and outcome is dependent upon dozens of people, many of whom you will never see or hear from. Simply stated, hospitals mostly are places of healing and care, but they are also places of deaths, mistakes, and breakdowns. Even the best hospitals are riddled with hazards. One of your jobs as a patient (and of your advocate and loved ones) is to be vigilant in observing, understanding, and knowing what is going on at all times. The hospital is full of people who can impair your recovery just as well as save your life or facilitate your recovery. Your health is in the hands of the lead doctors to be sure. It also is in the hands of other treating, consulting, on-call doctors, radiologists, pathologists, and the list goes on. You will be surprised how many names appear on the hospital bills. Your outcome also is in the hands of nurses (and no one is more valuable than a good nurse), orderlies, medical records people, technicians of various types, janitors, pharmacists, and staff. Your health and comfort is dependent upon the weakest link as well as the strongest.

As laypeople, we tend to assume that doctors and healthcare providers know best and are doing their job properly. In the final analysis, the levels of competence, commitment, cleanliness, professionalism, compassion, ability to communicate, and attitudes run the gambit just as in society as a whole. Further, the jobs are demanding and many feel overworked, underpaid, and underappreciated. They deal with patients and their family members during stressful times when people are not at their best. They deal with doctors who may not always be clear in their directions or pleasant. Hospitals are highly departmentalized with multiple shift changes and are rife with opportunities for miscommunication and non-communication. You get the picture.

The medical institutions vary considerably. Some are better than others. Some are cleaner. Some have a lot of experience in treating particular cancers and performing particular procedures. Experience in the particular procedure is an important variable in the outcome. Considering reputation is always important, but it is not always reflective of the current reality as applied to your hospital stay or procedure.

A 2013 study suggested "the numbers range from 210,000 to 440,000 deaths per year associated with medical error. The latter number would make it the third leading cause of death after heart disease and cancer. However, these numbers can only be estimated because medical records are often inaccurate and providers might be reluctant to disclose mistakes. . . . One of the 1999 IOM report's main conclusions is that the majority of medical errors do not result from individual recklessness or the actions of a particular group. More commonly, errors are caused by faulty systems, processes, and conditions that lead people to make mistakes or fail to prevent them . . . . The most common medical errors in the United States by occurrence are: adverse drug events, catheter-associated urinary tract infection (CAUTI), central line-associated bloodstream infection (CLABSI), injury from falls and immobility, obstetrical adverse events, pressure ulcers, surgical site infections (SSI), venous thrombosis (blood clots), ventilator-associated pneumonia (VAP), wrong site/wrong procedure surgery (most common basis for quality of care violations), and the following five most mis-diagnosed conditions: cancer related issues; neurological related issues; cardiac-related issues; timely responding to complications during surgery and post-operatively; and urological related issues." https://www.ncbi.nlm.nih.gov/books/NBK430763/

Medication errors are common. The FDA receives more than 100,000 reports associated with medications each year. A large number of patients are impacted by medications errors each year. Medication errors are common in other health care settings and at home. Wrong medicines, wrong doses, improper administration, filling errors, failure to follow instructions are among the errors. https://www.singlecare.com/blog/news/medication-errors-statistics/.

Notwithstanding errors and risks, most hospitals render outstanding care to most patients most of the time. We would be a lot worse off without them. We are not trying to add to your stress or anxiety, but you must know the dangers to avoid their adverse consequences. By understanding the risks, patients and their caregivers can take affirmative steps to prevent errors from happening.

Research the hospital: There are several sources available to get information on hospitals. For example, you can search the Hospital Locator, a database of more than 1,400 cancer hospitals that meet the guidelines and reporting standards of the American College of Surgeons' Commission at www.web.facs.org. You can investigate the performance of your local hospital and other healthcare facility with information from the Joint Commission on Accreditation of Healthcare Organizations at www.jcaho.org or www.qualitycheck.org. The Association of Community Cancer Centers website provides basic information about the cancer programs at their more than 500 member institutions at www.accc-cancer.org/cancer/cancen_cplocator.asp. The institutions designated by the National Cancer Center as comprehensive cancer centers or clinical cancer centers are usually solid choices!

We generally prefer large teaching hospitals to local community hospitals and we limit exposure to poking and prodding by medical students and interns by specific instruction. Although size can have pitfalls, some estimates suggest hospital death rates are in the range of 40% higher at hospitals with less than 100 beds than at those in larger hospitals. This may, in part, be a function of greater hospital capabilities or of doctors treating more patients with a specific illness at larger facilities.

There are various publications and groups that rate hospitals. For example, US News & World Report ranks hospitals. Here are the best 10 cancer hospitals overall according to its 2020 report: University of Texas M.D. Anderson Cancer Center (Houston); Northwestern Memorial (Chicago); Memorial Sloan-Kettering Cancer Center (New York); Johns Hopkins Hospital (Baltimore); Mayo Clinic (Rochester, MN); Dana-Farber Cancer Institute (Boston); Cedars Sinai (Los Angeles); Cleveland Clinic (Cleveland); University of Washington Medical Center (Seattle). https://health.usnews.com/best-hospitals/rankings/cancer. These are overall rankings and you should be more interested in the rankings with respect to your type of cancer and treatment.

You have to consider the organization, the rating methodology, and the particular types of cancer and treatments rated. Unquestionably, the above hospitals are outstanding institutions. There are a lot of other fine institutions. Through the National Cancer Institute's Cancer Centers Program, which was created as part of the National Cancer Act of 1971, NCI recognizes cancer centers around the country that meet rigorous standards for transdisciplinary, state-of-the-art research focused on developing new and better approaches to preventing, diagnosing, and treating cancer. Currently, there are 51 Comprehensive Cancer Centers. As previously stated, these institutions generally are excellent choices. You can locate these centers on the NCI website at: https://www.cancer.gov/research/infrastructure/cancer-centers/find.

Select a hospital experienced with the procedure that you are undergoing: When possible, select a hospital experienced in the procedure you are undergoing and investigate their success rate and rate of complications.

Get in and get out: Whatever hospital you ultimately select, you should enter the hospital with the most positive attitude that you can muster, have loved ones present to look out for you, get the treatment that you need, recover sufficiently, and then get the hell out of the hospital as soon as possible. The hospital is dangerous even for people with fully functioning immune systems. They are particularly risky places for patients with compromised immune systems and many patients fall into this category, particularly when undergoing treatment for cancer.

Get a private room: In some hospitals, this may not be possible, but in many hospitals it is possible and the cost difference generally is only a few dollars a day. You will be more comfortable, not subject to catching infections from roommates, better able to communicate with family, and able to watch the television channel of your choice without interference. You will only be disturbed when doctors and staff come to attend to you and not when they seek to torment your roommate. Rest is very important for recovery and healing and hospitals often are very difficult places to get large chunks of uninterrupted sleep.

Avoid weekends and holidays: Like most other places, senior people and top performers have preferences on scheduling. Intuitively and statistically, you are better off to have procedures done on weekdays rather than weekends or holidays. You cannot always pick the time, but when you can, select the periods when the best, most experienced staff are on duty.

Be a germaphobe: Simply stated, hospital-borne infections are a major concern. A few years ago the CDC reported that one out of twenty-five United States hospital patients will get one. Some studies show higher numbers. These infections are prevalent, dangerous, and every precaution must be taken to avoid them. Some are antibiotic resistant. Germs are opportunists, they pick on people when their immune systems are low, and they look for any opening and port of entry. Being on the lookout for germs is difficult since you cannot see them. As a cancer patient, there is a sign on your head saying "germs, come and get me."

Cleanliness is next to Godliness: To the extent possible, wash your hands, avoid eye, ear, and nose contact with anything, keep any sores or skin breaks clean and covered. Insist that those who visit you do the same. Also, insist that doctors and every staff member who touches you or touches anything that touches you washes thoroughly (not just a quick rinse), wears gloves (and, where appropriate, masks and other protective gear). Make sure that everything that penetrates you is sterilized. This means making sure ports, needles, and catheters are cleaned, changed, and sterilized. Do not assume that doctors and staff wash enough or scrub thoroughly. They may get annoyed, but ask them kindly to wash their hands, use another needle, and so forth. The previously-referenced msn.com article reported that one study showed doctors only washed their hands 44% of the time if nobody was looking and 61% of the time if they knew they were being watched. Regardless of how accurate these numbers are, doctors sometimes fail to wash their hands and, by our observations, we suspect the number is higher for other hospital personnel that come in connect with patients. Another habit of healthcare providers is to wash their hands or put on gloves and then make contact with contaminated objects, so you must watch what they do between the time they scrub or put on gloves and touch you. Hopefully, the COVID-19 pandemic has caused an improvement among doctors, heath care providers and the population as a whole that will be sustained. Remembering to wash your hands constantly is not always easy even for those in the habit of doing so. This means to remind the healthcare providers in a pleasant way to scrub. Make sure your guests adhere to the same standards and avoid having people who have or may have an infection visit you.

Know your treatment plan and procedures: Know your treatments plan, the procedures that you are there for and, if there are any inconsistencies or deviations, insist on a prompt and thorough explanation. If you do not get a satisfactory answer, ask someone else.

Be a stickler for proper identification: Make sure the doctors and staff refer to you by name, look at the label on the drug itself, and make sure things are properly labeled. Patient, record, drug, and procedure mix-ups are a major problem. The HIPPA privacy regulations have only exasperated this problem. You do not want to take the wrong medicine or dosage or have something you want to keep amputated.

Obtain and review test results: Make sure that you get test results in a timely manner. Review the results yourself or have your advocate do it. This is a way to make sure that you have the correct results and that you know the results. To the extent possible, review your hospital records routinely and contemporaneously. They are your records and contain your information. Some hospitals and nurses are more forthcoming than others. Do not assume that all of the healthcare professionals and staff have properly documented things, have fully read and comprehended what is in the records, or even that the records are complete or relate to the right patient. Having the staff aware that you are reviewing records keeps them on their toes. Reviewing your medical records will alert you to issues and provide information that you may not otherwise receive and will afford you the opportunity to ask questions and correct misinformation. Request, review, and ask questions.

Sometimes you have to fire a heath care provider from your team: If you don't feel that a doctor or staff member is competent, caring, or providing the proper care, politely but firmly remove them from your healthcare team. Do not allow yourself to be a human guinea pig or a practice field.

Have an advocate present at all possible times: A good advocate is more than someone who cares about the patient. He or she is someone who will learn the treatment plan, ask questions, double check, and speak up. The mere fact that doctors and staff know that someone is around observing and is present to advocate for the patient provides some level of protection in and of itself. The point is not to have an adversarial relationship with health care providers, but to help them render outstanding care by alerting them to patient needs, patient conditions, and to things needed to avoid error.

Take notes and ask questions: It is helpful to have a notebook of questions and to take notes. Make sure that all of your questions are answered to your satisfaction and in terms that you understand. Do not be afraid to repeat questions, ask follow-up questions, and press for answers. We have included space in Appendix "G" to write down questions, answers, and record other important information.

Understand the medications you take and will receive: Know the medication, names, and dosages of your medications as well as the reasons you are taking them. Know their potential side effects and drug interactions. You should double check to be sure that you are being given the correct medications, in the correct dosages, and at the proper intervals. The *Physician's Desk Reference* is a standard source of reliable information and there is a corresponding website as well.

Confirm all details and procedures: Make sure that any part of your body that is being operated on is marked. Make sure that you know who will be doing the operating and speak directly with the surgeon before surgery. To the extent possible, you or your advocate must confirm every possible detail.

Bring comfortable clothing for your hospital stay (such as sweats and slippers): Except when undergoing tests or procedures, you should not be forced to parade around in those stupid robes that serve only to provide free shows and pathways for infection and germs. Bring comfortable and protective clothing.

Bring lists: Depending upon the length of your stay, you will be asked between 5 and 1,000 times what medications you are taking, what your medical conditions and history are, what you are allergic to, and what insurance you have. This will happen whether you pre-register, post-register, or announce it on national television. Bring multiple copies of a list containing medications (type, dose, and times of day taken), medical history, medical procedures, food allergies, dietary limitations, and insurance information. Have one copy placed in your medical records (even though it might get lost) so that inquiring minds can find it, and have one that you can show to people as they ask you the questions. This will make it easier on you and make it more likely the information is accurately provided and recorded. Also, have a contact list for the benefit of the hospital and for your benefit. There may be times when you are experiencing pain or discomfort or when you are medicated and may not recall the phone number you need. Appendix "G" is the patient medical information notebook and it provides a useful way to record and retain medical information. Appendix "I" is a place to keep contact information.

Inform the hospital of any allergies or special conditions: Make sure you inform hospital staff and doctors of any allergies to medicine, any prior adverse reactions, and any other allergies or specific conditions or needs that you have.

Bring medical and personal care items that you need: We learned the hard way that the hospital may not have the medical items you need. If you wear contacts, bring your glasses because at some point they will find a reason to make you take your contacts out. Bring the items you need. There are some personal items and comfort items you can bring and use. Be sure that your treating physician knows so that you are not taking or doing something deleterious to your health. You would be surprised at the poor quality of toilet paper at some hospitals. The last thing you need is scratchy toilet paper. Ask about any limitations on the use of these items in advance.

What not to bring: Ladies should remove nail polish. Hospitals generally will ask you to remove it so that health care providers can check your blood circulation. Leave jewelry and other valuables at home. There are people in and out all of the time and you may be moving around. You do not need the burden of looking after valuable items that may be lost or stolen.

Have a cell phone with you: We have been told many times by doctors that the notion that cell phones interfere with medical equipment and procedures is utter nonsense. Many hospitals used to limit cell phone use. Now, however, almost all hospitals allow cell phones. You need to have ready access to the outside world. Make sure that you have your cell phone, charger, and related equipment.

Repeat and remind: When possible, put instructions and requests in writing so that they make it into your medical records. Regardless of whether your requests, needs, and wishes are provided orally or in writing, you will need to repeat and remind personnel and check to ensure instructions have carried out.

Have a screening procedure in place: We all need to know our family and friends care. Hospitalizations can be lonely and scary. We would be devastated if family and friends abandoned us while we were in the hospital. Yet, make sure that people who are sick or may be battling a cold, virus, or infection stay home. Their presence—best intentions aside—can be harmful to you and other patients. Also, there are times you may need rest or do not have the mental or physical energy to talk on the phone. Always thank people for caring and calling, but have a screening procedure in place whether it is taking the phone off the hook or assigning someone to act as your receptionist. There were times after the surgery in the hospital and at home while recovering from surgery or in the middle of chemotherapy when Scott did not have the desire to talk or the energy to repeat the bad or good news of the day or go over his history. Charlene took command of the phone and would tell people Scott's diagnosis, condition, prognosis, and inform people of developments. If Scott was up to it (which he generally was), he would get on the phone for a couple of minutes to talk to people so that they could connect. Scott could tell them he was alright and could extract some direct sympathy and energy. There are also websites that enable people to connect, communicate, and get updated information. One such site is www.caringbridge.org. This site allows you or your advocate to post information, maintain a diary, and allows people password access to stay updated on your condition and communicate with you.

Be careful about social media posts: Many people now post information about hospitalizations and medical conditions on social media. This information can be used by bad actors to take advantage of people and even target people for crime. Information about medical conditions can be used against people in a variety of ways. In the past, many people resented learning about major health conditions of friends and family via social media, but such postings appear to be the new norm. Also be respectful of privacy when posting information about the health of others.

Don't eat the hospital food: If you like or can hold down the hospital food, you may be more sick than you thought. Many times, you may not feel like eating because you are too sick or can only manage to eat a little. In such circumstances, you may be able to survive on ice cubes, Jell-O, and popsicles. If you have an appetite, but do not like the food at the hospital, within the confines of what the doctors allow you to eat, consider having something delivered to the hospital or have someone cater to your appetite and culinary needs by bringing you the food items you like or think you may be able to keep down. We are not saying ignore the diet requirements, we are saying that traditionally the words "hospital" and "food" rarely belonged together. We must point out that many hospitals have improved their food and menus considerably in recent years. The couple of times when Scott felt he could eat something from the outside world and the nurse objected, we asked the doctor if he preferred that we order in or that Scott eat nothing—the answer was to order food.

Be courteous, respectful, and appreciative: Many healthcare professionals work hard, genuinely care about patients, and deliver outstanding service. Remember to compliment, thank, and show genuine appreciation when warranted. Be respectful of health care personnel, their time, and the realities that they are confronting. It may be difficult to remember sometimes, particularly when you are sick, scared, or tired, but it is important to act professionally and respectfully as a patient and advocate. Make sure that you give credit where credit is due and thank people for their efforts.

Obtain and understand discharge instructions: Most people who leave the hospital are so glad to get out of there that they do not pay adequate attention to the discharge questions. Many of the rest are too sick, flustered, or incoherent to think of, much less obtain, all of the information needed. Keep a running list of questions. You need to know about the prescription and non-prescription medications you will be taking, care for incisions, dressing, ports, and surgery sites, activities you should do and limitations on activities, likely side effects and what to do about them, symptoms and signs that require prompt attention, follow-up physician appointments, how to contact your doctor in the event of an emergency. Go to the emergency room may be a correct response, but usually there should be an alternative to reach your doctor or his office directly. Sometimes arrangements may be needed for in-home care or other medical services.

Let people know what they can do to help: One of the polite and proper things to say to cancer patients or hospital patients is, "let me know if there is anything I can do to help." One of the common responses is "no" or "thanks, but just knowing that you care means so much to me." Such responses are appropriate when you actually do not need help. But if you do need help, take people up on these invitations and request help.

Here are a few suggestions as to how people may help. Even if you have a caregiver, advocate, or multiple family members there for you, sometimes they could use a break. Consider asking people to: drive or accompany you to doctor appointments or chemotherapy or radiation sessions; help out while you are at the hospital; take care of some chores or errands, such as getting groceries, medicines, laundry, or medical supplies; make preparations for your return home; spend some time in the hospital to spell other friends and family members; allow you to unburden yourself by listening or advising you on issues for which you are not getting adequate feedback or advice from family members; and the old taboo of asking for financial assistance.

For those of you who really want to help someone with cancer, keep in mind that the "anything I can do" offer is often difficult for the patient to tackle. Think about what the patient needs or could benefit from and make specific offers or volunteer for specific things.

Follow cogent medical advice: We have focused on asking questions and being active in your care. Make sure you are comfortable with the medical advice you are receiving. However, it is critically important to follow cogent medical advice. Many patients suffer as a result of failing to follow their health care team's orders and recommendations. If you have questions or think the recommendations need modification, discuss the matter with your health care team.

Follow cogent medical advice: This message is worth repeating, so we repeat it. Having the best doctors and getting the best medical advice does little good if you do not listen to the doctor's directives.

CHAPTER 17

YOUR SURVIVAL RATE, PROPERLY ADJUSTED, MAY BE 100 PERCENT (AN ILLUMINATING APPROACH TO CONQUERING CANCER).

As a cancer patient or someone who loves one, you want to know: what type of cancer it is; what are the treatment options (benefits and risks); are you in capable hands in terms of physicians and treatment centers; and what impact will this disease have on your life. We are told that some patients want to know about prognosis and others do not. Our approach always has been that we want to know prognosis, survival rates, and statistics and we routinely asked these questions. To us, inquiring minds want to know about their future and want to be able to weigh treatment options cogently. We want to know exactly what we are dealing with and how to defeat it. We understand that other patients may not want to know and their wishes should be honored.

Often doctors will not volunteer this information and you have to press them for the information. At the other extreme are those doctors who do not convey this information in an accurate or sufficiently positive tone. It seems that some doctors take pleasure in conveying bad news. Usually, it is simply a failure to appreciate the message from the perspective of the patient. Others think they are invincible in terms of their predictions.

Many doctors do not understand or have forgotten the fundamental importance of "hope" and the power of positive thinking. A doctor who cannot provide hope, optimism, and inspiration to a cancer patient should retire, no matter how experienced or technically sound the doctor claims to be. Similarly, a patient under the care of such a physician should find another doctor quickly. Cancer patients already are riddled with fear, doubts, and apprehension. They need to receive good medical care and an approach that is nurturing.

Everyone talks about the importance of the patient and advocate staying positive. The doctors and healthcare providers must also provide a genuine environment of hope and positive thinking. Hope and positive thinking are not the same as denial and are not at odds with reality or objective facts of cancer. They should be an important element of that reality in the treatment environment. Let's know exactly what we are dealing with and then come up with a positive plan for remedying the situation and conquering cancer.

Survival rates: At the outset, let's make sure that we are on the same page with respect to survival and survival rates. Cancer survival rates tell us the percentage of people who survive a certain type of cancer for a specific amount of time. Cancer statistics often use a five-year survival rate. Sometimes ten-year rates are used, but five-year survival rates, by far, are the most commonly used figures. For example, if the five-year survival rate for non-Hodgkin lymphoma is 70 percent. For every 100 people diagnosed with non-Hodgkin lymphoma, 70 survive for at least five years after diagnosis. Conversely, 30 people out of the 100 with non-Hodgkin lymphoma will die within five years. By now you know that there are dozens of forms of non-Hodgkin lymphoma and the survival rates vary considerably so more probing is required.

An overall survival rate includes people of all ages and health conditions diagnosed with that type of cancer, including those diagnosed very early and those diagnosed late. Overall survival rates do not specify whether cancer survivors still are undergoing treatment at five years or whether they are cancer free (achieved remission) at some point. Disease-free survival rate reflects the number of people who achieve remission. This means they no longer have signs of cancer in their bodies. Progression-free survival rate is the number of people who still have cancer, but their disease is not progressing.

You are considered a survivor from the day that you are diagnosed with cancer, not the date on which your active treatment is complete. So the doctor may correctly (although not appropriately) say, "congratulations, you are a cancer survivor" at the moment you are diagnosed. Reaching the five-year survival period does not mean that a person is cured. Many forms of cancer can recur after five or even ten years. For other types of cancer, recurrence is overwhelmingly likely to happen within five years and being a five-year survivor may be tantamount to being cured. As a general matter, the longer you go without a recurrence, the less likely you are to have a recurrence.

A couple of important lessons can be learned from the 1960's *2,000-Year Old Man* comedy albums of Mel Brooks and Carl Reiner. Reiner, as the straight man, interviewed Brooks who started out in the first record being 2,000 years old. In one album, when asked by Carl Reiner how he lived so long, the 2,000 year old man responded, "will to live." Carl Reiner follows up with something along the lines of, "ah the will to live." To which the 2,000 year old man retorted, "no, Doctor William Tolive."

Where there is life, there is hope. It used to be that, if a cancer patient lived two or three more years, they lived two or three more years. But with cancer research and breakthroughs, living another year or two or three could mean discovery of another treatment that will extend life or actually cure the disease.

The second lesson involves Mel Brooks, as the 2,000 year old man, speaking of life in the cave and about the biggest, toughest caveman who the others worshiped. His name, of course, was "Phil." One day "Phil" was struck dead by a bolt of lightning and the others recognized that, "there's something bigger than Phil!" You probably could fill up every professional sports stadium in the country with people who have survived cancer years after their doctors advised them "to get their affairs in order" and still have more survivors standing in line for seats. It is a common event that people whose doctors predicted would be dead live significantly longer or beat cancer altogether. With all due respect to doctors and modern medicine, you should not follow your doctor's orders or expectation to die. Crush these orders or expectations and continue to live. Please re-read this paragraph because the point bears repeating! When doctors tell patients that they consider terminally ill "how long they have," they are guessing. It may be an educated guess, but it is a guess. There are ranges for survival even for forms of advanced cancer. Although one famous cancer patient was told he had only months to live after being diagnosed with mesothelioma, he lived 20 years and died from something else. There is no cancer that has a survival rate of zero. Where there is life, there is hope. Don't let any doctor ever take away your hope.

We recall asking an accomplished heart surgeon questions regarding survival rates before Mary had a heart valve replaced with a porcine (pig) valve. The surgeon's response was that, for the individual patient, survival rates are meaningless. The answer is either 100% or zero. He then discussed the procedure he was going to do, the risks, the alternatives (including doing nothing), and the benefits. He said there are no guarantees, but he was entirely confident that Mary would survive the surgery and do well with her new value. He did not directly answer the question, but he provided us with the information and confidence we needed. All Mary needed was for us to tell her that she would be fine.

Nonetheless, it is important that people put this information in proper context, understand those things that will increase their own survival rate, which the surgeon correctly pointed out is either zero or 100%, and adopt the warrior attitude and approach that their survival rate is 100%. Believing that you will beat the disease can make it so.

Another helpful approach is to use the survival rate, whatever it is, as the baseline and make the appropriate upward adjustments based upon existing circumstances and circumstances that you can control. Survival rates include elderly patients, patients with other conditions and diseases, ignorant people without medical knowledge who do not take an active role in their care, people without caring families, people who die from infections and side effects, people who never get any medical care or get improper care, and people who lack the will to live. Accordingly, as a cancer patient, you should take steps to increase your chances of survival and adjust the survival percentages to reflect credits to which you are entitled as a matter of science and common sense. Just as one school of medicine looks at "real age" as opposed to biological age, we recommend looking at your "real survival rate."

Will to live: One of the most important determinants of beating cancer is "the will to live." Sure, it may be accompanied by a positive attitude. But it also may be accompanied by meanness, stubbornness, defiance, outrage, and anger. Whatever qualities you need to exhibit, make sure to muster, draw upon, fill up with, emit, and ooze the "will to live." Those that do should increase their survival rate by double digits.

Family and loved ones: Studies show that people with family, friends, and loved ones around them do considerably better than those who do not have such support. We suspect the reasons are multi-fold. These people have reasons to live and people to live for, reasons not to die, advocates and advisors by their side, and bubbles of love, care, and attention. Cancer patients should draw upon those that love and care for them during these times. People should go out of their way to befriend and genuinely care about a cancer patient. Do not let someone battle this disease and go through the treatments alone, no matter how strong or independent they appear. To the extent possible, keep people who annoy or aggravate you completely out of the picture. Lose any vexations to the spirit. Add some points for having loved ones around.

Draw on your faith or acquire some: We are not here to push any particular religion, but numerous studies show the medical benefits of religion and faith. People of faith do better on average than those without faith. Pray and then add points for faith to your survival rate.

Be a knowledgeable patient that is active in your own care and decision-making or have an advocate that fills this role: You will select the optimum treatment, and reduce the chances of being victimized by neglect, inattention, malpractice, and misfeasance. Add points to your survival rate.

Practice cleanliness and germaphobia: Many cancer patients succumb to the side effects of treatment or infections. Make sure you are not one of them. Wash frequently, carry antibiotic wipes, and avoid airplanes and sick people. Mask up where and when appropriate. Add some more points to your survival rate.

Secure the best doctors, treatments, and treatment facilities you can: For obvious reasons, do these things and add points to your survival rate.

Insurance: Maintain insurance or other provisions to allow you access to proper healthcare. The survival rates include people without insurance and with bad insurance. The better your insurance and ability to obtain optimal treatment, the more points you should add to your survival rate.

Youth and general good health: Add points if you are in good general health or if you are reasonably young. Survival rates include the elderly and ill. These factors can limit available treatments and adversely impact the patient's ability to withstand the rigors of treatment.

Proper diet and exercise: Not only can proper diet and exercise prevent some cancers, proper diet and exercise after diagnosis can improve health and survival in many cases. Add points for proper diet and exercise. Survival rates include people in poor shape and with poor dietary habits. If your habits need improvement, the diagnosis of cancer is a good time to improve your dietary and exercise habits.

Medical improvements: Over time, cancer treatments improve, new treatments are developed, and there are better therapies to treat, minimize, and eliminate side effects. Survival rates are based upon historic numbers and do not reflect recent advances in medicine. Because we believe that medicine is improving and there are important developments, the survival rate should be adjusted in an upper direction to account for this factor. As previously discussed, the pace of cancer research and developments has picked up considerable in recent years due in part to the Human Genome Project.

Offset the pessimistic aspects of medicine: Most professionals have strong egos. As a former corporate executive and as a lawyer, we have egos. Doctors have egos and enjoy hero potential. The lower the survival rate or worse the prognosis, the more likely the doctor is to emerge as a hero when you do survive. Additionally, doctors generally are not fans of lawyers. We know it is difficult to believe, but there are factions of society that are not fond of lawyers. Doctors want to avoid malpractice suits and nothing invites a suit more than a family displeased that their loved one with a readily curable form of cancer (let's say with a 95% survival rate) died at the hands of a doctor. Sarcasm aside, we believe that survival rates often are understated and points should be added to your survival rate to offset this bias. Unfortunately, some people do have cancers with poor survival rates. Even then, it is important to remember that there is no type of cancer with a survival rate of zero. Bearing all of these things in mind, we hope that you can see and believe that you will defeat cancer. The cancer warrior will make the appropriate adjustment to even an otherwise poor prognosis. This makes an important difference and further demonstrates that you will beat cancer. The forgoing discussion also helps to refocus you on the things that you can control and steps that you can take to help yourself.

CHAPTER 18

CANCER DIAGNOSES AND STAGING, UNDERSTANDING TESTS, AND OBTAINING SECOND OPINIONS (THE IMPORTANCE OF A PROMPT AND PROPER DIAGNOSIS)

Everyone by now should understand the importance of a prompt and proper diagnosis. Often the earlier cancer is diagnosed, the better the chances of survival. Sometimes an early diagnosis can result in a treatment that is less invasive or less toxic than that required for later stage disease. Early diagnosis, however, is more important for some types of cancer than others. There are some indolent forms of cancer where, even after being diagnosed, the treatment is simply "watch and wait." Some forms of cancer are difficult to diagnosis early because the symptoms do not present themselves until the disease is advanced. Sometimes cancer is discovered fortuitously in the course of routine or annual physical examination, routine testing, or testing for something else. Timing of diagnosis generally is important. You usually can help yourself immeasurably by going to the doctor promptly if symptoms are experienced. Still, there are many forms of cancer that can be treated effectively even at a more advanced stage.

Knowing one's body is important. People often know when something is wrong and those who pursue the cause diligently may save their lives. Many times people go to the doctor with complaints of pain or abnormality only to have those complaints dismissed by the doctor. We cannot tell you how many times we have heard stories about people going undiagnosed for months or years after they brought relevant complaints to the attention of their doctors only to have the complaints dismissed or attributed to something other than the cancer that existed. This points out the importance of not only bringing complaints and conditions to the attention of your doctor, but also pursuing things further with that doctor or with another doctor until you are satisfied. The patient errors of late complaints and dismissal of complaints without pursuit of medical attention can be costly. The doctor's failure to timely diagnose cancer also can be costly.

There are several warning signs commonly associated with various cancers that patients and doctors should consider. We discussed common symptoms associated with blood cancer previously. Speaking more generally about potential signs or symptoms of cancers, they may include: unusual bleeding or discharge; a lump that persists; skin that is itchy, red, scaly, dimpled, or puckered; a sore that does not heal within a couple of weeks; change in bladder or bowel habits; trouble urinating or pain when urinating; blood in the urine; bleeding or bruising for no known reason; blood in the stools; persistent cough or hoarseness; pain after eating such as heartburn or indigestion that does not reside; difficulty swallowing; belly pain; change in appetite; change in a mole; a cold or flu that persists; an infection that does not go away; a swollen lymph node not associated with pain or a cold; white or red patch on the tongue or in the mouth; headaches; vision changes; hearing changes; seizures; unexplained fever; severe or lasting fatigue; or night-sweats. There are many other possible signs. Importantly, having any of these signs does not necessarily mean you have cancer. There are be a variety of other causes for each of these signs.

What is needed is not simply a prompt diagnosis, but a prompt and accurate diagnosis. A prompt, inaccurate diagnosis may have some benefit in treating symptoms. If the cause of the symptoms is cancer, the prompt, inaccurate diagnosis can be disastrous even if some symptoms are treated. Usually the best chance to cure cancer is the first time you treat it.

There may be some circumstances in which part of the blame for an improper diagnosis lies with the patient. By being an accurate historian (relating the conditions, complaints, and symptoms accurately), you can increase the likelihood of a prompt and proper diagnosis. Be accurate and be sure to not leave out or understate your symptoms.

In the final analysis, the responsibility of an accurate diagnosis generally lies squarely at the doorsteps of the doctor and medical providers. This is of little assistance to the health and well-being of the misdiagnosed patient, so once again a burden falls upon the patient and advocate to make sure that the diagnosis is proper. We realize that the patient does not have the skill, knowledge, or expertise to diagnose medical conditions. We do not encourage patients to self-diagnose. As with other issues, the patient can read, go online, consider whether the diagnosis matches the symptoms, consider whether the correct tests are being conducted, ask questions and press the doctor and, if appropriate, go to another doctor.

Some of the major issues regarding diagnosis are whether the appropriate tests have been taken to diagnose the condition completely and accurately, whether the tests have been taken properly, and whether they were analyzed and interpreted properly. In the current climate, doctors are under considerable pressure and scrutiny by insurers with respect to testing and often are forced to endure questions, challenges, and non-payment for tests. Against this background, we provide some information regarding some of the testing to make a diagnosis of cancer or to rule out the diagnosis of cancer. We provide an overview of some of the common tests for background and so that you can ask your doctors appropriate questions to ensure you are properly diagnosed.

The National Comprehensive Cancer Network is a not-for-profit alliance of 21 of the world's leading cancer centers and sets guidelines for oncology practice in the United States. This is a great resource to see not only recommended treatment options, but also the testing and work-up recommended for diagnosing and staging various types of cancer. http://www.nccn.org. Let's discuss some diagnostic tests and tools.

It is worth repeating that, in this age of personalized or precision medicine, with greater frequency the unique molecular and genetic components of an individual's cancer can be identified and sometimes may be tested against potential treatments to determine the impact and response to particular treatments. In other words, more precise data may result in more effective treatment. It is important to note that diagnosis is not always a one-time event. A person's cancer may evolve over time and may evolve due to the impact of treatment.

Physical examination: Physical examination and clinical findings are important components of a diagnosis. Observation, palpation of masses, tumors, and lymph nodes and numerous other aspects of the physical examination form parts of the diagnostic picture.

Medical, work, family, and exposure histories: Medical history, work history, family health history, and history of exposures to potential carcinogens also are considered in rendering a proper and complete diagnosis. Sometimes they play an important role. Mesothelioma and asbestos exposure, for example, are closely linked, as are lung cancer and smoking.

Ultrasound: Ultrasound tests use high frequency sound waves to measure tissue density. Many types of cancer will show up with an ultrasound as an area of uneven density, often higher density tissue. There are some limitations to ultrasounds, including the inability to view the interior of bony structures and the waves being blocked by bone. Because the waves are not able to pass through air, ultrasound tests are not good at evaluating the digestive system. The clarity of an ultrasound attenuates as it passes through tissue, so ultrasound generally will not be useful for imaging deep within the body. The advantages to ultrasound are that such imaging does not harm tissue, and it is fast, inexpensive, and non-invasive. The technician basically waves a wand over the areas being tested.

X-Rays: X-rays use a form of ionizing radiation to generate two-dimensional images. They are very effective in imaging bone and dense tissue, but are not effective at imaging soft tissue. Sometimes the patient is given contrast (orally or intravenously) to make it easier to discern soft tissue. A mammogram is a form of x-ray used to look for signs of breast cancer. A limitation of x-rays is that the two dimensional nature of the images can produce false positives when an area of diffuse or stacked densities causes the appearance of "heaviness" in one section of the x-ray image. This is why technicians often take two images, one from the front and one from the side. X-rays are not accurate in distinguishing anomalies in dense tissue. X-rays are fast, relatively inexpensive, and easy to administer.

CT Scans: Computer tomography tests or CT scans take many more images than an x-ray in a precise and controlled fashion that permits the reconstruction of a 3-dimensional image. CT scans often are taken in "slices." The patient may be given oral and intravenous contrasts to enhance the imaging of soft tissue. Conventional CT scans take more time than an x-ray and require the patient to be somewhat immobilized during the scan. If the chest is being imaged, the patient may be told to hold his or her breath. Alignment problems between slices can sometimes result in missing a small mass that lies between slices. A conventional CT scan generally has a slice thickness of 8 mm to 10 mm. Higher resolution CT scans are quicker. Instead of scanning each slice with the patient bed stationary, the bed is moving continuously as the CT scanner scans around the body. It has a much higher resolution than conventional CT scans. A

HRCT scan has a slice thickness of 1 mm to 1.3 mm. At higher resolutions, more anomalies can be seen, but a much greater number of them turn out to be false positives. A limitation of CT scanning in general is an inability to view very fine details in soft tissue such as muscles or ligaments. Patient motion during a CT scan can cause the images to be blurry. Also, any metal in the body can cause streaks in the image. Scar tissue may also show up on a CT scan. CT scanning is slower and more expensive than x-rays and ultrasounds. The radiation exposure from a whole-body CT scan is approximately 100 times that of a chest x-ray. Modern machines are less confining (or closed) than the older machines used to be.

PET Scans: A positron emission tomography or PET scan uses an internal source of radiation (as opposed to use of an external source of radiation in a CT scan). About 45 minutes to two hours before the scan, the patient is injected with a form of radioactive sugar. After the sugar has had a chance to be absorbed by the body, the patient will be scanned in five to seven sections. Because the amount of radiation is very low, the PET scanner needs to focus on each section of the body for several minutes. The patient must not move during this time-period, and may be strapped in tightly. Hot spots on the PET scan show areas of metabolic activity. This can be useful in distinguishing active cancer from fibrotic (scar) tissue. False positives, however, can occur due to inflammatory lesions from recent surgery or chemotherapy. The patient cannot eat before the test and generally should not take any diabetic or glucose control medication before a PET scan.

Since PET scans and CT scans use similar equipment, it is possible to integrate them into a single PET-CT scanner. A PET-CT scan can yield more information than either scan on its own. PET scans may not be effective for identifying tumors that have a low metabolic rate, such as carcinoid tumors, mucinous cancers (such as ovarian cancer), and low-grade tumors (such as some lung cancers). PET scans are particularly useful in imaging the lungs and in measuring response to treatment for some cancers. Because of the length of time required to generate the image, patient movement and breathing can generate a blurry image. There is both a false positive and false negative rate to these scans as with other tests. The maximum resolution of a PET scan is 5 mm to 7 mm. As such, a PET scan is usually not used to identify smaller tumors.

MRI: A magnetic resonance imaging test or MRI uses strong magnetic fields to cause water molecules to resonate. It is very good at imaging soft tissue, such as the heart, lungs, liver, and other organs. An MRI cannot image calcifications and bone and cannot always distinguish between cancerous and non-cancerous anomalies. An MRI can image anomalies that are obscured by bone. Patients should notify the technician about any metal implants or foreign objects in their bodies.

Blood tests and tumor markers: Blood tests such as a CBC or complete blood count determine the number of red blood cells, white blood cells, and platelets and can be of diagnostic significance.

A tumor marker test detects chemicals produced by tumor cells (or other cells of the body) in response to the cancer found in the body and reflected in the blood, urine, or tissue. Some tumor markers identify a specific cancer, while others are not as specific. Remember that most markers are not definitive. Some of the more common tumor markers are: Alphafetoprotein (AFP) (liver or germ cell cancer); Beta Human Chorionic Gonadotropin (HCG); Cancer Antigen (CA) 19-9 (colon, rectum, stomach, bile duct, and pancreas); Cancer Antigen (CA) 15-3 (breast, ovary, lung, and prostate); Cancer Antigen (CA) 27-29 (breast, colon, stomach, kidney, lung, ovary, pancreas, uterus, and liver); Cancer Antigen (CA) 125 (ovary, uterus, cervix, pancreas, liver, colon, lung, and digestive tract); Carcinoembryonic Antigen (CEA) (breast, lung, prostate, pancreas, stomach, cervix, bladder, kidney, thyroid, liver, melanoma, and lymphoma); Immunoglobulins; Lactic Dehydrogenase (LDH); and Prostate Specific Antigen (PSA). There are many others.

Immunophenotyping: Immunophenotyping is a process used to distinguish among different types of cells (such as distinguishing normal lymphocytes from lymphoma cells) based on the presence of antigens (proteins on the surface of certain cells). Antigens are specific to different cell types and may be recognized by a specific type of antibody that locks onto that particular antigen. There are multiple methods of immunophenotyping, including flow cytometry or immunohistochemistry. Antibodies for a particular antigen are chemically modified in a laboratory so that they either emit fluorescent light (flow cytometry) or show color (immunohistochemistry) when they attach to their corresponding antigens. These modified antibodies are then mixed with cells from the patient's body. If they light up or change color, that indicates that the cells being studied have the antigen on their surface. Cytogenetic analysis involves looking at chromosomes from lymphoma cells under a microscope to look for any abnormalities in structure or number. The results often help doctors determine the type and subtype of NHL. Sometimes both immunohistochemistry and flow cytometry are needed for accurate immunophenotyping.

Chromosome immunohistochemistry: IHC involves the pathologist examining the slides under a microscope to look for the visible color change that happens when the antibodies attach to the antigens. Abnormalities can contribute to the development of lymphoma either by damaging or removing genes that regulate lymphocyte growth, or by adding genes that fuel lymphocyte growth. Either of these changes can cause the lymphoma to grow uncontrollably. Some of the most common types of chromosome abnormalities that occur in lymphoma are: translocation (parts of two different chromosomes break off and switch places with each other); deletion (part of a chromosome is missing); trisomy (the cell contains an extra copy of an entire chromosome); and amplification (a portion of a chromosome is repeated one or many times).

Genetic tests: A variety of tests may be employed to provide genetic information to better understand the genetic abnormalities in a patient or the subtype of disease present. For example, fluorescence in situ hybridization (FISH) uses fluorescent markers to identify changes in the genetic sequence along a chromosome. DNA sequencing: identifies variation in the DNA that could contribute to disease RNA sequencing identifies expression levels of genes that can help identify abnormal patterns of expression that may contribute to disease. There are numerous other tests.

"Scopes" and other tests: Other tests such as urinalysis, fecal occult stool tests, and a variety of "scopies" or scopes in which an optimal instrument (such as endoscopies, bronchoscopies, colonoscopies, cystoscopies, or laparoscopies) is inserted in various locations for viewing and/or removal of tissues.

Bone marrow biopsies: Bone marrow biopsies are used to determine the extent of the disease and whether there are cancer cells in the bone marrow.

Biopsies and pathology: In the final analysis, the pathology generally determines the diagnosis of cancer and type of cancer. Pathologists view the cells from biopsy samples of tumors, surrounding tissue and lymph nodes or the masses and body parts surgically removed or removed by biopsy (excision, core needle, fine need aspirate or otherwise). The accuracy depends upon the accuracy of the pathologists' review of the cells provided. But obtaining a sufficient sample also is imperative. For example, if the sample is too small or does not include all relevant parts, the diagnosis may be inaccurate, incorrect, or incomplete, even if the pathologist correctly interprets the sample in front of him. Because the pathology is critical to the diagnosis, you should talk to your doctor in detail about the pathology report to make sure that he understands it and that you do. You also should have the biopsy examined by another pathologist.

The pathology report will tell you the gross description of the tumor (color, weight, etc.) and the microscopic description; the size of the tumor; tumor stage (involvement of lymph nodes); tumor margins (whether or not it was found in the edges of the removed tissue); and type of tumor. The biopsy of an enlarged lymph node is a common diagnostic procedure. Many times, the diagnosis under a microscope is clear cut. But not infrequently, the biopsied lymphoid tissues pose challenging diagnostic problems. To solve them requires the careful observation and recognition of histologic alterations combined with the selective use of the many technologies available in the modern laboratory.

Dr. John P. Leonard of Weill Cornell was quoted a few years ago in the *NY Times* saying "even experts have trouble agreeing on the specific subtype. To give you an idea: if I got the 10 best lymphoma pathologists in the world together and they reviewed the same cases, they would disagree maybe 5 to 20 percent of the time. It's not uncommon for patients to be referred to another specialist and find out that they have a different form of non-Hodgkin's lymphoma than what they thought they had. That's why it's so important to get a second opinion that includes an expert look at the pathology." We agree with Dr. Leonard that it is important for people diagnosed with blood cancer to have their biopsies reviewed or confirmed by a hematopathologist. Hematopathology is the branch of pathology studying diseases of hematopoietic cells, including blood cancers. Hematopathology is a board certified subspecialty.

There are many other tests and diagnostic tools, but we wanted to provide you with some of the most common tests. Before undergoing tests, you should ask your physician about the test, any risks and alternatives, and what the tests can and cannot determine.

Prognostic factors: The health care team must determine the patient's general health status (performance status or functional status) to see how well a patient feels, what treatments the patient can tolerate, and whether the treatment is working, Performance status (PS) is a numerical rating of patients' general health and their ability to carry out normal daily activities (such as getting washed and dressed, going to work, and doing chores). PS is graded on a scale of 0–4, with the lower numbers indicating better health. Grade 0 is a patient who is fully active and able to carry on all pre-disease activities without restriction.

Grade 1 is a patient who cannot perform taxing physical activities, but is ambulatory and able to carry out light work do things that can be done while seated. Grade 2 is a patient who can move around and take care of oneself, up and about for more than half of awake hour. Grade 3 is someone who can partially take care of his or herself, but is confined to a bed or chair for more than half of awake hours. Grade 4 is a patient who is completely disabled – requiring others to care for him or her and completely confined to a bed or chair. Favorable or good prognostic factors tend to be associated with better outcomes, while unfavorable prognostic factors tend to be associated with worse outcomes. It is important to understand prognostic factors, but not to be discourage or become complacent by them.

Various prognostic indices have been developed for different forms of lymphoma. The International Prognostic Index (IPI) was first developed for aggressive (fast-growing) lymphomas such as DLBCL. The IPI is based on five factors represented by the acronym APLES: age, performance status (PS), lactate dehydrogenase (LDH) level, number of extranodal sites, and stage.

First, age reflects the statistics that all other things being equal younger adults usually are better able to tolerate treatment and are less likely to have co-morbidities than older adults. Second, performance status discussed above is considered. Third, involves LDH. Lactate Dehydrogenase and Beta-2 Microglobulin tests often are performed. High blood levels of the protein lactate dehydrogenase (LDH) are associated with fast-growing lymphomas. LDH can also be abnormal due to conditions other than lymphoma, such as muscle damage, liver disease, or bone marrow disease. False positive results can occur where red blood cells are destroyed when blood is drawn and transported to the laboratory. The last two factors consider the number and locations of sites impacted by lymphoma and the stage at diagnosis.

The Follicular Lymphoma International Prognostic Index (FLIPI) is based on the original IPI but excludes PS and adds hemoglobin level as a risk factor. Other indices have been developed for mantle cell and marginal cell lymphoma. Beta-2 microglobulin ($\beta 2M$) is another molecule that may indicate a worse prognosis when its blood levels are elevated in NHL patients. Testing for Hepatitis Virus, HIV, and HTLV1 may be conducted because the presence of these viruses in the body may affect the type of treatments given.

Before beginning some types of treatment, the doctor may measure the patient's baseline heart function to make sure that the patient's body can withstand treatment. This is especially important because some treatments can occasionally make heart function worse. Depending on the treatment used, the patient's heart function may be evaluated again during treatment to make sure the heart is tolerating the treatment.

Some treatments can put stress on the lungs. For this reason, the doctor may order pulmonary (lung) function tests (PFTs) before beginning treatment and again during treatment to make sure the patient's lungs are working properly

Review your test results: Although a patient may not be qualified to fully understand the test results, the significance of the results, or how the results fit into the entire picture (including symptoms, clinical findings, and other tests), we still think it is important for the patient or the advocate to review the results. We already have discussed the potential for mixing up patients and records. Asking for and reading the test results lets the doctors and staff know that you are involved in your treatment and may cause them to pay more attention in terms of obtaining the results in a timely manner and reviewing them more closely. Also, the results may cause you to ask questions and raise issues that otherwise may not be raised because the doctor did not pick up on something, was not aware of something that you or other doctors know, or does not disclose or discuss with you for any reason. In any event, it is another occasion for you to be active and informed in your mission of beating cancer.

Precise type of cancer: The first important component of the diagnosis of cancer is the type of cancer. Obviously, there are many varieties of cancer (lung, pancreatic, breast, etc.). Appendix "B" is a listing of cancer types. But many cancers have several forms. In the case of lymphoma, for example, it is not enough to know whether it is Hodgkin or non-Hodgkin, you must know what type it is (such as large, diffuse, B-cell non-Hodgkin or Mantle cell). The type can impact prognosis and treatment. Accordingly, it is important to know the exact type of cancer that impacts you. Precision is important. For many kinds of cancers the precise type of cancer is a moving target as additional research allows for further sub-dividing. It is also important to obtain proper analysis of any markers not only as an indicator of survival, but also because it could impact the treatment.

Staging: When cancer is diagnosed, the doctor generally must determine the stage or extent of the disease. The stage often impacts the patient's prognosis. Knowing a patient's stage also helps the surgeon, oncologist, or radiologist-oncologist make recommendations about the best course of treatment.

To determine the stage of a cancer, generally doctors look at the entire picture of the patient, including results from the physical exam, diagnostic tests including x-rays, ultrasound, biopsies, computerized tomography scans, magnetic resonance imaging, positron emission tomography, bone marrow tests, blood tests, and other tests combined to ascertain where the cancer is located, the size of the tumor or tumors, the areas and organs impacted, and whether the cancer has spread. Cancer staging applies to almost all solid tumors and to many blood cancers. Each type of cancer is staged according to specific characteristics.

There are a couple of cancer-staging systems that are commonly used. One is an overall stage grouping that uses Roman numerals and the other is the TNM system created by the American Joint Committee on Cancer.

Under the first system, stage I cancer is cancer that is diagnosed early and has not spread. "In situ" cancers are cancers that have been diagnosed at the earliest possible stage. Stage II cancer has spread into surrounding tissues, but not beyond the location of origin. Stage III cancer has spread to nearby lymph nodes. Stage IV cancers are cancers that have metastasized or spread to other parts of the body. The lower the stage, the better. But even many forms of cancer in stage IV can be treated successfully.

The TNM Staging System is based on characteristics of the tumor, lymph nodes, and metastasis. Each of these is categorized separately and classified with a number to give the total stage. The higher the number, the greater the degree of cancer involvement identified. "T" classifies the extent of the primary tumor, and is normally given as "T0" through "T4," with "T0" representing a tumor that has not even started to invade the local tissues ("in situ") to "T4" representing a large primary tumor that has probably invaded other organs. N classifies regional lymph node involvement. Regional lymph nodes are those draining the area around the primary tumor. "N0" means no lymph node involvement, while "N4" means extensive involvement. "M" is either "M0" if there are no metastases, or "M1" if there are metastases.

Second opinions: Because a prompt, accurate, and complete diagnosis is critical to correctly assessing the condition and treating the disease, a patient should almost always obtain a second opinion that encompasses the diagnosis, prognosis, treatment options, benefits and risks, and treatment recommendations. A second opinion that is predicated upon review of the medical and test reports alone is usually insufficient. It is better to have the other doctor and institution review the pathology, interpret the scans and tests, run critical blood work, conduct a thorough physical examination, and take a complete medical history. This way, your second opinion will not only reflect interpretations of the second doctor from the tests, but also will detect possible errors in the pathology, blood work, and imaging testing or reading. Providing the medical records and the other doctor's diagnosis and recommended plan has the advantage of providing information to the second doctor and eliminating duplication, but it also can influence the second opinion. We also believe it sometimes makes sense to select the doctor rendering the second opinion yourself (with input from other sources) as opposed to going to someone recommended by the first doctor.

Not only do we recommend obtaining a second opinion, the American Cancer Society and the American Society of Clinical Pathologists recommend a second opinion for every cancer diagnosis. The effort and expense necessary to obtain a consultation can be rewarded by the comfort of knowing that an original diagnosis was indeed correct. When a second opinion produces a different diagnosis or treatment recommendation, it provides options to the patient and may identify a misdiagnosis or incomplete diagnosis or produce a better treatment plan. Conversely, it may cast doubt upon the earlier diagnosis or treatment recommendations that were well-taken. As such, it may interject some uncertainty. Nonetheless, cancer presents too great a danger to not get a second opinion. Where there are conflicting opinions or recommendations or if you are not comfortable with the opinions that you have received, you may want to seek the opinion from yet another doctor. Most insurance plans cover second opinions, but check your plan out to make sure it is covered and to ensure that you comply with any requirements and obtain any necessary approvals.

Usually it is best to obtain a second opinion from a second institution to avoid bias and to have another team review your pathology, diagnosis, and treatment options. In selecting treatment options, consider any discipline bias that may exist. Physicians specializing in stem cell transplants, for example, may be more inclined to recommend a stem cell transplant. Make sure that you have explored your treatment options sufficiently before embarking upon treatment. Many patients have cancer that is a chronic condition. In view of the pace of developments, it is important to review options and obtain consultations periodically to ensure that you have up-to-date information.

Many medical institutions have tumor review boards and panels in which cases are presented to a group of doctors to obtain their input and thoughts regarding diagnosis, further work-up, and treatment.

Once you are confident in the diagnosis, you have to make determinations regarding what treatment or treatments to undergo.

CHAPTER 19

AN OVERVIEW OF CANCER TREATMENTS (SELECTING THE MOST EFFECTIVE TREATMENT FOR YOUR CANCER)

Obtaining the proper treatment for your cancer is critically important. There is no responsible way that we could attempt to make any recommendations as to what treatment or treatments you should undergo. It depends upon so many factors unique to you, including: the type of cancer you have; the stage of the cancer; your medical history; your general health and other conditions; predictive markers; the symptoms you are experiencing; your age; your preferences and those of family members and doctors whose input you value; other treatments available to you; side effects and your tolerance and ability to endure them; insurance and financial conditions; and so many other variables.

There also is no way that we can catalogue all of the potential treatments in this book and there are meaningful developments regarding treatment options and efficacy of treatments on a continuous basis. Appendix "C" contains a wealth of organizations, resources, and online sources from which you can obtain detailed and updated information on your type of cancer, available treatments, and clinical trials. Your health care team, of course, will be your primary source of information.

That being said, we have a few general opinions that we will offer. First, if there are treatments for your disease that have proven to be effective, you should seriously consider undergoing those treatments instead of undergoing unproven or experimental treatments. This seems to be obvious, yet many patients understandably are afraid of chemotherapy or radiation and may attempt to avoid these treatments in favor of treatments they believe to be less toxic. The same scenario presents itself when the patient is afraid of surgery. These fears and concerns are understandable. We all have them. But the consequences of failing to undergo treatments that have proven to be effective can be life threatening.

The experimental treatment may fail, may cause severe side effects, and you may wind up undergoing the traditional treatment anyway. Or worse, you may have lost the opportunity to undergo the traditional treatment at all or in time for it to be effective or to have the same chance of success. In considering treatments, you must find out the full range of options and what treatment opportunities may be lost as a result of the treatment you undergo. As we previously stated, treating cancer the first time around usually provides the best opportunity for eradicating the disease.

These days there are a variety of clinical trials that warrant serious consideration. However, where traditional treatments are not a satisfactory option and you cannot get into a clinical trial, you may consider alternative treatment, experimental treatment, or treatment available only in other states or countries. Hopefully, it will not be boiled wombat pee or black widow tablets. Fortunately, we did not have to go that route because effective conventional treatment was available. We have helped several patients get into clinical trials and treatments not available in their geographical area and can report some wonderful examples in which departure from standard regimens proved to be very successful. But careful, investigation is imperative.

Obviously, the likelihood of success of the treatment is an important consideration. However, other factors such as whether the treatment would limit or eliminate future treatment options should be considered.

There are several resources to obtain information on available treatments and clinical trials and to help you evaluate your options. Doctors, cancer patients, organizations, chat groups, and websites top the list. We thought it would be helpful to provide some information on some of the forms of treatment. Once again, more current and complete information on treatments for the various forms and stages of cancer can be found through the various organizations and resources listed in Appendix "C." As we have emphasized, it is important that the treatment plan be tailored to the individual patient and to his or her particular cancer.

The National Comprehensive Cancer Network is a not-for-profit alliance of 21 of the world's leading cancer centers and sets guidelines for oncology practice in the United States. Its guidelines for the diagnosis and treatment of cancer by site is a very useful resource. http://www.nccn.org. Below is a summary of the cancer treatment armamentarium. We have divided the array of treatments into three broad categories: conventional and current treatments; cutting edge treatments; and maintenance therapy and clinical trials. Keep in mind that, although some treatments that may be discussed under cutting edge treatments at the time of preparing this book, they may be conventional by the time you read this book. Indeed, many of these "newer" treatments already have a proven track record.

CONVENTIONAL AND CURRENT TREATMENTS

Conventional treatments are put forth as standard of care by the National Comprehensive Cancer Network (NCCN), an alliance of 31 leading cancer centers devoted to patient care. This alliance provides a consensus in the form of NCCN clinical practice guidelines, outlining standard of care treatments to provide the best patient outcome. Here are some of these conventional treatments.

Surgery: Surgery is the oldest form of cancer treatment. Often, surgery offers the greatest chance for cure of many types of cancer, particularly if the cancer is localized. Debulking surgery is done to remove some, but not all, of the tumor. It is done when removing the entire tumor would cause too much damage to an organ or nearby tissues. In such cases, the doctor may remove as much of the tumor as possible and then try to treat what is left with radiation therapy or chemotherapy. Supportive surgery is used to help with other types of treatment. For example, installing a vascular access device such as a catheter is supportive surgery. Reconstructive surgery also is common such as breast reconstruction after mastectomy or the use of tissue flaps, bone grafts, or prosthetic materials after surgery for oral cavity cancers. Surgery, in the form of biopsies, plays a key role in diagnosing cancer and cancer staging. Fine needle aspiration uses a very thin needle attached to a syringe to pull out a small amount of tissue from a tumor. Advances in surgical techniques have resulted in less invasive operations in a number of instances. Robotic surgery, for example, has been used with increased frequency.

Chemotherapy: Chemotherapy simply means chemical or drug therapy. It involves the use of drugs to destroy cancer cells. It is a systemic treatment, as opposed to a localized treatment, meaning it goes wherever the bloodstream carries it and can impact cells and organs all over the body. In addition to the site of the original or primary tumor, it also will attempt to kill cancer cells that may have spread to distant organs and tissues. Chemotherapy works because cancer cells grow more quickly than normal cells. During growth periods, the cell is the weakest. But some normal cells, such as hair and the intestinal lining, also grow rapidly and also may be damaged by chemotherapy. That is why some of the common side effects of chemotherapy include nausea, diarrhea, constipation, mouth sores, and hair loss.

There are many varieties of drugs and different types of drug actions that impact the tumor cells in different ways, to prevent cell division (*e.g.*, cyclophosphamide and doxorubicin), starve the cancer cells (*e.g.*, 5-fluorouracil), or even paralyze them (*e.g.*, vincristine). Certain hormones and hormone-substitutes are also used as hormonal therapy to complement chemotherapy (*e.g.*, tamoxifen). Sometimes a single drug is used, but more commonly there is a regimen of multiple drugs used in combination. Combinations are used to improve the chances of destroying cancer cells at different points in their life cycles.

Chemotherapy can be used for different goals, including curing the cancer. Chemotherapy given after surgery (as adjuvant chemotherapy) is done to try to decrease the recurrence of the cancer. Sometimes, chemotherapy can slow or stop the spread of cancer. Or it can kill cancer cells that have spread to other parts of the body. It can be used to relieve symptoms caused by the size of the cancer. Chemotherapy can be used to shrink a tumor before surgery or radiation therapy. The National Cancer Institute's website (www.cancer.gov) is a good source for information on chemotherapy regimens.

In this face-paced world of cancer research and treatment developments, the options are evolving quickly and patients and physicians must consult current sources. Further, we are moving toward more of an individualized phase of cancer research and treatment, in which particular cancers may be treated differently even for the same broad type or subtype of disease. At the same time, sometimes better treatment options are derived by turning to older drugs such as Bendamustine.

Radiation: Radiation therapy is another common treatment for cancer. Speed of cell division makes cancer cells more sensitive to radiation. Radiation can come from a source outside the body (external beam radiation) as either a low-energy or high-energy beam. Radiation sources can also be placed inside the body, using small seeds or beads of radioactive material placed in or around the tumor area. Radiation therapy is applied close to the tumor and, as such, is a localized treatment. Yet, sometimes full body radiation is used. Certain cancers, such as leukemia, lymphoma, skin cancer, and many reproductive organ cancers often are treated with radiation therapy. Many solid tumors with good blood and oxygen supplies can be treated with radiation therapy as well. If you have a tumor that is not very well supplied with blood and oxygen, higher doses of radiation may be required to kill those cells. Radiation therapy has improved in some ways in recent years with an increased ability to target and increase the dosage of radiation to the desired site and decrease the radiation received in surrounding areas by a variety of means.

Two delivery methods that were originally used to reduce radiation side effects are dose fractionation, or splitting the total dose of radiation therapy into multiple doses, and physical shielding with lead blocks to reduce the area of exposure. Currently, most radiation treatments are administered daily, 5 days a week—strictly for the convenience of maintaining a normal work week. The 24-hour interval and the 2-day interval between doses allow for recovery of normal tissue between doses; cancer cells, in general, have less recovery ability. There is no doubt that using fractionation has reduced side effects compared with single-dose delivery used half a century ago. Although cancer cells tend to be less resilient than normal tissue, there is a chance that the intervals between fractionated doses of radiation may allow cancer cells to recover. Some recent findings suggest that some cancers are best treated by reducing the 24-hour interval between doses to 6 to 8 hours to enhance the toxic effects on cancer cells while still preserving an adequate time interval for the recovery of normal cells. This technique, called hyperfractionation, has been used to treat a variety of cancers. Hyperfractionation requires sophisticated equipment, so it is important for patients to be treated at specialty medical centers that have experience and staff trained in this technique.

Intensity-modulated radiation therapy (IMRT) delivers varying intensities of radiation with a rotating device. The intensity is varied by the placement of "leaves," which either block or allow the passage of radiation. The rotating component of this technique allows for more specific targeting of the cancer, sparing normal tissue from damage caused by radiation exposure. In conventional radiation therapy, the beam is usually delivered from several different directions, up to 5 or 10. The greater the number of beam directions, the more the dose will be confined to the target cancer cells, sparing normal cells from exposure. IMRT delivers radiation from every point on a helix, or spiral, rather than only a few points.

Three-dimensional conformal radiation therapy (3-D CRT) is a promising approach for the treatment of some cancers. Using CT and other scans, radiation oncologists have developed methods of determining the tumor size and shape in three dimensions. This allows high-dose external beam radiation therapy to be delivered primarily to the cancer with less damage to normal cells. For example, three-dimensional conformal radiation has allowed radiation oncologists to reduce the amount of radiation to the breast by 50 percent, which should decrease the risk of secondary breast cancer. It is important for conformal radiation to be administered at special cancer centers with sophisticated equipment and trained staff.

Proton therapy is an advanced form of radiation that has received considerable press. At this point it remains experimental and protons are of questionable value.

Combination therapy: Combination therapy is commonplace. Often patients undergo a combination of surgery, chemotherapy, immune therapy, and/or radiation and the order may vary.

Hormonal treatment: Hormonal treatment is used for cancers that depend upon hormones to grow. Some treatments add hormones, others remove them. These treatments generally are given either orally or by injection.

Cryosurgery: The idea of cryosurgery is simple—freeze the cancer cells to death. Cryosurgery with liquid nitrogen has long been used to treat tumors on the surface of the body. With the development of the cryoprobe, a slender wand with circulating liquid nitrogen, internal tumors can now be frozen as well. Live ultrasound pictures help to avoid damage to nearby healthy tissue and are used to monitor the location and placement of the probe. Cryotherapy has been effective for some retinoblastomas (cancer of the retina), cancers of the skin, and cancer of the cervix. It has been subject to investigation for the treatment of prostate and liver cancers. It is a localized form of therapy.

Stem cell and bone marrow transplantation: Stem cell transplantation involves the infusion of healthy stem cells into the body. A stem cell transplant can help your body make enough healthy white blood cells, red blood cells, or platelets, and reduce your risk of life-threatening infections, anemia, and bleeding. It is effectively giving the patient a new immune system. Stem cell transplants can use cells from your own body (autologous) or they can use stem cells from donors (allogeneic). There are risks associated with transplantation such as graft-versus-host disease in the case of allogeneic stem cell transplants, where a donor's transplanted stem cells attack your body. Often before the transplant, patients undergo high dose chemotherapy and possibly radiation to destroy cancer. Mini stem cell transplants involve less intense conditioning. High dose chemotherapy is difficult and there are complications including infection that patients must consider. This can be a difficult process to go through, but there have been improvements that have reduced mortality associated with transplants and it can result in a cure. Stem cell transplantation is a cellular therapy. You can watch our interview with Dr. Henry Fung discussing stem cell transplantation on *Battling and Beating Cancer*.

FDA Approved Cancer Drugs: The National Cancer Institute website contains a listing of FDA approved drugs by cancer type. You can review the list by visiting: https://www.cancer.gov/about-cancer/treatment/drugs/cancer-type. We summarize the listings for lymphoma below by way of example.

For Hodgkin Lymphoma the FDA approved drugs include (as of October 2020): Adcetris (Brentuximab Vedotin); BiCNU (Carmustine); Bleomycin Sulfate; Brentuximab Vedotin; Carmustine; Chlorambucil; Cyclophosphamide; Dacarbazine; Dexamethasone; Doxorubicin Hydrochloride; Keytruda (Pembrolizumab); Leukeran (Chlorambucil); Lomustine; Matulane (Procarbazine Hydrochloride); Nivolumab; Opdivo (Nivolumab); Pembrolizumab; Prednisone; Procarbazine Hydrochloride; Vinblastine Sulfate; and Vincristine Sulfate. Drug combinations (regimens) include: ABVD; ABVE; ABVE-PC; BEACOPP; COPDAC; COPP; COPP-ABV; ICE; MOPP; OEPA; OPPA; STANFORD V; and VAMP. The listing also identifies the drugs that comprise the regimens.

The long list of drugs approved for non-Hodgkin lymphoma (as of May 2021) include: Acalabrutinib; Adcetris (Brentuximab Vedotin); Aliqopa (Copanlisib Hydrochloride); Arranon (Nelarabine); Axicabtagene Ciloleucel; Beleodaq (Belinostat); Belinostat; Bendamustine Hydrochloride; Bendeka (Bendamustine Hydrochloride); BiCNU (Carmustine); Bleomycin Sulfate; Bortezomib; Brentuximab Vedotin; Brexucabtagene Autoleucel; Breyanzi (Lisocabtagene Maraleucel); Brukinsa (Zanubrutinib); Calquence (Acalabrutinib); Carmustine; Chlorambucil; Copanlisib Hydrochloride; Copiktra (Duvelisib); Crizotinib; Cyclophosphamide; Denileukin

Diftitox; Dexamethasone; Doxorubicin Hydrochloride; Duvelisib; Folotyn (Pralatrexate); Gazyva (Obinutuzumab); Ibritumomab Tiuxetan; Ibrutinib; Idelalisib; Imbruvica (Ibrutinib); Intron A (Recombinant Interferon Alfa-2b); Istodax (Romidepsin); Keytruda (Pembrolizumab); Kymriah (Tisagenlecleucel); Lenalidomide; Leukeran (Chlorambucil); Lisocabtagene Maraleucel; Loncastuximab Tesirine-lpyl; Methotrexate Sodium; Mogamulizumab-kpkc; Monjuvi (Tafasitamab-cxix); Mozobil (Plerixafor); Nelarabine; Obinutuzumab; Ontak (Denileukin Diftitox); Pembrolizumab; Plerixafor; Polatuzumab Vedotin-piiq; Polivy (Polatuzumab Vedotin-piiq); Poteligeo (Mogamulizumab-kpkc); Pralatrexate; Prednisone; Recombinant Interferon Alfa-2b; Revlimid (Lenalidomide); Rituxan (Rituximab); Rituxan Hycela (Rituximab and Hyaluronidase Human); Romidepsin; Selinexor; Tafasitamab-cxix; Tazemetostat Hydrobromide; Tazverik (Tazemetostat Hydrobromide);Tecartus (Brexucabtagene Autoleucel); Tisagenlecleucel; Treanda (Bendamustine Hydrochloride); Trexall (Methotrexate Sodium); Truxima (Rituximab); Ukoniq (Umbralisib Tosylate);Umbralisib Tosylate; Velcade (Bortezomib); Venclexta (Venetoclax); Venetoclax; Vinblastine Sulfate; Vincristine Sulfate; Vorinostat; Xalkori (Crizotinib); Xpovio (Selinexor); Yescarta (Axicabtagene Ciloleucel); Zanubrutinib;Zevalin (Ibritumomab Tiuxetan); Zolinza (Vorinostat); Zydelig (Idelalisib); Zynlonta and (Loncastuximab Tesirine-lpyl). Approved regimens include: CHOP; COPP; CVP; EPOCH; Hyper-CVAD; ICE; R-CHOP; R-CVP; R-EPOCH; and R-ICE.

This will provide you with an idea of the number of approved drugs. Obviously, not all of these drugs are appropriate for all sub-types and all patients. Similar listings can be found for leukemia, multiple myeloma, and many solid tumors on the website.

CUTTING EDGE TREATMENT OPTIONS

Some of the newer treatment options are discussed below. Although newer, these treatments are starting to be used extensively.

Chimeric Antigen Receptor (CAR) T-cell Therapy: CAR T therapy is a type of personalized immunotherapy in which a patient's T cells are enhanced by the addition of an engineered gene. The patient's blood is collected, the T cells are separated out and the rest of the blood is returned to the patient. The T cells are genetically modified to produce special receptors on their surface called chimeric antigen receptors (CARs), allowing them to recognize and kill malignant cells. The patient is given chemotherapy to reduce the number of immune cells in the body. Then the patient receives the CAR T-cell therapy via IV infusion. The genetically modified cells grow in number and amplify the immune response by directly attacking the cancer cells. The CAR T cells can survive for long periods of time and provide ongoing tumor control and protection against recurrence through replication of the modified cells. In 2017, the first CAR T-cell therapy, axicabtagene ciloleucel (Yescarta), was approved by the FDA to treat diffuse large B-cell lymphoma (DLBCL); a second CAR T-cell therapy, tisagenlecleucel (Kymriah), was approved in 2018 to treat DLBCL, and a third therapy, brexucabtagene autoleucel (Tecartus), was approved in 2020 to treat mantle cell lymphoma (MCL). Several other CAR T-cell therapies are being studied. Many of the common side effects of CAR T-cell therapy are similar to those experienced by patients taking other lymphoma therapies, such as fatigue, decreased appetite, chills, diarrhea, fever, infection, nausea, cough, vomiting, and constipation. Patients may also experience neurological effects. These symptoms usually occur the first two to three days after receiving the CAR T cells and include altered mental state (encephalopathy), headache, tremor, dizziness, speech problems (aphasia), delirium, insomnia, and anxiety. Cytokine release syndrome (an intense systemic inflammatory response) is a unique side effect in response to the activation and growth of a patient's CAR T cells and will be monitored. A medication called tocilizumab (Actemra) was approved by the FDA in 2017 for the treatment of CAR T-cell–induced severe cytokine release syndrome.

Adoptive cell therapy: This is a type of immunotherapy in which T cells (a type of immune cell) are given to a patient to help the body fight diseases, such as cancer. In cancer therapy, T cells are usually taken from the patient's own blood or tumor tissue, grown in large numbers in the laboratory, and then given back to the patient to help the immune system fight the cancer. Sometimes, the T cells are changed in the laboratory to make them better able to target the patient's cancer cells and kill them. Types of adoptive cell therapy include chimeric antigen receptor T-cell (CAR T-cell) therapy discussed above and tumor-infiltrating lymphocyte (TIL) therapy. Adoptive cell therapy that uses T cells from a donor is being studied in the treatment of some types of cancer and some infections. Also called adoptive cell transfer, cellular adoptive immunotherapy, and T-cell transfer therapy.

Targeted therapies: Targeted therapies attack lymphoma cells in a more specific way than chemotherapy drugs. FDA-approved targeted therapies used in the treatment of NHL include: histone deacetylase (HDAC) inhibitors belinostat (Beleodaq), romidepsin (Istodax), lenalidomide (Revlimid) Belinostat (Beleodaq) and vorinostat (Zolinza); proteasome inhibitor bortezomib (Velcade); the PI3K inhibitors copanlisib (Aliqopa), idelalisib (Zydelig), and duvelisib (Copiktra); Bruton tyrosine kinase (BTK) inhibitors acalabrutinib (Calquence), ibrutinib (Imbruvica), and zanubrutinib (Brukinsa); Bcl2 inhibitor venetoclax (Venclexta); EZH2 inhibitor tazemetostat (Tazverik); nuclear export inhibitor selinexor (Xpovio).

Photopheresis/Extracorporeal Photochemotherapy: A fraction of the patient's blood is removed from the body, treated with a chemical that makes lymphocytes more likely to die when exposed to ultraviolet radiation, and re-infused back into the patient. This therapy has been approved by the FDA for the treatment of one cancer. It may also be effective in the treatment of graft-versus-host disease, a potential complication following an allogeneic (donor) stem cell transplant.

Biological or immune therapy: These are more recent modalities of treatment that provide important options for a number of patients and types of cancer. This type of therapy uses drugs, vaccines, immunotherapy, and monoclonal antibodies to boost your immune system in its effort to fight off the cancer cells. Because the body is capable of making these materials in small amounts to fight cancer, additional amounts that are made in the laboratory and given to patients may destroy the cancer cells. Immune boosters also stimulate the body to repair tissues or make new healthy cells after chemotherapy. There are several types of immune therapy.

Nonspecific immunomodulating agents stimulate the immune system to increase the production of invasion-fighting blood cells and chemicals. For example, Bacillus Calmette-Guerin, developed as a vaccine against tuberculosis, also is used to treat superficial bladder cancer after surgery to prevent recurrence. A solution is held in the bladder for a short time and then emptied during urination. Biological response modifiers help the body change the way it interacts with cancer cells. The biological response modifiers include interferons, interleukins, colony-stimulating factors, monoclonal antibodies, and vaccines. They work by a variety of mechanisms including stopping or slowing the growth of cancer cells, facilitating the destruction of cancer cells by the immune system, boosting immune system cells to destroy cancer cells, blocking or reversing the changes in a normal cell that makes it cancerous, improving the body's repair and replacement abilities after normal cells have been damaged or destroyed by treatments, and preventing cancer cells from spreading. The modifiers can be combined with each other, or with radiation therapy or traditional chemotherapy. Side effects vary from patient to patient, but can include rashes at the site of injection, fatigue, bone pain, flu-like symptoms with fever, chills, nausea, vomiting, loss of appetite, and various allergic reactions.

Colony-stimulating factors stimulate the bone marrow to produce larger populations of red and white blood cells and platelets, after radiation therapy or chemotherapy have affected the bone marrow. They allow doctors to increase doses of chemotherapy drugs, because the bone marrow will be producing large amounts of cells needed to fight any infections, avoid anemia, and reduce bleeding tendencies. G-CSF and GM-CSF, for example, improve the white blood cell counts and stem cell production. Erythropoietin stimulates red blood cell production to help avoid anemia and the need for transfusion during chemotherapy. Oprelvekin is a platelet booster, and may help you avoid platelet transfusions if you are receiving high-dose chemotherapy. Colony-stimulating factors are being studied for the treatment of some leukemias, metastatic colorectal cancer, melanoma, lung cancer, and other types of cancer.

Immunotherapy is a major development in the treatment of cancer, with the range of approved immunotherapies growing. Multiple types of immunotherapies have been approved by the FDA for treatment of non-Hodgkin lymphomas, antibodies, antibody-drug conjugates, radioimmunotherapy, novel agents, and cellular therapy. Plasma cells are specialized B lymphocytes that make proteins called antibodies. Antibodies help fight infection by recognizing and sticking to viruses, bacteria, or other foreign substances in the body. Each antibody is naturally designed to recognize one specific antigen (protein on the surface of certain cells). Monoclonal antibodies are molecules that have been engineered in a laboratory to attach to one specific target (antigen) on the surface of cancer cells and they are effective for patients with cancer cells expressing that specific antigen. Antibodies generated in the laboratory are all identical in their protein sequence and are made from one "mother" B lymphocyte. Hence, the reason they are called monoclonal (one clone). Once injected in the patient, the monoclonal antibodies travel through the blood and attach themselves to the cells that have antigens they recognize. This can either stop or slow down the growth of cancer cells that have that specific target, or it can trigger an "alarm" that harnesses an immune reaction to recognize and destroy the cancer cell. In addition to Rituxan which was the first approved monoclonal antibody approved back in the late 1990s, obinutuzumab (Gazyva), and ofatumumab (Arzerra) are direct at the CD20 antigen. used to treat non-Hodgkin lymphomas. Tafasitamab-cxix (Monjuvi) binds to the CD19 antigen on B lymphocytes to promote cell death. Some cancer cells have large amounts of PD-L1 protein, which helps them "hide" from immune cells. The monoclonal antibody, pembrolizumab (Keytruda), is a checkpoint inhibitor which targets PD-L1 to allow the body to attack the lymphoma cells. In recent years, we have seen the FDA approve immunotherapy drugs like Ketruda to treat more and more cancer types. Most recently, it was approved for advanced triple-negative breast cancer; a cancer type that otherwise has very little in the way of treatment options. Mogamulizumab-kpkc (Poteligeo) is a monoclonal antibody that disrupts lymphocyte movements through the body. So-called biosimilars have been approved as well. Brentuximab Vedotin (Adcetris) targets CD30. Polatuzumab vedotin-piiq (Polivy) Polatuzumab vedotin-piiq is a combination of the small toxic drug monomethyl auristatin E (MMAE or vedotin) attached to a monoclonal antibody targeting CD79b (polatuzumab), a component of the B-cell receptor.

Radioimmunotherapy: Monoclonal antibodies are one of the great recent advances. We call these smart drugs because they target the cancer cells and leave healthy cells alone. Sometimes they have been described as seeking out and destroying their cancer-counterpart antigens. In actuality, they harness an immune response from the body. Some monoclonal antibodies have been approved by the Federal Drug Administration. A couple of notable examples are rituximab (Rituxan) for the treatment of some lymphomas and trastuzumab (Herceptin) for the treatment of some breast cancers. Bevacizumab (Avastin) and cetuximab (Erbitux) are approved for the treatment of colon cancer. Rituxan is part of the treatment for so many patients with non-Hodgkin lymphoma that it has been called by many "vitamin R." Others have been approved and research is ongoing for the application of monoclonal antibodies to additional types of cancers and to come up with additional monoclonal antibodies.

Monoclonal antibodies can be combined with radioactive isotopes to form a powerful treatment. The monoclonal antibodies target and trigger an immune response to the cancer cells and they carry with them a dose of radiation that kills the cancer cells. Zevalin and Bexar are a couple of examples of such drugs.

This is an appropriate place to elaborate on a few points because we are familiar with Zevalin and Bexar (no longer available) as these therapies are used for some lymphomas. We know several people who have had success with them and we have had involvement in trying to keep them available. Monoclonal antibodies in combination with other regimens of traditional chemotherapy and with radioactive isotopes are important weapons in the arsenal of doctors and patients for some cancers. Monoclonal antibodies illustrate that meaningful advances in treatment do come with investment in research. Scott went through chemotherapy before rituximab was available. He was given a regiment known as CHOP. Had he gone through chemotherapy in more recent years, the monoclonal antibody rituximab would have been included as part of his regimen. Also, in the case of some follicular lymphomas, traditionally thought to be treatable (and for which patients could be put in remission for years) but not curable, it appears that RIT may be curative or at least dramatically extend the time of the remission for many patients. We know patients who failed other treatments and have been in complete remission after RIT for 23 years and counting! Since being used for cancer, the Federal Drug Administration has approved rituximab for some forms of arthritis, illustrating that the investment of research in one area can produce positive results in another and highlighting the importance of determining the role of the immune system in cancer and other diseases.

Cancer impacts people differently—even the same type of cancer can have a different course for different individuals. For example, we have been in meetings discussing lymphoma where two patients have been diagnosed with the same type of lymphoma. At the time, one was diagnosed about 12 to 14 before and had not undergone any treatment. Watch and wait has been this patient's approach and we suspect this person will never require active treatment for lymphoma. Another patient diagnosed with the same type of lymphoma exhausted the existing treatments without obtaining a meaningful remission within a couple of years after diagnosis. She had a wonderful doctor, who is one of the top lymphoma doctors in the country and a wonderful man. He went to bat for her and got her into a clinical trial involving Zevalin and she has been cancer-free ever since. This illustrates the importance of research and medical developments for sure. To our minds, it also raises questions as to whether the difference in the patients relates to their immune responses or whether there are more breakdowns or significant factors currently unknown that distinguish their cancers.

The ability to subdivide cancers is somewhat of a mixed blessing. The positive side, which outweighs the negative, is that it allows for distinctions in treatment regimens, research, and individualized treatments. One adverse reality is that drug companies, for obvious reasons, focus their research activities on the larger market segments and people with rarer forms of cancer may not reap the same benefits of research and introduction of new therapies.

Returning to Zevalin and Bexar, there was considerable debate as to whether these treatments, which have been curative for many patients, are being under-used and under-prescribed. How could that be the case? Because of the radioactive isotope aspect, many community hospitals are not equipped to provide the treatment. Some patients were advised of the treatment by their doctors and referred to major treatment centers in the area. Others were not. Is it the lack of education about the drugs on the part of the doctors, the desire to keep the business, or other factors accounting for this reality? These are all fair questions to ask.

This is an example of a curative treatment on the market that the incompetence of government bureaucrats has threatened to make unavailable to patients by reason of its Medicare and Medicaid reimbursement policies.

In the November 13, 2007 edition of Newsweek, Jonathon Alter wrote as follows:

> Several clinical trials have shown that the drugs work for most patients. Some seem to have been cured (we won't know for sure for a few more years), and almost all have seen their lives prolonged, often significantly. According to one clinical trial, patients with follicular lymphoma who received standard treatment achieved remission 36 percent of the time. When Zevalin was added, the figure was 89 percent. Bexxar produced at least some response in 97 percent of patients in one study. Particularly for older patients who cannot handle a stem cell transplant, these are essential treatment options . . . .
>
> You would think all of this would mean booming sales for Bexxar and Zevalin and cheering from the government, which has approved precious few drugs in recent years that actually show success in treating cancer.

Wrong. The fathers and mothers and husbands and wives and sisters and brothers who are living longer because of RIT [radioimmunotherapy] are apparently of no (that's right: no) concern. Maybe these doctors and bureaucrats would feel differently if someone in their family had lymphoma.

The first reason RIT is in trouble has to do with doctors who work in offices or small hospitals that are not equipped for what is known as "nuclear medicine." Administering RIT requires special licensing and special equipment. Because most oncologists not affiliated with major cancer centers don't have that particular board certification or technology, they aren't likely to recommend that their lymphoma patients go for RIT at a big hospital. If they do, the doctors are more likely to lose patients and reimbursements, because once these oncologists send their patients to a doctor certified to administer RIT, as one specialist told me, "they don't come back." Not all of these office-park oncologists are greedy; some have good reasons to prescribe another treatment. It depends, of course, on the individual patient. But generally speaking, Bexxar and Zevalin are being dramatically underutilized, even though they have already saved thousands of lives.

With sluggish sales, the future of these wonder drugs is uncertain, as The New York Times explained in a front-page article last summer. But what the Times and the rest of the press has missed is that Washington is now poised to deliver the *coup de grâce* to RIT.

CMS [Centers for Medicare and Medicaid Services], the most powerful federal agency you've never heard of, has total authority over which treatments Medicare and Medicaid will cover. Smelling weakness in the RIT market, it announced in August that it will reimburse hospitals less than 50 percent for Bexxar and Zevalin. Because hospitals can't be expected to pick up the other half (the drugs cost more than $25,000), this will mean the effective end of these life-saving treatments.

Even if a wealthy individual wants to pay out of pocket for RIT, it won't be available, because CMS says it will "terminate the provider agreement of any hospital" that administers the treatment to some patients but not to "Medicare patients who need it."

The absurdity of this defies belief. Here's the government acknowledging that many cancer patients "need" the treatment, but warning that if hospitals offer it, they will "terminate" their indispensable Medicare funding for the hospital!

We engaged in public policy efforts years ago to keep the treatments economically viable. The effort of patients, small non-profits, and patient advocates have led the effort and have at least been successful in keeping one of the two treatments alive. The manufacturer of Bexxar cut back production several years ago without notice or consultation with patients or advocates. It lost its effort to have CMS properly reimburse the drug and subsequently took Bexar off the market. This illustrates the political, institutional, and other battles cancer champions must fight even where an effective therapy has been brought to market. We have written on this topic and conducted an extensive interview with Dr. Mark Kaminski, one of the pioneers of Bexxar. This is a very useful source of information about RIT and you can listen to the interview at blogtalkradio.com/battling-and-beating-cancer.

MAINTENANCE THERAPY AND CLINICAL TRIALS

This last category runs the gambit from maintenance therapy some of which involves traditional treatments, to clinical trials which are studies that often add a new agent to standard of care treatments (but can include more novel therapies, to experimental agents (which usually are called for where no effective, proven treatment exists).

Maintenance therapy: Maintenance therapy refers to the ongoing treatment of patients whose disease has responded well to treatment. The purpose of maintenance therapy is to enhance response to prior therapy and to improve the duration of remission. Maintenance therapy typically consists of drugs given at lower doses and longer intervals than those used during initial therapy. Depending on the type of NHL and the drugs used, maintenance therapy may last for weeks, months, or even years. Rituximab (Rituxan, Rituxan Hycela) or rituximab biosimilars (Truxima, Ruxience) or obinutuzimab may be used as maintenance therapy for CD20-positive B-cell NHLs following a good initial response to the drug in patients with indolent (slow growing) lymphomas.

Clinical trials: Fortunately, there is a variety of promising research and additional treatments in the works. In the absence of effective, approved treatment, patients should explore clinical trials. There are even some instances when a patient may consider and benefit from a clinical trial even where other viable options exist. Although your oncologist is the first resource for information on clinical trials, he or she is not the only resource. Once again, several organizations, internet sites, and fellow patients can provide a wealth of information on clinical trials and many of them are listed in Appendix "C." Just like seeking the best conventional treatment for a patient's individual cancer is important, the same applies for seeking clinical trials. Patients and doctors should come to some consensus not only about pursuing a clinical trial, but pursuing the best one for the patient's cancer. Patients should be open to the possibility of exploring clinical trial options anywhere.

We thought it would be helpful to provide an overview of how clinical trials work. Clinical trials are research studies on people to determine the safety and efficacy of a new treatment, therapy, or medical device under controlled conditions. Clinical trials are constantly in progress all over the world. A clinical trial is one of the final steps of a long research process. The experimentation does not start on people. Before the clinical trial, there should be extensive review of safety and effectiveness done in the laboratory and on animals. If a treatment is not safe or effective on rats, mice, and other laboratory animals, it does not make it to a clinical trial. If the results show potential benefits that exceed the risks or side effects, human studies may be carried out. Clinical trials often require large numbers of participants to properly evaluate effectiveness and long-term safety of a drug or device.

Clinical trials should follow strict protocols. Protocols may require a treatment to be examined alone or compared with a sugar pill (placebo) or a treatment that already is in use. Alternatively, a trial may be designed to determine whether an existing treatment may have additional uses. Protocols also describe who may participate in the trial, the schedule of tests, procedures, medications and dosages, and the length of the study. Patients participating in a trial are examined regularly by doctors and researchers who monitor their health and follow the safety and effectiveness of the treatment.

Clinical trials of a new drug typically go through four phases. Phase I is primarily designed to determine safe doses and the best modality of the drug or treatment (should it be given by mouth, injection, or inhalation). Phase II continues to test the safety of the drug and how well it works. Phase III involves giving the drug to an even larger number of people over a longer time period, and often compares the drug or treatment being studied against known treatments. Phase IV involves ongoing monitoring of large patient groups after a drug or treatment has been approved and marketed.

Although you may want to participate in a given clinical trial, the trial may not want you. You must satisfy specified criteria to participate. Because each clinical trial looks for answers to different questions, each trial has specific guidelines regarding who is qualified to participate. The guidelines describe characteristics that may include such things as age, type of disease, medical history, and medical condition. For example, it may require that you tried and failed another specified treatment or that you have not undergone other treatments. You must meet these characteristics to qualify for participation in the study. You may not understand the criteria and the criteria do not always make sense from the standpoint of pure treatment of patients. First and foremost, however, clinical trials are studies. We are aware of instances where people who did not satisfy the criteria for a clinical trial have nonetheless been allowed to participate in a clinical trial. Accordingly, it pays to be persistent and to have a physician that is an effective advocate.

Assuming you qualify, the ultimate question is whether you should participate. Before entering a trial, your "informed consent" is required. You will be told such things as: what the trial will consist of (regimen, testing, length of time); why the research is being conducted; what the researchers seek to accomplish; what the risks and benefits are; what other treatments are available; and your right to exit the trial at any time. They will make you sign consent forms.

By now you know that you will not sign any consent form until you are comfortable that you wish to participate. How can you be sure it makes sense to participate in the trial? Speak with the doctors and researchers. Do your own research and speak with your own doctor and confidants. Before any trial is carried out with human participants, the protocol is reviewed, approved, and monitored by an institutional review board that follows government guidelines and includes safeguards that purport to protect you and ensure the risks are as low as possible. This board is a fancy name for a group of doctors, statisticians, community members, and clergy that is supposed to ensure the clinical trial is ethical and protects the rights of patient participants. Research centers involved in human research are required by federal law to have such a board in place to approve and review a trial during the time it is active. Board members are not paid.

You should know that other players are involved in these clinical studies. Drug companies, hospitals, insurers, and governmental agencies sponsor clinical trials. The trials generally take place in a university teaching hospital, a local hospital, a clinic, or a doctor's office. It is always a good idea to "follow the money." We all have heard about doctors being paid based on containing costs by not ordering tests, not prescribing treatments, or otherwise having a financial incentive that may conflict with the interests of the health of a doctor's patient. With clinical trials, doctors and researchers may be paid for enrolling each participant in a study. In evaluating whether to participate, you may be interested in whether someone urging you to participate is making a commission.

Keep in mind, you are not guaranteed to receive the treatment being tested. You may be a member of the "control group." Members of this group usually get a placebo or the standard treatment instead of the experimental drug to measure whether there is a mental or emotional element impacting the study or so the drug or treatment being studied can be compared with a baseline. Participants will not know if they are in the control group or the experimental group. Participants in a blinded or masked study are not aware of which treatment they are receiving. When neither the participants nor the research team knows which participants are receiving treatment or placebo, the study is called a double blind study, because everyone is unaware of who is receiving the drug or therapy being tested. This type of study is designed to try to remove both the patients' and the doctors' expectations of the results from impacting the study.

Whether or not to participate in a clinical trial depends first and foremost on whether or not there are better treatment options available to you. In some cases, the study may be complementary and not preclude other treatments. Clinical trials offer advantages—the main one is access to new treatments or drugs that are not available to the public. It also may provide a level of care and monitoring the patient may not otherwise be able to afford or have access to. There always is the altruistic motive of benefiting medical science in the hope of helping other patients. Clinical trials are an important part of making new treatment available. Potential risks include the side effects or adverse reactions to medications or treatments. There may be considerable inconveniences associated with trips to the study sites, complex dosage, or monitoring requirements that may not exist with other treatment. The clinical trials we have in mind are do not make patients guinea pigs. Patients receive the standard of care and also may receive additional agents that have shown some efficacy. Our radio show on clinical trials featuring Dr. Julie Vose, Chief of the Division of Hematology Oncology and Professor of Medicine, University of Nebraska Medical is available at www. blogtalkradio.com/battling-and-beating-cancer.

Your health care team as well as many non-profits can be a good source of information on clinical trials. Also, you can locate clinical trials supported by the National Cancer Institute at: https://www.cancer.gov/about-cancer/treatment/clinical-trials/search. The National Cancer Institute's Cancer Information Service can also provide a tailored clinical trials search that you can discuss with your doctor. To reach them call 1-800-422-6237. The US National Library of Medicine website contains a listing of over 388,000 publicly and privately funded studies throughout the world. Visit: https://clinicaltrials.gov/.

Vaccine therapies: There has been much written about using vaccines to treat cancer. Cancer vaccines are generally made to boost the immune response in the presence of cancer in order to defeat it. Cancer vaccines are specific to a type of cancer and are made from cancer cells themselves. They are given to help the body remember the cancer type and fight off any possible recurrence in the future. We have a friend who, in his 30s, received vaccine treatments for late stage melanoma and has done magnificently for years. Instead of a 20% five-year survival rate under traditional interferon treatment, early studies showed the vaccines achieved an 80% five-year survival rate. Twenty years later, our friend is doing very well and we look forward to receiving holiday cards from him, his wife, and beautiful daughter. However, the current reality is that vaccines remain experimental and are not used at this point as a standard treatment for cancer.

The Human papillomavirus (HPV) vaccines exemplify an approach in preventing cancer. These are vaccines that prevent infection by some types of human papillomaviruses. Available HPV vaccines protect against either two, four, or nine types of HPV. All HPV vaccines protect against at least HPV types 16 and 18, which cause the greatest risk of cervical cancer. The CDC recommends that not only women, but males also should receive HPV vaccines. Males need to be concerned about HPV for at least two reasons. First, they can be carriers of HPV and can infect their partners. Second, males are at risk for several HPV-associated cancers such as anal cancer, penile cancer, and throat cancer.

Right To Try Act: The Right to Try Act, or the Trickett Wendler, Frank Mongiello, Jordan McLinn, and Matthew Bellina Right to Try Act, was signed into law on May 30, 2018. This law provides a way for patients who have been diagnosed with life-threatening diseases or conditions, such as cancer, who have tried all approved treatment options and who are unable to participate in a clinical trial to access certain unapproved treatments. The Right to Try Act permits eligible patients to have access to eligible investigational drugs. The U.S. Food and Drug Administration's role essentially is limited to receipt and posting of certain information submitted regarding Right to Try use.

An eligible patient is a patient who has: (1) been diagnosed with a life-threatening disease or condition; (2) exhausted approved treatment options and is unable to participate in a clinical trial involving the eligible investigational drug (this must be certified by a physician who is in good standing with their licensing organization or board and who will not be compensated directly by the manufacturer for certifying); and (3) has provided, or their legally authorized representative has provided, written informed consent regarding the eligible investigational drug to the treating physician.

An eligible investigational drug is an investigational drug: (1) for which a Phase 1 clinical trial has been completed; (2) that has not been approved or licensed by the FDA for any use; (3) for which an application has been filed with the FDA or is under investigation in a clinical trial that is intended to form the primary basis of a claim of effectiveness in support of FDA approval and is the subject of an active investigational new drug application submitted to the FDA; (4) whose active development or production is ongoing, and that has not been discontinued by the manufacturer or placed on clinical hold by the FDA.

If you are interested in Right to Try, you should discuss this with your physician. Companies that develop and make drugs, in this context called sponsors, can provide information about whether their drug/biologic is considered an eligible investigational drug under Right to Try and if they are able to provide the drug/biologic under the Right to Try Act. Ultimately, sponsors developing drugs for life-threatening diseases or conditions are responsible for determining whether to make their products available to patients who qualify for access under the Right to Try Act.

Side effects: There are many potential side effects associated with the various treatments. These vary from patient to patient and from treatment to treatment. Some of these include anemia, loss or change of appetite, bleeding, constipation, depression, diarrhea, hair loss, hormone changes, fever, mouth sores, lesions, nausea, vomiting, infection, aches and pains, sleeping difficulty, fatigue, rashes, swelling in your hands and feet and other symptoms and conditions. Secondary cancers, heart conditions, and other serious side effects are possible. Peripheral neuropathy may be caused by some chemotherapy drugs and radiation. This involves damage to peripheral nerves or nerves that control the sensations and movements of arms and legs. The symptoms depend mostly on which nerves are involved, but common symptoms include pain, burning, tingling, weakness, and numbness. It can be a short term or long-term issue and there are preventatives and treatments available in many cases.

Weight changes are common with chemotherapy. Although many expect to lose weight while undergoing chemotherapy, many people instead gain weight because of steroids or anti-nausea drugs. Water retention may increase as well.

There is another condition that some patients will experience that we want to mention because it does not receive sufficient attention and it can be distressing to patients, particularly if they are not alerted to it. Many patients experience a mild cognitive impairment that has been called "mental fog," "brain fog," or "chemo brain." Cancer survivors have worried about and been frustrated by the mental cloudiness they notice before, during, and after chemotherapy for some time, but only recently has any meaningful research been done on this. The cause is not known, but some drugs can cause changes in the brain that impact memory, planning, processing, and other functions. Usually, this is only temporary and the brain recovers over time.

We detailed our adventures with side effects in Part 1. Appendix "K" includes some information regarding some of the side effects and includes some suggestions. The best thing to do is discuss the potential side effects with your medical providers and have a plan for addressing those that can be addressed, if you experience them.

Potential results of therapy: The range of potential outcomes of treatment varies considerably. Complete cure is the result that all patients hope to achieve. Some treatments provide a period of remission or are otherwise beneficial. In some instances, treatment can leave the patient worse off. Sometimes there is a series of treatments planned for the patient. Other times, options are tried in a particular order to offer the best chance of success, to minimize side-effects, or to leave future treatment options available. Thus, the results of a particular treatment must be viewed from the perspective of the entire treatment plan and range of available outcomes. Because there often is confusion about the terms used to describe the results of treatment, we discuss some of the terms commonly used.

Cure is the term used by doctors to describe the situation in which there are no current signs of cancer and the length of time is sufficient to believe that the cancer is in complete remission and unlikely to return. Many types of cancer, including some subtypes of lymphoma and lymphoma are curable.

Complete response is when all signs of cancer have disappeared after treatment. It does not mean that the cancer is completely cured, but it suggests that the symptoms have disappeared and the cancer cannot be detected using current tests. Where complete remission is maintained for a long period, it is called a **durable remission**.

Partial remission is the term used where the cancer has responded to treatment and shrunk to less than one half of its original size.

Minor response is where the tumor has shrunk following therapy, but still is more than one half of its original size.

Minimal residual disease refers to a small number of cells that remain in the blood or bone marrow after the completion of treatment.

Stable disease means the cancer has not gotten better or worse following treatment.

Disease progression means the cancer has grown or spread during therapy or observation.

Relapse refers to disease that reappears or grows again after a period of remission.

Refractory disease refers to cancer that does not respond to treatment or in which the response to treatment does not last very long.

The above discussion illustrates the broad range of therapies now available to treat cancer and shows the armamentarium has expanded considerable in recent years due to research. No doubt important progress has been made. It is important to point out that there is more to the equation of available treatments than medical advancement. The discussion of RIT above illustrates regulatory, pricing, and reimbursement issues can threaten otherwise available and effective treatments. Another major issue is drug shortages.

The problem of drug shortages: While we are fighting for new and better treatments, keeping the supply of many long-standing drugs proven effective for cancer and other conditions has been a struggle in recent years. For example, Cytarabine first received Food and Drug Administration approval in 1969. It is a critical component in the treatment for many patients with acute myeloid leukemia or AML. Used in combination with antibiotics, it has a cure rate of 40 to 50 percent. For several years, there was a shortage of this drug. Some major cancer and academic medical centers rationed the drug and other hospitals ran out. Two of the three companies that make Cytarabine had production difficulties, and the third company could not fill the void. The problem apparently was the formation of crystals. Although doctors are most concerned about restoring the supply of Cytarabine for AML patients, they are also concerned about the long-term effects on clinical research. Cytarabine is not the only drug in short supply. In 2010, there were 211 shortages, up from 58 six years earlier. Shortages of chemotherapy drugs such as cisplatin and bleomycin, as well as certain antibiotics, heart medications and pain killers, have all been reported.

A more recent example involves ALL. About 15% of children with the most common type of childhood cancer, acute lymphoblastic leukemia, develop an allergic or other immune reaction to the chemotherapy drug Pegaspargase, which has been an important part of treatment regimens for ALL.

An alternate form of the drug, Erwinia asparaginase, may be substituted if a patient develops an immune reaction to pegaspargase. However, manufacturing problems have led to global shortages of Erwinia asparaginase. Children who do not receive a full course of asparaginase are at greater risk of their cancer relapsing. On June 30, 2021, the FDA approved a new form of asparaginase, erwinia chrysanthemi (recombinant)-rywn (Rylaze), which was developed to address the ongoing shortages of Erwinia asparaginase.

In May 2021, ASCO's *Journal of Clinical Oncology* reported that drug shortages "are a clear and growing challenge. Prominent shortages included oncology medications and supportive care products essential for the care of cancer patients. Oncology drug shortages often result in disruptions in the timing of chemotherapy treatments, alterations in the dose or regimen administered, or even missed doses when alternative agents are unavailable." This was based upon a survey that was distributed by the Hematology Oncology Pharmacy Association to its members. A total of 68 organizations completed the survey, with 63% of the institutions reporting one or more drugs shortages a month. Most experienced increased costs from oncology drug shortages and some experienced reimbursement issues when they switched to brand name therapies due to shortages. Treatment delays, reduced doses or alternative regimens were reported by 74.63% of respondents. The most common cancers implicated by drug shortages were acute lymphocytic leukemia, lymphoma, and myeloma with dose reductions noted in 36.36%, 36.36 and 15.91%. The top five oncology drugs on shortage included Epirubicin, flutamide, decitabine, mechlorethamine, dactinomycin with the top 5 supportive care drugs on shortage being noted as hydrocortisone, bivalirudin, promethazine, mycophenolate sodium and scopolamine. Some medication errors were attributed to oncology drug shortages. The conclusion was that oncology drug shortages occurred frequently in 2020. Shortages led to delays in chemotherapy and changes in treatment or omission, complicated clinical research and increased the risk of medication errors and adverse outcomes.

Recent events associated with the COVID-19 pandemic have underscored the importance of having medications and medical devices and protective gear produced in the United States.

The future of personalized cancer treatments and the relentless pursuit of the best patient outcome: After years of the promise of personalized cancer treatments, we are now beginning to see the groundbreaking impact on patient outcome. The genetic role of cancer was revealed by the innovative work of Dr. Janet Rowley (discussed below) and others. The Human Genome Project fueled personalized medicine and immunotherapy has represented one of the major categories in this cancer treatment revolution. Immunotherapy now is widely used for many cancers and is the subject of numerous future studies.

Over the years the identification of sub-types of cancers has led to matching patients with more effective treatments resulting in better outcomes. For many patients and some cancers, doctors and researchers are now able to go beyond this and account for individual genetics and molecular structure of a person's cancer to formulate a personalized treatment plan. Studies of human genes and the genes in different cancers have not only helped researchers design more effective treatments, they have also helped to develop and advance tests for cancer and ways to prevent it. Applications of personalized cancer medicine can not only result in more effective treatments for a patient, but also in treatments with fewer side effects. Simply stated, a personalized treatment aims to affect healthy cells less and cells involved in cancer more. In many instances, your doctor may work with you on a personalized cancer screening, diagnosis, or cancer treatment plan. This may include learning about your chances of developing cancer and choosing screening tools to lower the risks, matching the treatment to your genes and your cancer's genes, and predicting how likely the cancer is to recur.

Today, you may still have the usual treatment for your type and stage of cancer. However, your doctor may personalize treatment based on information about your genes and the cancer's genes. With increasing frequency, personalized medicine is becoming part of conventional treatments and significantly optimized for clinical trials. As mentioned before, the leading examples of personalized cancer medicine are targeted treatments, including immunotherapies. A targeted treatment targets specific genes and proteins that allow a certain cancer to grow and survive. Researchers are discovering new targets for more cancers each year. Then, they create and test new drugs for these targets. Cancers with targeted treatment options for some patients include some: bladder cancers, brain cancers, cervical cancers, colorectal cancers, endometrial cancers, esophageal cancer, head and neck cancers, kidney cancers, leukemias, liver cancer, lymphomas, lung cancers, melanoma, multiple myelomas, neuroblastomas, pancreatic cancers, prostate cancer, stomach cancers, and thyroid cancers. The goal is to determine patient-specific targeted drug treatments for a particular type of cancer.

Today, understanding the genes important for cancer initiation and disease progression is not enough. Pharmacogenomics also has an important role to play. Pharmacogenomics involves the study of how your genes affect your response to drugs. For example, you may process a certain drug faster than most people do such that it goes through your system more quickly. This may mean you may need a higher dose for the drug to work as well as it does for most people. Alternatively, you might process a drug more slowly than most people such that it stays in your bloodstream longer than usual. You might have more side effects or need a lower dose. This informs the important decision of dosing and could also inform frequency of treatments.

Technologies, platforms, and artificial intelligence (AI): Technologies, platforms, and AI have revolutionized the approach to personalized medicine and applications of them already are exploding in biomedical research and clinical decision-making. AI excels at recognizing patterns in large volumes of data, extracting relationships between complex features in the data and identifying characteristics in data that cannot be perceived by people. It has already produced results in radiology. The Food and Drug Administration approved the first AI-based software to process images rapidly and assist radiologists in detecting breast cancer in screening mammograms. Integration of AI technology in cancer care could improve the accuracy and speed of diagnosis, aid clinical decision-making, and lead to better patient outcomes.

The National Cancer Institute, for example, reported that its investigators have developed a deep learning approach for the automated detection of precancerous cervical lesions from digital images. Another group of NCI intramural investigators used a computer algorithm to analyze MRI images of the prostate. Historically, standard biopsies of the prostate did not always produce the most accurate information. Starting 15 years ago, clinicians at NCI began performing biopsies guided by findings from MRI, enabling them to focus on regions of the prostate most likely to be cancerous. MRI-guided biopsy improved diagnosis and treatment when utilized by prostate cancer experts. There is greater potential for the use of MRI-guided biopsy. New AI algorithms under development now aim to surpass the capabilities of well-trained radiologists by enabling the prediction of patient outcomes from MRI.

Currently, it is fair to say that the use of AI in cancer research and care is in its infancy. Yet, AI already is being used in many ways in research for new cancer treatments. AI is being used to identify specific gene mutations from tumor pathology images instead of using traditional genomic sequencing. For instance, the NCI reported AI accurately distinguish between two of the most common lung cancer subtypes (adenocarcinoma and squamous cell carcinoma) and could predict commonly mutated genes from the images and also has been used to identify mutations in brain cancer using noninvasive techniques. AI also is being used to detect proteins or nucleic acids that are important in cancer growth, to make predictions for new drugs to target those molecules, and to help evaluate the effectiveness of those drugs. Research is also being conducted to identify novel approaches for creating new drugs more effectively.

So far, most decision support for technologies have focused on machine learning and AI platforms that are unidimensional, relying on lone tumor parameters, such as genetics or tumor imaging to predict patient response to therapy and outcome. We know that there is more to understanding tumor behavior and patient response to therapy than just one lone parameter. Thus, there is a need for technologies to integrate multimodal tumor and patient characteristics defined at the time of diagnosis and understand how they synergistically contribute to a patient's tumor behavior and response to therapy. By doing this, clinical support can go beyond mass population statistics not only to ensure that patient's receive treatments that are best suited for their cancer but to ensure that they avoid those with toxic side effects. Beyond utility for clinical decision making, there is also a need for tools to organize patient-specific data in meaningful ways that can be presented and provided value towards improving the patient's experience. Such tools would help patients better understand and navigate their cancer, something very much needed in this day and age.

As you can see, cancer research, diagnosis, and treatment will continue to evolve and improve in these days of personalized treatment. Patients should be looking for personalized treatment plans to beat cancer, increase survival, and minimize side effects of treatment.

CHAPTER 20

EMPLOYING A COMPLEMENTARY/ INTEGRATIVE APPROACH (CONVENTIONAL MEDICINE CAN USE A HELPING HAND)

We are no more dieticians, physical trainers, industrial hygienists, or lifeologists than we are physicians. We realize many cancer patients look carefully into vitamins and supplements, anti-cancer diets, physical exercise programs, and adjunctive therapies of various types. This is not only appropriate, but can be very helpful to a patient's recovery, overall health, and even cancer survival.

At the outset, it is important to distinguish between complementary medicine and alternative medicine. Complementary medicine is used along with standard medical treatment, but is not considered by itself to be standard treatment. One example is using acupuncture to help ease some side effects of cancer treatment. Alternative medicine is used instead of standard medical treatment. One example is using a special diet to treat cancer instead of chemotherapy. Complementary medicine often can be helpful. Alternative medicine is something patients should exercise particular caution before using.

You should consult with your physicians and other health professionals about diet, lifestyle, and exercise issues to ensure that you are not doing anything that will interfere with your treatments or recovery. Some doctors are very knowledgeable about these issues and will provide important information or at least send you in the right direction. Many doctors, however, fail to counsel their patients on diet, exercise, and complementary therapies. There are several reasons for this: it may not be their areas of interest, knowledge, or comfort; they may not have the time; they may not believe that it is their role; or they may not believe that these issues are significant to the patient's recovery. Accordingly, many patients are left to fend for themselves on these issues. There are many good books and resources available. But careful, research and scrutiny is required.

We do not believe that any of the following are a substitute for conventional treatment for cancer, but these are some things that may help prevent some instances of cancer, promote recovery, and in conjunction with appropriate medical treatment may increase survivorship or reduce or delay recurrence of the disease. Here are some of our thoughts on the subject of healthy lifestyle issues.

Avoid occupational exposures and air pollution: Most of us have to earn a living, but many jobs involve extensive or frequent exposure to toxic chemicals. It is best to avoid occupations that present exposure to such chemicals altogether. At a minimum, understand your occupational exposures, seek to avoid them, wear appropriate protective equipment, and adhere to proper safety and industrial hygiene practices. Keep in mind, white collar positions, like blue collar positions, may involve exposures to cancer-causing agents.

Protect against exposure to toxic chemicals at home: Toxic chemicals are not limited to the work place. Protect yourself against exposure to toxic chemicals at home by avoiding and minimizing exposure to various cleaning products, pesticides, and insecticides. Choose your personal grooming products, hair care products, skin care products, dyes, and make-up carefully to minimize risks. Also, some recommend airing out your dry cleaning before you bring it in the house. Know what chemicals you are using and, where possible, substitute potentially harmful chemicals with safe alternatives.

Keep a clean house and practice good personal hygiene: There are associations between certain bacterial and viral infections and cancer. Also, while you are undergoing treatment your immune system may be compromised and you do not need to add an infection to the list of elements you are fighting. Hand washing, avoiding contact with people who are sick, and practicing good hygiene should become a way of life.

Avoid unprotected exposure to the sun: There are some healthy aspects to exposure to the sun, such as the creation of vitamin D. Prolonged, unprotected exposure, however, generally should be avoided. When undergoing treatment, it often is best to avoid sun exposure altogether.

You should check with your physician before exposing yourself to the sun's rays. Say no to tan beds and tan sprays.

Eat a well-balanced diet to the extent possible and stick with "anti-cancer" foods: A diet that includes fish (salmon, mackerel, anchovies, sardines, and white albacore tuna); organic meat and omega-three eggs (in low quantities); lentils, peas, and beans; olive oil, flaxseed oil, omega-three butter, cod-liver oil; multigrain and sourdough bread; wheat; whole-grain rice; oatmeal; power vegetables (cabbage, asparagus, bananas, brussels sprouts, cauliflower, broccoli, carrots, sweet potatoes, tomatoes, beets, and some varieties of mushrooms); parsley, mint, basil, rosemary, garlic, onion, leeks, chives, and ginger; the pretty rainbow of fruits (strawberries, raspberries, blueberries, blackberries, cranberries, cherries, apricots, oranges, lemons, and grapefruit); natural yogurt; walnuts, pecans, and almonds; and dark chocolate is generally what the literature suggests. We do not particularly care for eating fish and think that there are countervailing concerns related to pollution warranting concern. In terms of dealing with issues of appetite and nutrition, visit: https://www.cancer.gov/about-cancer/treatment/side-effects/appetite-loss/nutrition-pdq

Engage in exercise and physical activity: Stay active and, when in doubt, check with your physician about your routine. There are many books and materials on exercise, so we will not add to the dialogue in this book.

Drink safe water: It is not only important to drink a sufficient quantity of water, but to know that the water you are drinking is safe. Testing the source of your tap water and using appropriate filters is one way. Drinking mineral or spring water from a known and reliable source is another.

Avoid excess consumption of alcohol: Although there are reports that drinking red wine (in moderation) is not harmful to most people and may be helpful, avoiding excess consumption of alcohol is part of a cogent lifestyle and anti-cancer plan.

Make sure your doctors know what supplements you are taking: You have to be careful regarding the vitamins and supplements you are taking and make sure that your doctors know what you are taking. A recent example makes the point well. Many people advocate drinking green tea either to promote health or to help with symptoms of chemotherapy. Yet, in February 2009, researchers at the University of Southern California reported that green tea renders a cancer drug used to treat multiple myeloma and mantle cell lymphoma completely ineffective in treating cancer. The study found that a component of green tea extract called EGCG destroys any anticancer activity of the drug Velcade in tumor-bearing mice. The finding was unexpected and the researchers reported, "[o]ur hypothesis was that GTE or EGCG would enhance the anti-tumor effects of Velcade, and that a combination of GTE with Velcade (or EGCG with Velcade) would turn out to be a superior cancer treatment as compared to treatment with Velcade alone." This did not turn out to be the case.

Promote your mental and emotional health and have a strong will to live: We have discussed elsewhere that physiology is associated with good mental health and the importance of the will to live, but this is very important. Along those lines, surround yourself with helpful, positive people and keep the negative naysayers at bay. Have people around that you can talk to. Acknowledge your emotions, fears, anxieties, anger, and even depression and address these feelings. If you would benefit from counseling or professional assistance, get it.

Empower yourself and adopt a warrior mentality, not a victim mentality: Arm yourself with knowledge of the disease, the treatment options and be an active participant in your treatment and health care. Adopt the mentality of a warrior or conqueror, not a victim.

Remain a "no-smoking" zone: The risks of smoking and second-hand smoke are well known. Tobacco use is the single biggest cause of cancer in the world, responsible for more than a quarter of all cancer deaths, including cancers of the lung, mouth, throat, nose and sinuses, liver, pancreas, stomach, cervix, breast, bowel, kidney and bladder.

Avoid exposure to infectious agents: Although cancer is not contagious, exposure to certain viruses such as HIV can increase the risk of or cause cancer.

Keep current, but avoid blindly following fads or the latest study: The pace of science and studies—including studies on the causes of disease, the effectiveness of treatments, and on health and nutrition—is amazing. Every day new studies and reports come out. It is important to keep current. It also is important not to blindly adjust your course based upon a new study or report. You need to be educated and have good sounding boards (including doctors) to help you evaluate the information.

Promote your spirit and health through appropriate complementary therapies: There are several adjunctive therapies or treatments that cancer patients undergo that also are sensible. Acupuncture, massage, visualization, hypnosis, meditation, relaxation, martial arts, yoga, herbal therapy, and a host of other things are used by cancer patients and have been reported to ease pain, promote healing, or otherwise make positive contributions. As long as your doctors are informed and approve, such adjunct therapies can be beneficial. A list of clinical trials looking into the efficacy of such therapies can be located at: https://www.cancer.gov/about-cancer/treatment/clinical-trials/cam-procedures.

Scott's Mind Power Therapy: The adjunctive therapy that Scott employed was "Scott's Mind Power" or "SMP." We understand the power of the mind and Scott employed SMP, which is a visualization technique Scott used when he was undergoing chemotherapy and radiation. Scott ceased using SMP a few weeks after his radiation therapy was completed.

We know that you hardly can wait to learn about SMP and promise that you will not read about it anywhere else, so here it goes. Scott knew that lymphoma involved white blood cells known as lymphocytes. So he would visualize his defective white blood cells as containing dark spots on them. In his mind, he would run his white blood cells through a Scott-O-Meter, which was a tube about two inches in length and green in color. On the left side of his mind the white blood cells had dark spots. In the center they would pass through the Scott-O-Meter and when they came out on the right side, they were spotless, healthy white blood cells. There was no schedule or pre-determined time for turning the meter on. Scott would visualize this often, sometimes while undergoing chemotherapy, sometimes in the waiting room, sometimes in bed, and sometimes while watching television or thinking. There are some clear advantages to the treatment. First, we have just taught the treatment to you and you now have the ability to undergo the treatment at no cost. Second, there are no known side-effects. Although Scott believed it to be useful, there is no scientific support for the efficacy of the Scott-O-Meter. Indeed, he did not tell Charlene that he was doing this at first because he thought that she may think that, on top of everything else, the conventional treatments he was undergoing were making him crazy.

We interviewed Dr. Janine Gauthier on both the *Battling and Beating Cancer* radio and television shows. If you are interested in learning more about integrative medicine, visit www.blogtalkradio.com/battling-and-beating-cancer. Many fine institutions, including Northwestern Memorial Hospital and Rush University Medical Center, put integrative medicine into action.

Again, there is an important difference between an integrative approach and unproven experimental claims. Quackwatch.org contains information about questionable cancer treatment claims and tips to protect patients from being victimized. The National Center for Complementary and Alternative Medicine website, nccam.nih.gov, from the National Institutes of Health, lists clinical trials and information on complementary and alternative therapies.

Alternative treatments: For many forms of cancer and many patients, there are effective treatments with proven track records. Where a patient has a proven treatment available, he or she must think long and hard before going with an experimental or unapproved treatment, merely because of unsubstantiated claims or promises or because they seek to avoid the short term anticipated torture of treatments such as chemotherapy or radiation. We are very sympathetic about the desire to forego the pain and suffering associated with some traditional treatments. Still, we have seen some people forego a conventional treatment that offered a promising outcome in favor of some form of "pie in the sky" therapy only to suffer anyway and, in the process, lose the time and opportunity for a cure or extensive remission.

We do believe that patients should be aggressive and seek the best available treatment and opportunity for a cure. In fact, we have worked with patients to find such treatments even where they involved inconvenience or traveling a good distance. The fundamental elements driving the determination included solid information and statistics about the results of the treatment suggesting it substantially improved survival chances, the considerably more extensive side effects of the conventional treatment, and the ability to revert back effectively to the conventional treatment in the event the alternative treatment was not successful. We understand that, where conventional treatment is not a viable option and there is an experimental treatment in a clinical trial that shows some promise, patients may choose the route that affords some potential benefit. FDA approval can be a slow process and often effective treatments are available in other countries before they are available in the United States. Once again, research into the treatments and facilities is critical, but we know several patients that, after doing their research, elected to undergo treatment in other countries.

Often patients from the United States go to Europe for treatments not available in the United States. The Tufts Center for the Study of Drug Development reported that cancer patients in the United States get faster access to more oncology drugs to treat their disease than patients in Europe, but Americans have to pay more for the treatments. They found that new oncology drug approvals in the United States outpaced European approvals by 33% between 2000 and 2011 (40 drugs versus 30).

The bottom line is that most cancers—even those with high cure rates—are life threatening. If there are proven treatments available, go with them. False starts, bad choices, bad doctors, and unwarranted delay can mean lost opportunities for effective treatment. Where experimentation means lost opportunity for a cure or substantial remission, generally it should be avoided. If there is a treatment option that is more favorable or less toxic and undergoing such treatment will not delay or preclude proven treatments or impact their efficacy, such options should be explored. Consider clinical trials when making your treatment decisions. Make sure that you have all of the available information and make the decision that is best for you.

Having received optimal treatment from the best available doctors and having adopted a healthy lifestyle and a warrior mentality, you will beat cancer. Now you can focus on being a cancer warrior and helping win the war against cancer.

CHAPTER 21

THE SUPERHIGHWAY TO CURING CANCER (A STRATEGY FOR CURING CANCER AND A NATIONAL CALL TO ACTION)

The United States of America waged war on cancer fifty years ago as we outlined previously. The war was started belatedly and there has not been enough progress, at least for the millions of Americans who have since died of cancer. It is time that we finish the war on cancer because a victory will save millions of lives.

The prior chapters have dealt with important issues: Scott's survival which was of paramount importance to us and your survival which is of paramount importance to you. In this chapter, we complete the circle by offering some views on what is necessary to cure cancer globally. It may be that it will take a long time to cure all forms of cancer, but the cancer patient must believe and hope that a cure for his or her cancer will come soon. Science, politics, and human nature present obstacles to curing cancer and a new approach may be in order.

Let's get on the superhighway to curing cancer (blood cancer research and the role of the immune system): By now you know our involvement with lymphoma and blood cancer education, awareness, advocacy and fundraising. You can consider for yourself any bias this may present. We observed that lymphoma was a much under-publicized disease considering more than half a million Americans are battling the disease, the rates of non-Hodgkin lymphoma have nearly doubled since the 1970s, and lymphoma is the third most common cancer in children. We quickly found that so many people did not know what lymphoma was or even that it was cancer. Yet, everywhere we went it seemed that someone had lymphoma or knew someone with lymphoma. The lack of sufficient funding for lymphoma research has hampered patients with many forms of cancer.

During our years of searching to cure cancer another reality keep hitting us in the face. Some people exposed to carcinogens get cancer, others do not. Cancer cells live inside of all of us. Why do they take hold in some and not in others? There is more to the cancer-forming process than exposure to carcinogens. After all, we are constantly being assaulted by external forces such as infectious agents, pollutants, and toxins that attempt to destroy or take control of our body. We also are under attack from within. When cells divide, errors in the genes (mutations) can result in abnormal cells that do not function properly. When abnormal cells grow in an uncontrollable fashion that the body's defenses cannot contain, such cells multiply and eventually form a tumor.

Despite attacks from outside and inside the body, most people remain reasonably healthy for most of their lives. Our ability to survive external and internal assaults depends largely upon our immune system. One of the reasons that most people remain healthy is, in part, due to immunosurveillance. Immunosurveillance refers to the monitoring process of the immune system to detect and destroy not only infected cells but normal cells that have transformed into cancer cells.

The immune system is a collection of cells, structures, and organs that exist to identify, contain, and destroy bacteria, viruses, and abnormal cells before or after they harm the body. The immune system can be thought of as warriors that are always "on guard" to protect the body. Invading organisms and abnormal cells generally are identified by the immune system through proteins known as antigens located on the surface of cells. Special receptors located on the immune cells lock on to these antigens. When an antigen and an immune cell lock together, the immune response begins and the body acts to destroy, remove, or wall off the foreign invaders or abnormal cells.

The lymph system is a critical part of the body's immune system. It consists of a series of thin tubes called lymph vessels that branch into all parts of the body. Lymph vessels carry lymph, which is a watery fluid that contains white blood cells called lymphocytes. Within the vast network of vessels are groups of small, bean-shaped organs called lymph nodes. These nodes are located throughout the body. Lymph flows through lymph nodes and structures including the spleen, thymus gland, tonsils, and bone marrow. Lymph nodes filter lymph fluid, removing bacteria, viruses, and other foreign substances.

Lymphocytes, as previously discussed, are types of white blood cell that fight infections. They are made in the bone marrow, develop in the thymus, and can be activated in the spleen and lymph nodes where they circulate and access the blood and the lymph vessels. Lymphocytes have incredible specificity, recognizing foreign cells and acting quickly to destroy them. There are two main types of lymphocytes: B-lymphocytes and T-lymphocytes. B-lymphocytes develop into plasma cells that produce proteins known as antibodies. Antibodies circulate in the blood and react with toxins, bacteria, and some cancer cells. The antibodies target only the antigen on the surface it has been programmed to attack. The body can then identify and remove these unwanted substances. However, some invaders can evade B-lymphocytes by growing inside the body's own cells. This is where T-lymphocytes come into play. They sense when the body's own cells have become infected and destroy them directly. T-lymphocytes help the body fight viral infections and destroy abnormal or cancerous cells. Once an invader has been destroyed, surviving B-lymphocytes and T-lymphocytes develop into specialized memory cells on guard in case the particular antigen is encountered again.

One of the non-profit organizations that we were involved with had a slogan that lymphoma research was the Rosetta stone, unlocking the mysteries of cancer. This is true, but we took an important additional step, stating that blood cancer research is the superhighway to curing cancer.

The evidence of history establishes that lymphoma and leukemia research has produced tremendous results in medical research that extend well beyond blood cancers. So many cancer treatments were developed through lymphoma and leukemia research. Stem cell transplantation, combination chemotherapy, monoclonal antibodies, vaccines, and other therapies used on lymphoma have proven to be successful with other forms of cancer. Even Tamoxifen, which did not prove to be effective for lymphoma, has been an effective form of treatment for some breast cancers. During clinical trials of Rituxan (a monoclonal therapy) on lymphoma patients, it was discovered that it was efficacious for rheumatoid arthritis. The FDA has since approved it for use in rheumatoid arthritis patients.

Fundamentally, blood testing and research has an advantage of accessibility over solid tumors. Additionally, the blood plays a central role in cancer development and eradication. Solid tumors—such as prostate cancer, colon cancer, and breast cancer often are readily treatable when localized. These tumors can spread or metastasize. As the American Association for Cancer Research Cancer Progress Report says, [m]etastasis is the spread of cancer from a primary tumor to other areas of the body where the cancer cells establish new tumors . . . It is the most lethal attribute of cancer cells that is responsible for more than 90% of the morbidity and mortality associated with cancer. Therefore, studying the fundamental properties of metastasis is essential to conquering cancer." www.aacr.org/Uploads/DocumentRepository/2011CPR/2011_AACR_CPR_Text_web.pdf.

How does cancer spread? The blood and lymph systems are major highways for cancer to spread. Conversely, if you can cut off the blood supply to tumors, the tumors may die. Once again, the role of the immune system in eradicating cancer cells before they spread cannot be ignored. Blood cancer research is critical.

There is more to the story. The white blood cells are the body's patrol warriors continuously identifying and killing bacteria, viruses, and cancer cells. The B and T lymphocytes require previous exposure to agents of disease in order to recognize and attack them. There are important cells that do not need prior exposure to a disease agent to mobilize against it. These cells are aptly named Natural Killer Cells or NK cells. They detect invaders, contact them, and attack the invaders by unleashing poisons. NK cells release perforin that forms a passageway through the cancer cell's membranes and granzymes that activate the cancer cell's self-destruction mechanism, causing the death of the cancer cells. The remains of the cancer cells are digested by the macrophages.

Inflammation also plays a role in cancer and immune cells play a role in inflammation. Immune cells gearing up to heal lesions produce inflammation. Cancer cells also need to produce inflammation to sustain growth. Growing tumors use the same inflammation substances that the immune cells use (cytokines, prostaglandins, and leukotrienes) to reproduce and spread. The over production of inflammation can neutralize the white blood cells. Some studies suggest that patients on anti-inflammatory medication (such as ibuprofen) may receive benefits in the form of decreased incidence of cancer.

The mind and body work together. At some level, we all understand that stress plays a role in bringing on cancer and hindering recovery from the disease. There are physiological reasons that account for the impact of stress and other emotions. Prolonged emotional stress, anger, despair, or feelings of helplessness can lead to chronic release of noradrenaline and cortisol which stimulate inflammation. The white blood cells of the immune system—NK cells, T lymphocytes, and B lymphocytes—appear to be hampered considerably by feelings of helplessness and the loss of the will to live. The will to live plays an important role in defeating cancer. The interaction of exposures and the body's immune response to them play a big role in cancer. The immune system plays a major role in understanding cancer, preventing cancer, treating cancer, and curing cancer. To be sure, there is synergy in cancer research. If you are battling or committed to defeating a particular form of cancer, support that research. But if you have blood cancer or are looking to make inroads to curing cancer in general, support blood cancer research. We believe that, empirically and intuitively, lymphoma and blood cancer research is the superhighway to curing cancer. Let's get on the superhighway to curing cancer.

We fully believe that our national plan for curing cancer must involve prevention, screening, fundraising, advocacy, research, and public policy for all of the hideous forms of cancer.

Prevention: Benjamin Franklin, the tenth son of a soap maker, had an extraordinary life. Printing, discovering electricity, engaging in politics, and providing enduring wisdom are among the achievements of this amazing man. Most of us learned Mr. Franklin's adage that "an ounce of prevention is worth a pound of cure" early in life from our parents. In turns out that Mr. Franklin's wisdom applies to cancer.

It is worth repeating that a substantial proportion of cancers could be prevented, including all cancers caused by tobacco use and other unhealthy behaviors. According to the American Cancer Society Cancer Facts & Figures 2021: "Excluding non-melanoma skin cancer, at least 42% of newly diagnosed cancers in the US – about 797,000 cases in 2021 – are potentially avoidable, including the 19% of cancers caused by smoking and at least 18% caused by a combination of excess body weight, alcohol consumption, poor nutrition, and physical inactivity. Certain cancers caused by infectious agents, such as human papillomavirus (HPV), hepatitis B virus (HBV), hepatitis C virus (HCV), and Helicobacter pylori (H. pylori), could be prevented through behavioral changes or vaccination to avoid the infection, or by treating the infection. Many of the more than 5 million skin cancers diagnosed annually could be prevented by protecting skin from excessive sun exposure and not using indoor tanning devices. In addition, screening can help prevent colorectal and cervical cancers by detecting and removing precancers in the colon, rectum, and uterine cervix. Screening can also detect these and some other cancers early, when treatment is often less intensive and more successful. Screening is known to reduce mortality for cancers of the breast, colon, rectum, cervix, lung (among people who smoke, or used to smoke), and probably prostate."

We must invest more in programs to reduce obesity in school children and educate and instill lifelong habits of proper diet and exercise. We have engaged in bringing about these important lifestyle changes as members of the National Board of Selectors of Jefferson Awards for Public Service.

Investing more money in cancer research: Over the years, many Democrats, Republicans, and Independents have been champions for people battling cancer. Many more have fallen short of the mark. Currently, our government's commitment to curing cancer—as opposed to the tremendous commitment demonstrated by so many dedicated patients, family members, advocates, physicians, and researchers—is underwhelming.

Our country always has been the world leader in so many important categories, including medical research and development. Given that one in two men and more than one in three women in America will be diagnosed with cancer during their lifetimes, "the bell" likely will toll for many people that you know and love on account of cancer. Devoting more resources to cancer research is the right thing to do because it will save lives and reduce suffering of all Americans. Devoting more resources to cancer research also is the sensible thing to do from the standpoint of saving taxpayers' money, encouraging growth and investment, and creating productive jobs. Now more than ever is the time for us to be Americans—not American's—with respect to cancer research.

This collection of more than 200 complex diseases with an untold number of subtypes that we generically refer to as "cancer" exacts a tremendous cost on the country and the world.

Cancer research has yielded a large return on investment. JAMA reports "investments in cancer R&D have been quite worthwhile—producing a value to society far in excess of costs—we estimated a consumer surplus of $1.9 trillion. Thus, even when increases in cancer costs are taken into account, cancer survival gains were of tremendous value to patients." http://jama.ama-assn.org/content/303/11/1084.short. Few areas of government spending can match the fabulous return on investment realized from cancer research.

Squeaky wheels get oiled and cancer patients, survivors, and those impacted by the disease are not squeaky enough. We must insist that the government prosecute the war on cancer more vigorously and put in place the resources for a prompt and complete victory. We also must do our part by raising money for cancer research. It is not enough to donate or fundraise for an organization. We must insist that the money is used wisely and efficiently on research with proper designs and on research that makes strategic sense.

A tangible example of how cancer research saves lives: Research has paid important dividends for cancer patients and there are many recent examples. Treatments that were in clinical trials a few years ago are live-saving staples today. Research is laborious, time-consuming, expensive, and can be hit or miss. But one development can spiral into lifesaving treatments for thousands of patients. Developing an effective drug is difficult, but is only part of the battle. You have to get a drug to market, keep it on the market, and prevent the government from defunding it out of existence. Criticize drug companies all you want, but they play a vital role. Praise governmental agencies all you would like, but often regulation is more of a detriment than a protector.

Ultimately, it is incumbent upon those of us impacted by cancer to make sure that the government, big "non-profits," and the drug companies focus on making life-saving treatments available. Life-saving treatments do not magically appear, they are the result of many false starts and failures, the investment of considerable money in cancer research (money that comes from pharmaceutical companies seeking money, government funding, and private donations), years of work, and the devotion of talented scientists. Now let's look at a real life example of how blood cancer research is the super highway to cancer research and why that highway runs through Chicago.

As we eluded to earlier, "Gleevec" has been a miracle drug for patients with chronic myelogenous leukemia or CML. According to the American Association for Cancer Research "a diagnosis of CML was akin to death sentence until 2001, when a novel drug, called imatinib mesylate (Gleevec), was approved by the FDA. Now, the 5-year survival rate for CML has climbed to 95%." The American Cancer Society previously reported that the 5-year survival rate from CML went from 31% for cases diagnosed during the period of 1990-1992 to 55% for those diagnosed from 2001-2007.

Chicago's Hyde Park was home to one of the world's leading cancer researchers. Dr. Janet Rowley rode her red bicycle from her Hyde Park home to her laboratory at the University of Chicago every day. Scott was interviewing one of the doctors at the University of Chicago for the radio show when he met Dr. Rowley for the first time. He was awestruck because he was well aware of her landmark work. "Just call me Janet" said this scientist who changed the face of cancer research. We had the privilege of dinning with Dr. Rowley and her husband Donald (a renowned doctor in his own right) on multiple occasions. Dr. Rowley's work established that cancer is a genetic disease. She proved that mutations in critical genes lead to specific forms of leukemia and lymphoma and she demonstrated that one can determine the form of cancer present in a patient directly from the cancer's genes. So what? The Philadelphia chromosome. This changed the way cancer was understood, opened the door to development of drugs directed at the cancer-specific genetic abnormalities, and created a paradigm that continues to drive cancer research. In short, Dr. Rowley was known as the matriarch of cancer genetic research. She opened the door to the age of individualized cancer treatment and targeted treatment. It did not happen overnight, her work dates back to the early 1960s, with major breakthroughs in the 1970s. Dr. Rowley's work resulted in the drug known as Gleevec discussed above and later to even more effective drugs. One development leads to another. Dr. Rowley was awarded the Presidential Medal of Freedom in 2009.

This story illustrates the importance of research and the major benefits resulting from the cogent investment of time and money with world class researchers such as Dr. Rowley. It also exposes fundamental flaws in our research grant system. Proven researchers such as Dr. Rowley should not have to spend so much time filling out grant forms—there should be fast track approval for established researchers. Finally, it proves what Charlene often says "one person can make a difference." You can watch or listen to our interview with Dr. Michelle Le Beau, Director of the University of Chicago Cancer Research Center, where we discuss leukemia research and Dr. Rowley's work and you can also watch Charlene's interview with Dr. Rowley – which was the last or one of the last substantive interviews of Dr. Rowley on our *Battling and Beating Cancer* shows.

Sharing information: Steps need to be taken to encourage and facilitate the sharing of information. The quest for money, informational superiority, and prestige factor into life at hospitals, non-profit organizations, medical centers, and research facilities and have repressed the sharing of knowledge. Having leading clinicians and researchers sharing knowledge, insights, and the results will reduce wasteful and duplicative efforts and accelerate the pace and number of breakthroughs. Through meetings and the internet, a cross-section of researchers, clinicians, and patients should communicate, share information, and make refinements. The vision of separate scientists locked up in their labs and maintaining secrecy is not acceptable. The stakes are too high. For this reason, we have worked hard to have researchers, institutions, and advocates collaborate. Collaboration among institutions now is becoming the norm rather than the exception.

Curing cancer plans: Doctors and scientists often point out that scientific research and developments do not lend themselves to business plans. Research and development of all sorts of products and industries are part of business plans. The various consortiums and scientific advisory boards for the various cancers must each come together with a plan for curing the type of cancers within their respective domains.

In 2003, the Director of the National Cancer Institute challenged the nation "to eliminate the suffering and death due to cancer by 2015." The strategic objectives to reach the outcome include preempting cancer at every opportunity by understanding the causes and mechanisms of cancer, accelerating progress in cancer prevention, improving early detection and diagnosis, and developing effective treatments and ensuring the best outcomes for all by understanding the factors that influence cancer outcomes, improving the quality of cancer care and life for patients and their families, and overcoming health disparities. You can obtain a copy of the NCI Strategic Plan on its website, www.cancer. gov. The date has come and gone, but the idea of setting a target date makes sense.

We believe that all of the organizations and institutes should set a goal of curing all cancers by 2040 and come up with very specific and detailed plans for curing the type of cancer or cancers they are involved in by that date. Adjustments can be made along the way.

We still have such a long way to go. In the aggregate, to defeat cancer we need to commit a lot more money to research, invest it in cogent research, have researchers "reach to the next level," and have the researchers share their results.

Educating cancer patients and the general population: Educational programming always is needed to teach and implement what we know about prevention, reduction of risk, optimal treatments, and the importance of early diagnosis.

Educating physicians and health care providers: Patients expect their "learned intermediaries" such as doctors to know all of the treatments options and make the best recommendations to them. Unfortunately, that is not always the case. Many times doctors simply do not have the necessary information or breadth or depth of experience.

Testing and screening: There are meaningful tests and screenings that are excellent (although not perfect) for detecting various forms of cancer and early diagnosis and treatment greatly increases the likelihood of a cure. People need to get the appropriate screenings. Loved ones need to pressure their family members to get the appropriate screenings. Healthcare providers must re-examine notions about screenings. For example, many women are getting breast cancer at ages significantly younger than the age recommended for initial mammograms. This is unacceptable. The criteria must be reviewed periodically and revised when warranted.

Hope: Where there is life, there is hope. It is important that organizations, government representatives, physicians, nurses, healthcare providers, and researchers provide the twin gifts of life and hope to cancer patients.

Urgency: It is also important that these same individuals and entities move forward with the urgency demanded as so many lives hang in the balance. It is time to make curing cancer a much greater priority. In our experience, the passion, energy, and commitment of volunteers invested in curing cancer makes volunteers much more effective than paid staff members of non-profit organizations. Professional staff have their role to play and can bring important skills to the equation. But committed volunteers must lead the effort. Let's be Americans, not Americants, when it comes to curing cancer. This is a national call to action to cure cancer and commit to taking the actions and dedicating the resources necessary to accomplish this mission.

As discussed in the final chapter, an approach of the magnitude and with the urgency as that employed for the COVID-19 pandemic should be used to eradicate cancer.

CHAPTER 22

THE IMPACT OF THE COVID-19 PANDEMIC

The impact of COVID-19 on people with cancer will not be known fully for several years. The pandemic may be winding down in some parts of the world, but is far from being in the world's rear view mirror. As we write new variants are emerging and substantial issues exist as to whether and to what extent COVID-19 will be a matter that the United States and the world will have to deal with for an extended period of time. Although data continues to roll in and considerable analysis and research remains to be done, it is not too early to begin examining the impact COVID-19 has had on the cancer world and to consider lessons learned as we move into the later part of 2021.

COVID-19 in people with cancer: One issue early on was whether people with cancer or undergoing treatment for cancer are more likely to acquire COVID-19 or are more likely to have severe disease or to die from the disease than people in the population at large. People with cancer are generally viewed to be more susceptible to infectious agents because of their impaired immune systems due to the cancer itself or its treatments such as surgery, chemotherapy, radiation, or immunotherapy. However, factors that have been most consistently linked with increased risk of severe disease and/or death from COVID-19 in patients with cancer mirror those in the general population. These appear to include male sex, age 60 and older, a history of smoking, obesity, hypertension, cardiovascular disease, and diabetes. The early data has been mixed.

The American Cancer Society has reported in its Cancer Facts and Figures 2021 that some early studies suggested that COVID-19 patients with cancer were at higher risk for severe complications or death than those without cancer, especially individuals with lung and blood cancers.

However, larger, more recent studies have produced conflicting findings. The American Cancer Society correctly points out that prospective studies with long-term follow up are needed to better understand the effects of COVID-19 in patients with cancer. In sum, though we know cancer patients have suffered mightily from the pandemic, additional time and studies are required to determine whether and to what extent cancer patients were adversely impacted as compared to the overall population as a direct result of contracting COVID-19.

It is beyond cavil that the COVID-19 pandemic has had numerous consequences that have adversely impacted the cancer community. Early in the pandemic health care resources were diverted away from cancer and other patients to address a rapidly growing number of individuals ill with COVID-19, to protect health care workers, and to protect healthy people from exposure to the virus. So-called "non-urgent" health care was delayed and even suspended and some of the treatments delayed may not actually have been "non-urgent."

Delays in cancer screening, diagnosis, genetic testing, and treatment due to reduced health care access likely will result in a short-term drop in cancer diagnoses, but certainly will be followed by increases in late-stage diagnoses and preventable cancer deaths. The intermediate and long-term impacts will be monitored closely. More people will die from cancer due to the pandemic.

Many individuals delayed and still continue to delay preventive care and symptom follow-up due to fear of exposure to COVID-19, loss of employment, and/or employer-based health care. At the onset of the pandemic, the American Cancer Society and other organizations recommended that routine cancer screenings and other elective medical procedures be postponed in order to prioritize urgent medical needs and reduce the spread of COVID-19. This guidance, along with fear of contracting the virus in health care settings and limited access at health care facilities, resulted in a steep drop in screening. One electronic medical record company reported an estimated 80% to 90% decline in screening for breast, colorectal, and cervical cancers among their patient population during March and April of 2020 compared to the same time period in 2019. Screenings for these cancers had risen by June of 2020, but was still down 29% to 36% from pre-pandemic levels. HPV vaccinations dropped 73% between February and April 2020, which could impact cervical cancer patients adversely through delayed diagnosis.

As we point out elsewhere, early and proper diagnosis of cancer saves lives. It also often results in a less rigorous course of treatment then the more intense treatments often associated with advanced disease. Alternative tests – such as in-home stool-based screening tests for colon and rectal cancers – have been used with increased frequency. One study of diagnostics data reported that, among people who received medical testing for any reason, there was a 46% decline in diagnoses of six common cancers (breast, colorectal, lung, pancreas, stomach, and esophagus) during March 1 to April 18, 2020, compared with January 6, 2019, to February 29, 2020, ranging from a 25% drop for pancreatic cancer to 52% for breast cancer.

Cancer treatments also have been delayed. The American Cancer Society Cancer Action Network began surveying cancer patients and survivors in late March 2020 to examine the influence of the pandemic on health care delivery. In May 2020, 79% of respondents in active treatment reported delays in their care, up from 27% in April. The most commonly reported delays were for in-person provider visits (57%), imaging services (25%), surgical procedures (15%), and access to supportive services (20%), including physical therapy or mental health care.

Additionally, behavioral changes during the pandemic and related shut downs, such as weight gain, physical inactivity, and alcohol consumption likely will present long-term health consequences. The increase in abuse, depression, mental disease, and suicide takes its toll on people and families with cancer as well. The financial stress and potential loss of health insurance also cannot be ignored.

In sum, the COVID-19 pandemic is expected to result in increased cancer mortality over the long term due to delayed diagnoses, interruptions or alterations in potentially curative treatment, the possibility that some adults will abandon prior patterns of preventive care, and other factors. The National Cancer Institute estimated a 1% increase in deaths from breast and colorectal cancer over the next 10 years, the equivalent of approximately 10,000 excess deaths due to the pandemic's impact on screening and treatment. The American Cancer Society suggests this may be an underestimate because models assumed a 6-month disruption in care followed by the return to routine care, which has since proven too optimistic. A similar study estimated that cancer diagnosis delays in England would result in additional deaths ranging from 5% for lung cancer to about 15% for colorectal cancer. Future studies and analysis will provide better insights into the impact of the COVID-19 pandemic on cancer patients.

Lessons learned and changes to health care delivery: The experience of the pandemic has taught us several lessons that may alter cancer treatment and result in some improvements for cancer patients. During the pandemic, health care providers transitioned many patient visits to virtual care, consisting of telephone or video consultations. Telemedicine allows receipt of many aspects of necessary care remotely while minimizing transmission of the coronavirus or other infectious agents to clinicians and patients. Telemedicine was not widely used prior to the pandemic, despite evidence of substantial patient interest, in large part due to restricted reimbursement. The landscape had begun to change in recent years because of increased passage by many states of parity laws that require private insurers to reimburse for telemedicine services. Changes in federal and state policy in March 2020 facilitated the rapid expansion of telemedicine by granting equal reimbursement and relaxing Health Insurance Portability and Accountability Act (HIPAA) requirements to allow for the use of video, telephone, and text-based applications and reducing the burden of multi-state licensing requirements for out-of-state providers. Although some of these changes may be temporary, one can envision benefits to cancer patients long term by being able to use telemedicine appropriately, particularly where travel presents difficulties or where exposure of immune compromised patients to a variety of infectious agents can be limited. It may expand access to additional consultations and provides greater flexibility to patients and health care providers alike. In short, the pandemic helped usher in the age of telemedicine.

In 2020. ASCO established the Steering Group on Cancer Care Delivery and Research in a Post-Pandemic Environment to evaluate the changes made in oncology care delivery, clinical research, and regulatory oversight in response to the COVID-19 pandemic as well as to make recommendations on how to proceed as the pandemic subsides. In December 2020, ASCO published its recommendations for adopting a broad set of reforms to improve patient access to high-quality cancer care and participation in clinical trials as well as how to address the pandemic's devastating effects on both patients and oncology health care providers. Many of the recommendations relate to simplifications of the delivery of health care and reducing regulatory and administrative burdens on health care providers and patients. Among the positive consequences of the pandemic were changes to research procedures that benefited patients, including allowing patients to virtually consent to trials and receive study-related treatment at local facilities. The FDA and the National Cancer Institute relaxed regulations and procedures in clinical trial participation while prioritizing the safety of trial participants and researchers during the pandemic. Many of these changes should be carried forward. Where possible, investigational oral drugs were shipped to patients' homes with greater frequency instead of having them travel to the trial site and with increased frequency patients have had lab work done in local facilities near their home. All of that enabled more patients to participate in clinical trials. Prioritizing patients with cancer for vaccination is another item many advocate. As of this writing the effectiveness of vaccines on patients undergoing certain forms of treatment is subject to study.

Appropriate reduction of regulatory and systemic burdens is a major lesson learned. Perhaps, the most important lesson learned from the pandemic is that a large investment in cancer research and a cooperative approach between the government and private sectors will save millions of lives. The impact of cancer – although it is more diffuse inasmuch as it involves hundreds of diseases – in terms of morbidity, mortality, and economic and humanomic costs is far greater than that imposed by the pandemic.

More aggressive government spending and public private partnerships needed to eradicate cancer. As previously stated, Operation Warp Speed resulted in multiple, effective vaccines being developed, brought to market, and administered to people in record time. Coordination, public/private partnerships, and government investment in research figured prominently in the success of that effort. Cancer research also figured prominently as it yielded the platform for the vaccines. Relaxation of regulation to allow for emergency use authorization of the vaccines and therapeutics was also important. A similar investment and sustained effort would have a major impact on eradicating cancer. Cancer advocates must make a hard push in the months and years ahead. Curing cancer in many ways is tougher and focusing a sustained effort may be more difficult because we actually are dealing with hundreds of diseases. We can and must make a much larger investment in cancer research – more money and now!

The importance of consulting with a doctor you trust. Unfortunately, some information about the virus, treatment options, vaccines, masks, and the pandemic is not accurate or complete. This situation still is evolving and there remains much to be learned. "Science" has been politicized far too much in the context of COVID-19.

In making decisions about your health and the health of your family, we urge people to do their own research, think critically, evaluate information carefully, and above all confer with a physician that they trust. It is particularly important for cancer patients to obtain input of their oncologists and other doctors regarding vaccines, precautions, and therapies. This will assist you in evaluating the information and undertaking the course of action appropriate for you in light of your medical history and conditions.

The importance of common sense infection control: Many of the points that we have made about handwashing, protective gear, staying away from people with infections, and staying home when you are or suspect you may be sick in the context of protecting yourself against infection as a result of a compromised immune system have taken on greater urgency due to the pandemic. Hopefully, people have learned and will apply these protective practices going forward.

COVID-19 continues to take lives and make people sick. New variants emerge as the virus transmogrifies. Vaccine boosters are becoming available as of the writing of this edition. Events will continue to unfold and new data and studies will continue to come in for an extended period of time. We will continue to learn much more about the pandemic over the next several years. We suspect that HCRF has not yet hosted the last episode of *Cancer & COVID Talks* with Dr. Platanias.

We would be remiss if we did not end this chapter by expressing our heartfelt sympathies for those impacted by COVID-19 and by remembering those lost to the pandemic. We also wish to thank all of the wonderful people who saved lives and helped people during the pandemic.

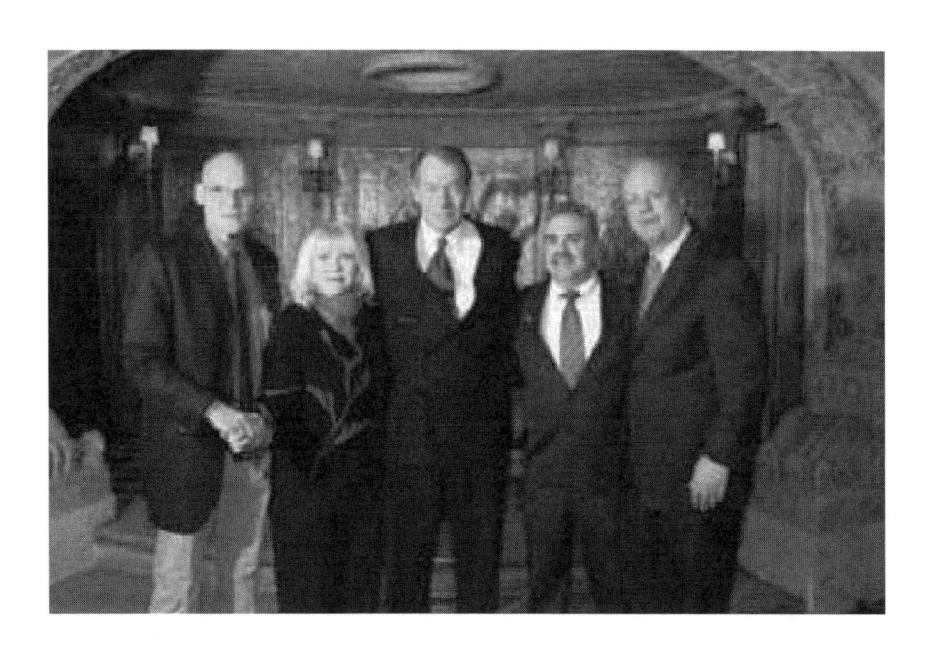

Charlene and Scott with James Carville, Charlie Rose, and Karl Rove. Curing cancer requires cogent strategy and commitment across the aisle.

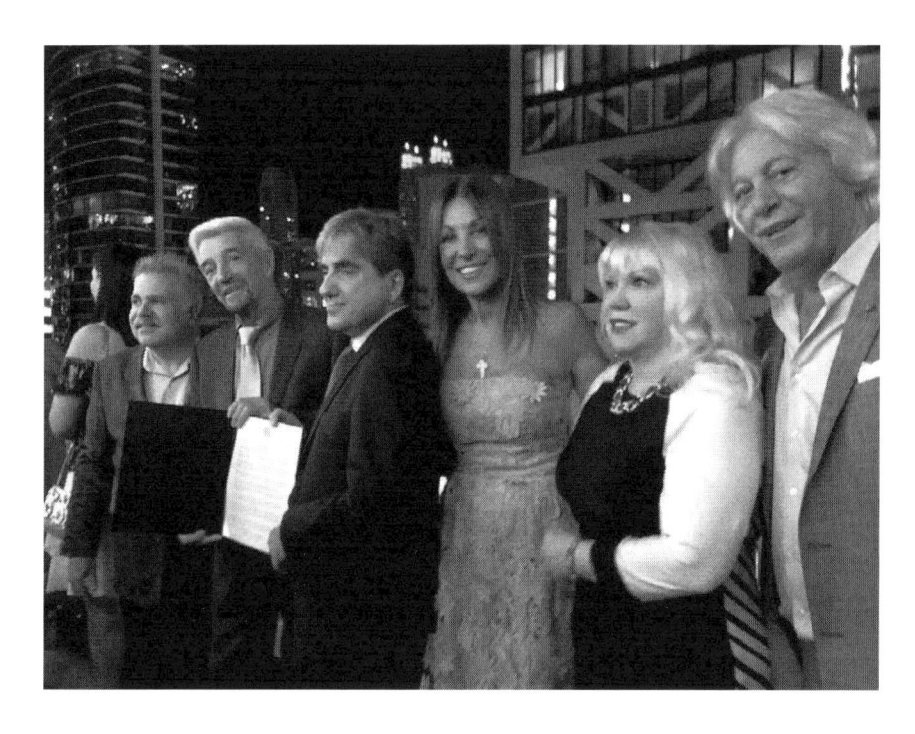

Presentation of Hippocratic Cancer Research Foundation Day Proclamation with Tom Dreesen, Dr. Platanias, Eleni Bousis, and Jimmy Bousis joining Charlene and Scott.

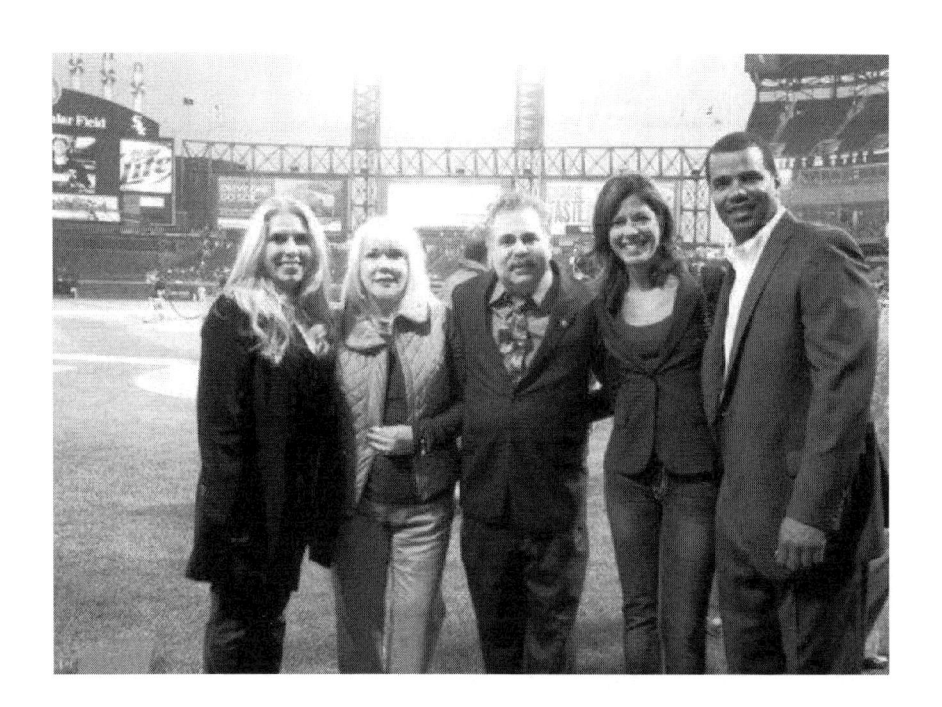

Charlene and Scott on US Cellular Field with CNN's Zoraida Sambolin and White Sox General Manager Kenny Williams.

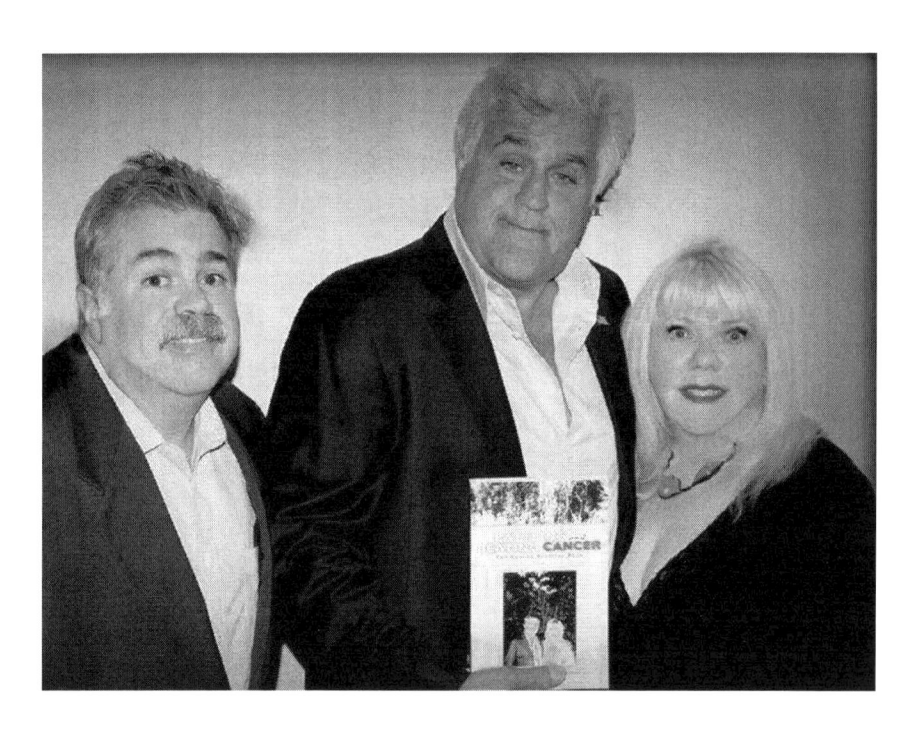

Charlene and Scott with Jay Leno.

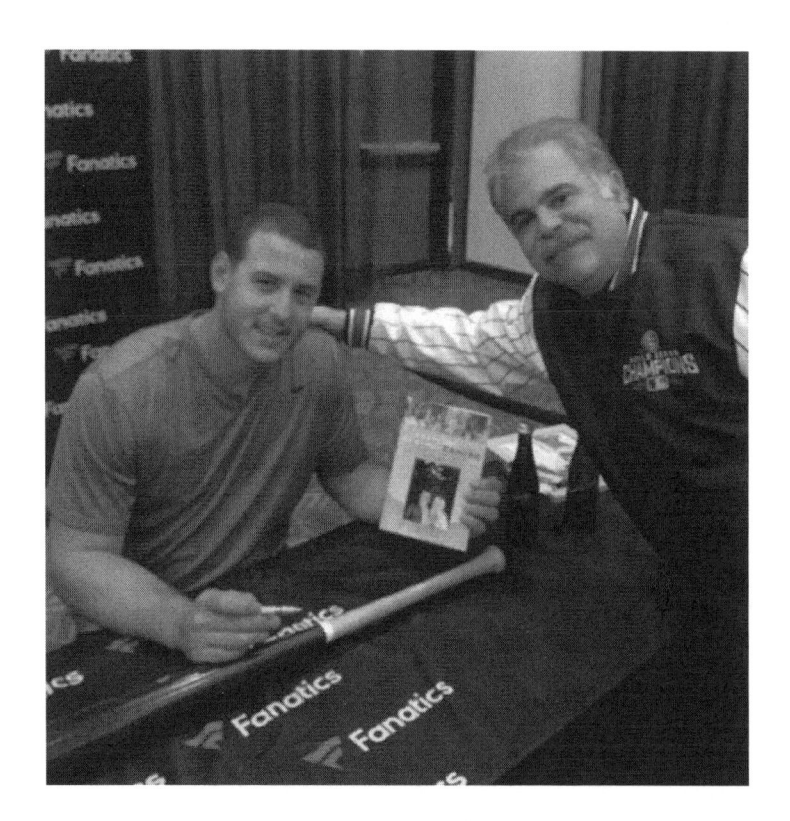

Former Chicago Cub and Lymphoma Survivor Anthony Rizzo.

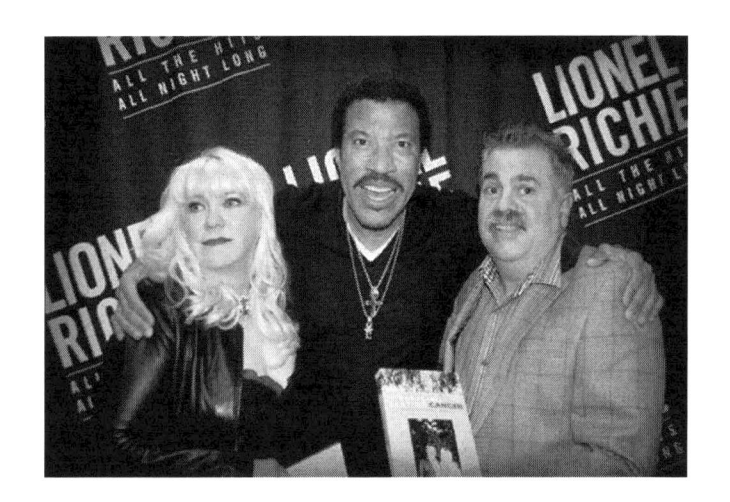

Charlene and Scott with Lionel Richie.

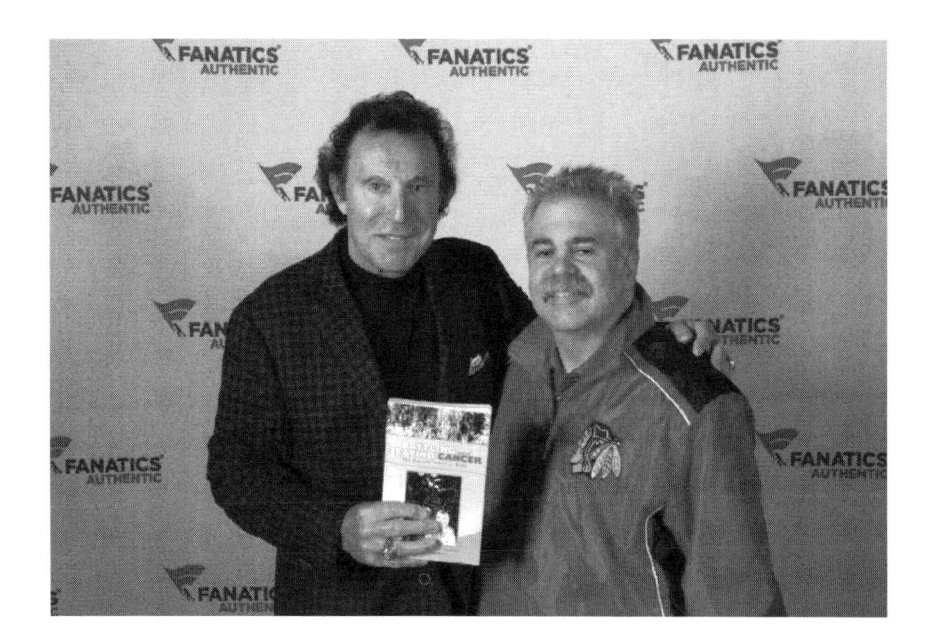

Blackhawk Hall-Of-Fame Goalie Tony Esposito recently died of pancreatic cancer.

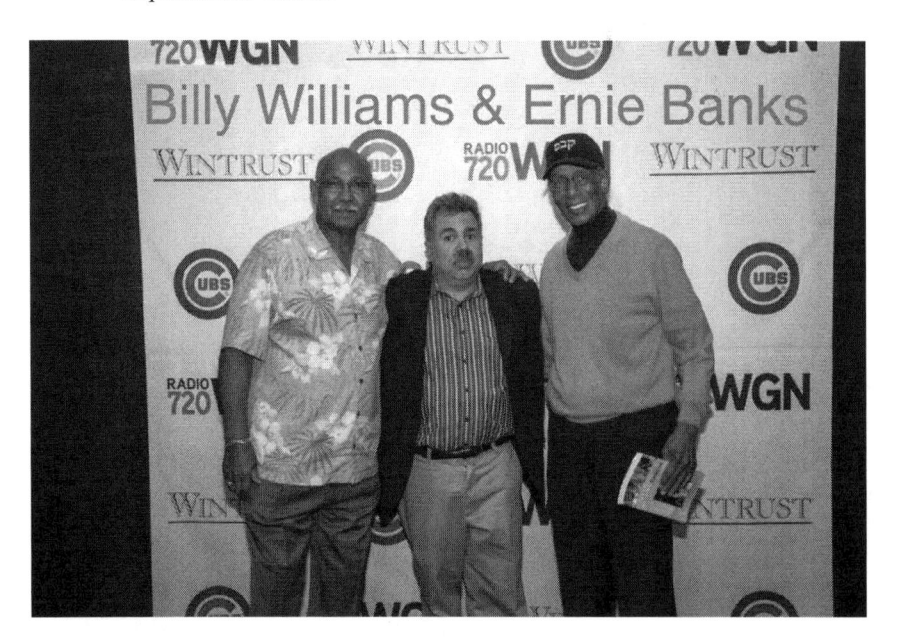

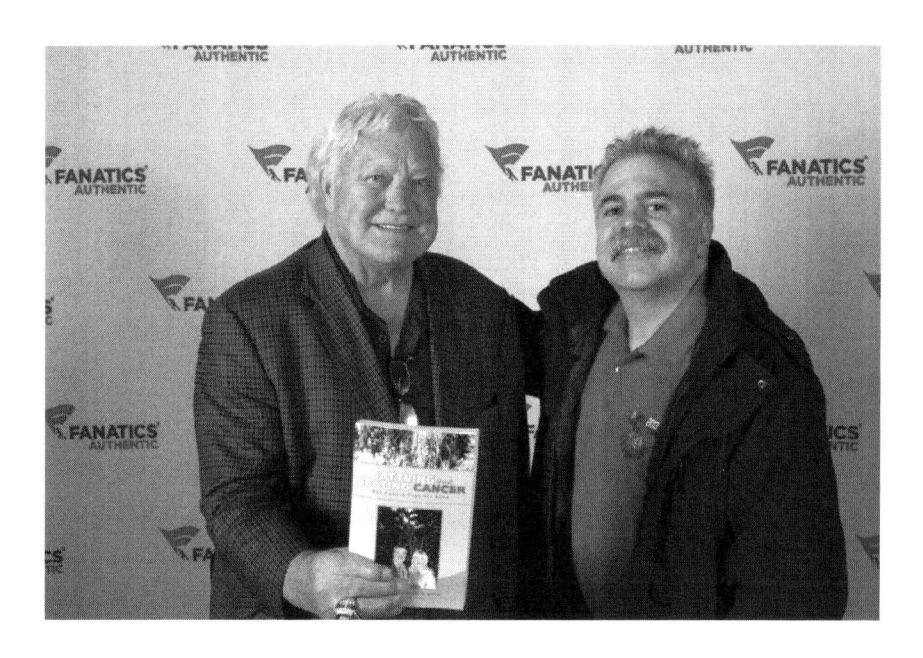

The Golden Jet Bobby Hull.

Charlene and Scott with Harry Connick Jr.

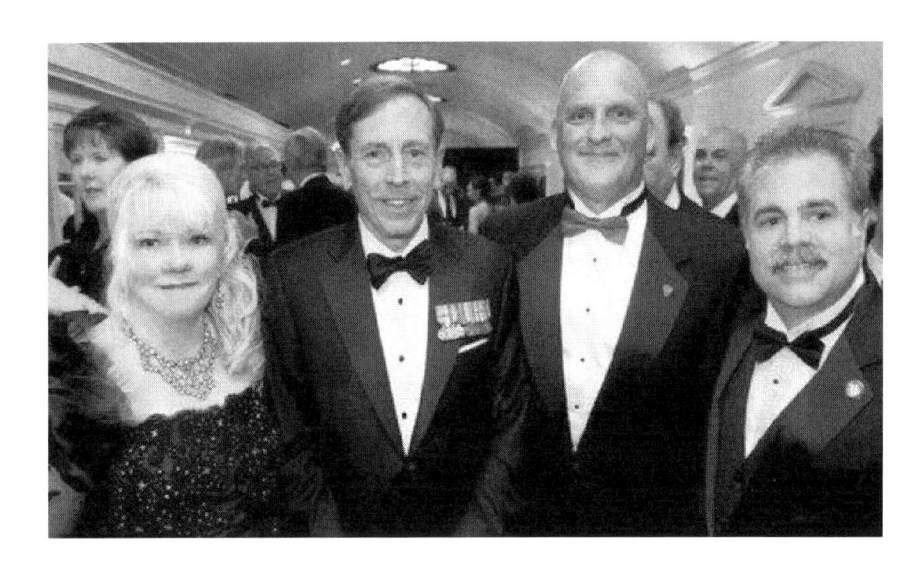

Charlene and Scott with General David Petraeus.

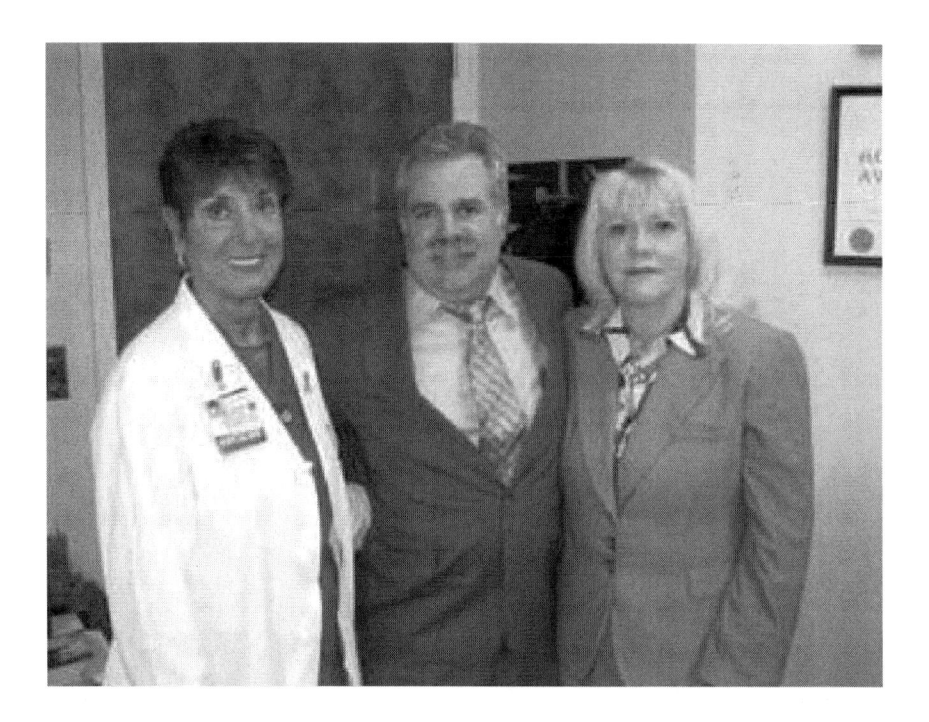

Charlene and Scott with Dr. Stephanie Gregory.

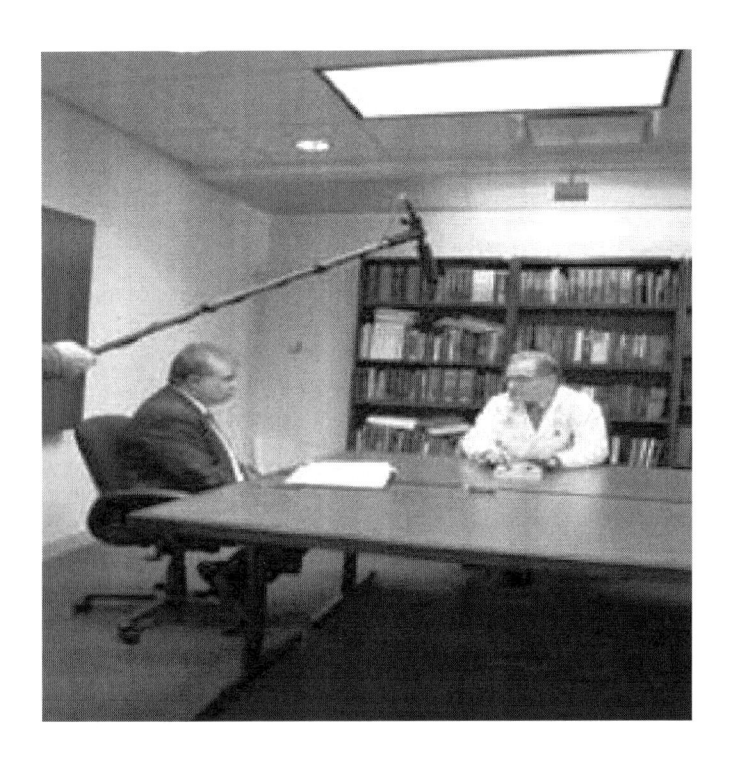

Scott interviewing Dr. Leo Gordon on the *Battling and Beating Cancer Radio Show*, airing on the Blog Talk Radio Network.

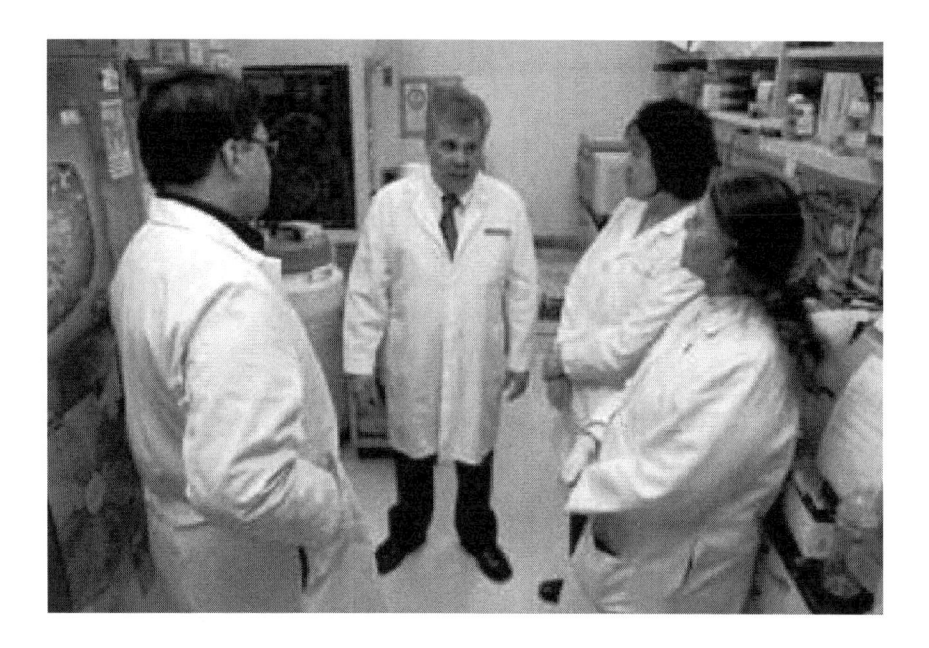

Scott talking with cancer researchers inside the lab.

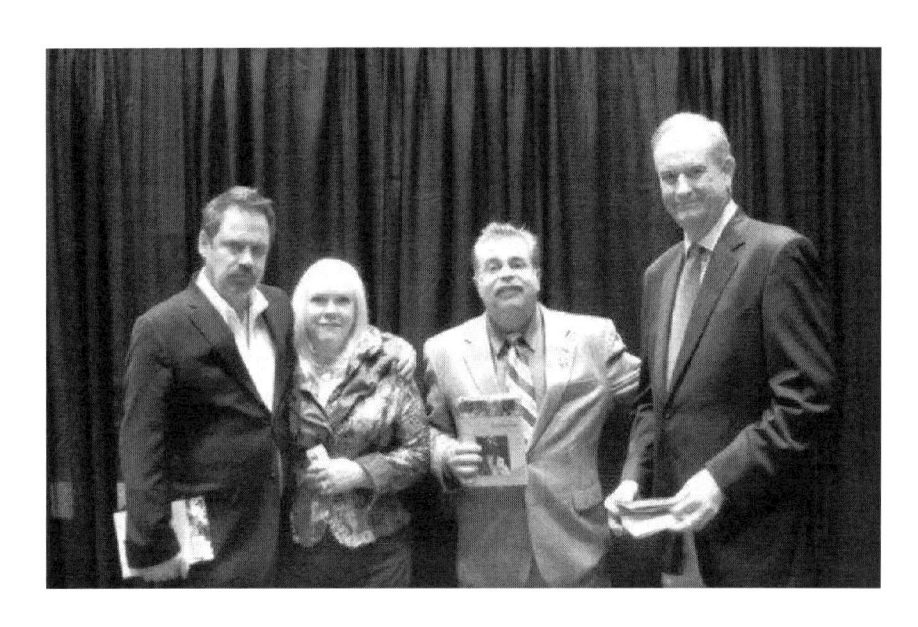

Charlene and Scott comparing notes with Dennis Miller and Bill O'Reilly.

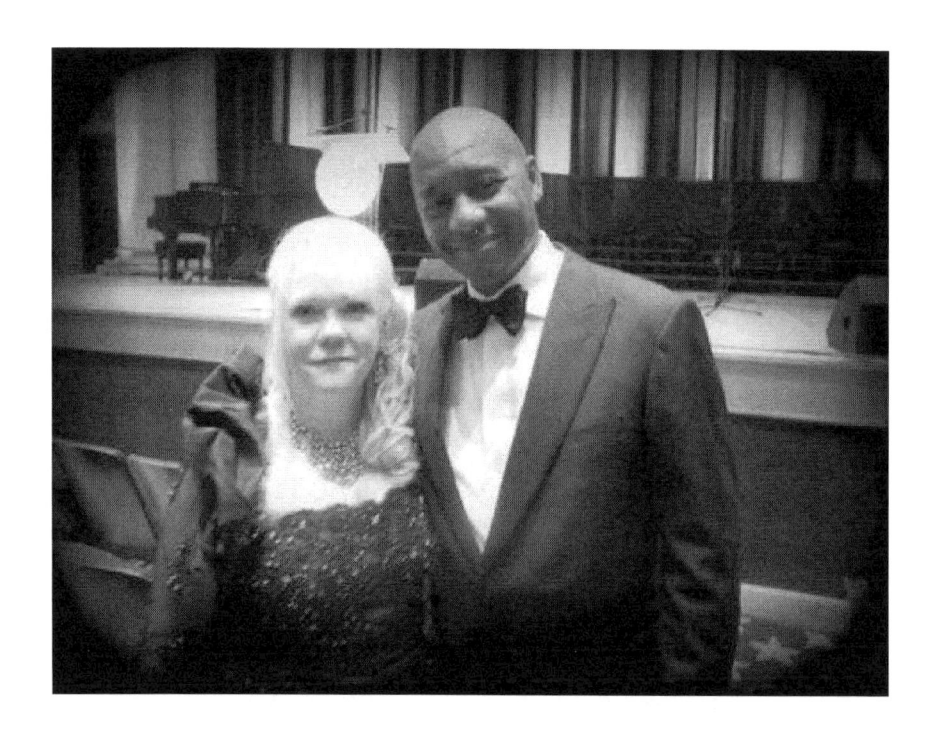

Charlene with Branford Marsalis.

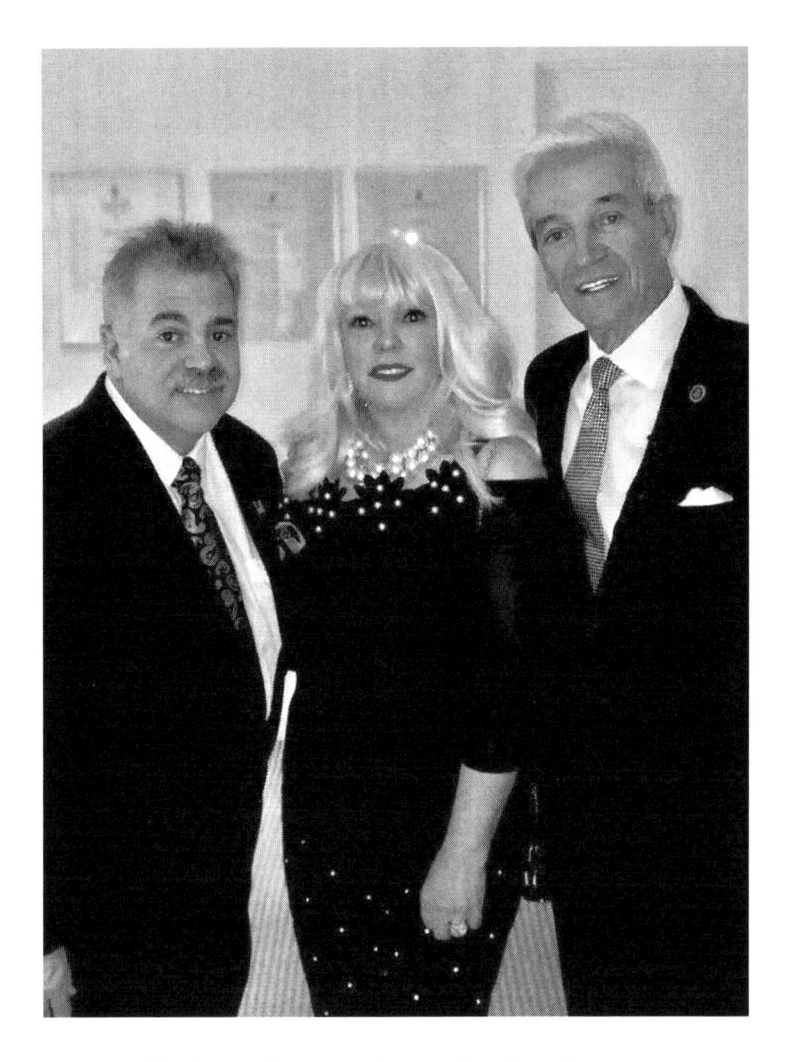

Charlene and Scott with comedian Tom Dreesen.

PART 3

PATIENT'S SURVIVAL COMPENDIUM APPENDICES OF INFORMATION, CHECKLISTS, AND A NOTEBOOK TO HELP YOU CONQUER CANCER

APPENDIX "A"

COMMON CANCER TERMS

DICTIONARY RESOURCES

There are many outstanding medical and cancer dictionaries that are readily accessible online. Accordingly, we have included only a limited number of common cancer terms below. Some of the dictionary resources that we have found to be useful include:

National Cancer Institute: (www.cancer.gov/publications/dictionaries/cancer-terms)
American Cancer Society glossary: (www.cancer.org)
Association of Cancer Online Resources: (www.acor.org)
Rare Cancer: (dictionary.rare-cancer.org)
Medline: (www.nlm.nih.gov/medlineplus/mplusdictionary.html)
MedicineNet: (www.medterms.com)
Stedman's Medical Dictionary: (www.stedmans.com)
Dorland's Medical Dictionary: (www.dorlands.com)

In addition, Gray's Anatomy of the Human Body, which is available online at www.bartleby.com/107, is a helpful resource containing illustrations and descriptions of the human anatomy.

COMMON CANCER TERMS

Adenosquamous carcinoma—a type of cancer that contains two types of cells: squamous cells (thin, flat cells that line select organs) and gland-like cells.

Adjunct therapy—another treatment that is used with the primary treatment for the purpose of assisting the primary treatment.

Allogeneic bone marrow transplant—the procedure by which a patient receives a bone marrow transplant from stem cells of a genetically similar, but not identical, donor.

B cell—a white blood cell that comes from bone marrow. As part of the immune system, B cells make antibodies and help fight infections.

Basal cell carcinoma—a type of skin cancer that arises from the small, round cells found in the lower part (or base) of the outer layer of the skin.

Benign—non-cancerous tumor.

Biopsy—the removal of cells or tissues for examination by a pathologist under a microscope.

Bone marrow—the soft, sponge-like tissue in the center of most bones. Bone marrow produces white blood cells, red blood cells, and platelets.

Bone marrow transplantation—a cancer treatment that involves a procedure to replace bone marrow that has been destroyed by treatment with high doses of anticancer drugs or radiation. Transplantation may be autologous (an individual's own marrow saved before treatment), allogeneic (marrow donated by someone else), or syngeneic (marrow donated by an identical twin).

Cancer—diseases in which abnormal cells divide without control. Cancer cells can invade nearby tissues and can spread to other parts of the body through the blood and lymph systems.

Carcinogen—a substance that causes cancer.

Carcinogenesis—the process by which normal cells turn into cancer cells.

Carcinoma—cancer that begins in the skin or in tissues that line or cover internal organs.

Carcinoma in situ—a group of abnormal cells that remain in the tissue in which they first formed.

CAT scan—a series of detailed pictures of areas inside the body taken from different angles created by a computer linked to an x-ray machine.

CBC—a blood test that checks the number of red blood cells, white blood cells, and platelets (complete blood count).

Chemotherapy—treatment with drugs to kill cancer cells that may be given orally or intravenously.

Complete remission or complete response—the disappearance of all signs of cancer in response to treatment, this does not necessarily mean the cancer is cured.

Debulking—surgical removal of as much of a tumor as possible either to increase the chance that chemotherapy or radiation therapy will kill the remaining cells, to relieve symptoms, or to increase the period of survival.

Diffuse—widely spread as opposed to localized or confined.

Disease-free survival—the length of time after treatment during which a patient survives with no sign of the disease.

Fibroid—a benign smooth-muscle tumor, often in the uterus or gastrointestinal tract.

Five-year survival rate—the percentage of people alive five years after they were diagnosed with or treated for a disease.

Germ cell tumor—a type of tumor that begins in the cells that give rise to sperm or eggs. Germ cell tumors can be located in most parts of the body and can be either benign or malignant.

High-dose chemotherapy—intensive drug treatment that kills cancer cells and destroys the bone marrow, which usually is followed by bone marrow or stem cell transplantation.

High-dose radiation—an amount of radiation that is greater than typical radiation therapy specifically directed at the tumor to avoid damaging healthy tissue.

Histology—the microscopic study of tissues and cells.

Hormonal therapy—treatment that adds, blocks, or removes hormones to stop or slow the growth of some types of tumors.

Immune response—the immune systems actions against foreign substances or antigens.

Incidence—the number of new cases of a disease diagnosed each year.

Indolent—a type of cancer that grows slowly.

Interferon—a biological response modifier that interferes with the division of cancer cells and can slow tumor growth.

Leukemia—cancers that begins in blood-forming tissue such as the bone marrow and causes large numbers of abnormal blood cells to be produced and enter the blood.

Lymphoma—cancers that begin in lymphocytes or the white blood cells of the immune system

Lymph node—a bean type tissue that is surrounded by a capsule of connective tissue. Lymph nodes filter lymph (lymphatic fluid) and they store lymphocytes.

Malignant—cancerous tumors capable of invading and destroying nearby tissue and spreading to other parts of the body.

Metastasis—the spread of cancer from one part of the body to another.

Multiple myeloma—cancers that begin in the cells of the immune system.

Neoplasia—abnormal and uncontrolled cell growth.

Oncology—the study of cancer.

PET scan—a test in which a small amount of radioactive glucose (sugar) is injected into a vein, and a scanner is used to make detailed, computerized pictures of areas inside the body where the glucose is used.

Plasma—the clear, yellowish, fluid part of the blood that carries the blood cells.

Platelet—a type of blood cell that helps prevent bleeding by causing the formation of blood clots.

Polyp—a growth that protrudes from a mucous membrane.

Radioimmunotherapy—a systemic radiation therapy in which a radioactive substance is linked to an antibody that locates and kills tumor cells when injected into the body.

Radiotherapy—a cancer treatment by which high-energy radiation from x-rays, gamma rays, neutrons, protons, and other sources kill cancer cells and shrink tumors. Radiation may come from a machine outside the body (external-beam radiation therapy) or it may come from radioactive material placed in the body near cancer cells (internal radiation therapy).

Sarcoma—a cancer of the bone, cartilage, fat, muscle, blood vessels, or other connective or supportive tissue.

Squamous cell carcinoma—cancer that begins in the thin, flat cells known as squamous cells that are found in the tissue that forms the surface of the skin, the lining of the hollow organs of the body, and the passages of the respiratory and digestive tracts.

Staging—determination of the extent of the cancer within the body for purposes of determining prognosis or treatment of the disease.

Stem cell—a cell from which other types of cells develop.

Stem cell transplantation—replacing immature blood-forming cells that were destroyed by cancer treatment to help the bone marrow recover and continue producing healthy blood cells.

Survivor—a patient who remains alive and continues to function during and after diagnosis. A person is considered to be a survivor from the time of diagnosis.

T cell—a type of white blood cell that attacks virus-infected cells, foreign cells, and cancer cells.

Thymoma—a tumor of the thymus, an organ that is part of the lymphatic system and is located in the chest, behind the breastbone.

Ultrasound—a test in which high-energy sound waves are bounced off internal tissues or organs and make echoes. The echo patterns are shown on the screen of an ultrasound machine, forming a picture of body tissues called a sonogram.

Vaccine—a substance or substances intended to cause the immune system to respond to a tumor or to microorganisms, such as bacteria or viruses. A vaccine can help the body recognize and destroy cancer cells or microorganisms.

APPENDIX "B"

CANCER TYPES

This listing is derived from the National Cancer Institute's Website.

A

Acute Lymphoblastic Leukemia, Adult
Acute Lymphoblastic Leukemia, Childhood
Acute Myeloid Leukemia, Adult
Acute Myeloid Leukemia, Childhood Adrenocortical Carcinoma
Adrenocortical Carcinoma, Childhood
AIDS-Related Cancers
AIDS-Related Lymphoma
Anal Cancer
Appendix Cancer
Astrocytoma, Childhood Cerebellar
Astrocytoma, Childhood Cerebral

B

Basal Cell Carcinoma
Bile Duct Cancer, Extrahepatic
Bladder Cancer
Bladder Cancer, Childhood
Bone Cancer, Osteosarcoma and Malignant Fibrous Histiocytoma
Brain Stem Glioma, Childhood
Brain Tumor, Adult
Brain Tumor, Brain Stem Glioma, Childhood
Brain Tumor, Central Nervous System Embryonal Tumors, Childhood

Brain Tumor, Cerebellar Astrocytoma, Childhood
Brain Tumor, Cerebral Astrocytoma/Malignant Glioma, Childhood
Brain Tumor, Ependymoblastoma, Childhood
Brain Tumor, Ependymoma, Childhood
Brain Tumor, Medulloblastoma, Childhood
Brain Tumor, Medulloepithelioma, Childhood
Brain Tumor, Pineal Parenchymal Tumors of Intermediate Differentiation, Childhood
Brain Tumor, Supratentorial Primitive Neuroectodermal Tumors and Pineoblastoma, Childhood
Brain Tumor, Visual Pathway and Hypothalamic Glioma, Childhood
Brain and Spinal Cord Tumors, Childhood (Other)
Breast Cancer
Breast Cancer, Childhood
Breast Cancer, Male
Bronchial Tumors, Childhood
Burkitt Lymphoma

C

Carcinoid Tumor, Childhood
Carcinoid Tumor, Gastrointestinal
Carcinoma of Unknown Primary
Central Nervous System Embryonal Tumors, Childhood
Central Nervous System Lymphoma, Primary
Cerebellar Astrocytoma, Childhood
Cerebral Astrocytoma/Malignant Glioma, Childhood
Cervical Cancer
Cervical Cancer, Childhood
Childhood Cancers
Chordoma, Childhood
Chronic Lymphocytic Leukemia
Chronic Myelogenous Leukemia
Chronic Myeloproliferative Disorders
Charlene McMann-Seaman & Scott Seaman
Colon Cancer
Colorectal Cancer, Childhood
Cutaneous T-Cell Lymphoma

E

Embryonal Tumors, Central Nervous System, Childhood
Endometrial Cancer
Ependymoblastoma, Childhood
Ependymoma, Childhood
Esophageal Cancer
Esophageal Cancer, Childhood
Ewing Family of Tumors
Extracranial Germ Cell Tumor, Childhood
Extragonadal Germ Cell Tumor
Extrahepatic Bile Duct Cancer
Eye Cancer, Intraocular Melanoma
Eye Cancer, Retinoblastoma

G

Gallbladder Cancer
Gastric (Stomach) Cancer
Gastric (Stomach) Cancer, Childhood
Gastrointestinal Carcinoid Tumor
Gastrointestinal Stromal Tumor (GIST)
Gastrointestinal Stromal Cell Tumor, Childhood
Germ Cell Tumor, Extracranial, Childhood
Germ Cell Tumor, Extragonadal
Germ Cell Tumor, Ovarian
Gestational Trophoblastic Tumor
Glioma, Adult
Glioma, Childhood Brain Stem
Glioma, Childhood Cerebral Astrocytoma
Glioma, Childhood Visual Pathway and Hypothalamic

H

Hairy Cell Leukemia
Head and Neck Cancer
Hepatocellular (Liver) Cancer, Adult (Primary)
Hepatocellular (Liver) Cancer, Childhood (Primary)

Hodgkin Lymphoma, Adult
Hodgkin Lymphoma, Childhood
Hypopharyngeal Cancer
Hypothalamic and Visual Pathway Glioma, Childhood

I

Intraocular Melanoma
Islet Cell Tumors (Endocrine Pancreas)

K

Kaposi Sarcoma
Kidney (Renal Cell) Cancer Kidney Cancer, Childhood

L

Laryngeal Cancer
Laryngeal Cancer, Childhood Leukemia,
Acute Lymphoblastic, Adult Leukemia,
Acute Lymphoblastic, Childhood
Leukemia, Acute Myeloid, Adult
Leukemia, Acute Myeloid, Childhood
Leukemia, Chronic Lymphocytic
Leukemia, Chronic Myelogenous
Leukemia, Hairy Cell
Lip and Oral Cavity Cancer
Liver Cancer, Adult (Primary)
Liver Cancer, Childhood (Primary)
Lung Cancer, Non-Small Cell
Lung Cancer, Small Cell
Lymphoma, AIDS-Related
Lymphoma, Burkitt
Lymphoma, Cutaneous T-Cell
Lymphoma, Hodgkin, Adult
Lymphoma, Hodgkin, Childhood
Lymphoma, Non-Hodgkin, Adult
Lymphoma, Non-Hodgkin, Childhood

Lymphoma, Primary Central Nervous System

M

Macroglobulinemia, Waldenström
Malignant Fibrous Histiocytoma of Bone and Osteosarcoma
Medulloblastoma, Childhood
Medulloepithelioma, Childhood
Melanoma
Melanoma, Intraocular (Eye)
Merkel Cell Carcinoma
Mesothelioma, Adult Malignant
Mesothelioma, Childhood
Metastatic Squamous Neck Cancer with Occult Primary
Mouth Cancer
Multiple Endocrine Neoplasia Syndrome, Childhood
Multiple Myeloma/Plasma Cell Neoplasm
Mycosis Fungoides
Myelodysplastic Syndromes
Myelodysplastic/Myeloproliferative Diseases
Myelogenous Leukemia, Chronic
Myeloid Leukemia, Adult Acute
Myeloid Leukemia, Childhood Acute
Myeloma, Multiple
Myeloproliferative Disorders, Chronic

N

Nasal Cavity and Paranasal Sinus Cancer Nasopharyngeal Cancer
Nasopharyngeal Cancer, Childhood Neuroblastoma
Non-Hodgkin Lymphoma, Adult
Non-Hodgkin Lymphoma, Childhood Non-Small Cell Lung Cancer

O

Oral Cancer, Childhood
Oral Cavity Cancer, Lip and
Oropharyngeal Cancer

Osteosarcoma and Malignant Fibrous Histiocytoma of Bone
Ovarian Cancer, Childhood
Ovarian Epithelial Cancer
Ovarian Germ Cell Tumor
Ovarian Low Malignant Potential Tumor

P

Pancreatic Cancer
Pancreatic Cancer, Childhood
Pancreatic Cancer, Islet Cell Tumors
Papillomatosis, Childhood
Paranasal Sinus and Nasal Cavity Cancer
Parathyroid Cancer
Penile Cancer
Pharyngeal Cancer
Pheochromocytoma
Pineal Parenchymal Tumors of Intermediate Differentiation, Childhood
Pineoblastoma and Supratentorial Primitive Neuroectodermal Tumors, Childhood
Pituitary Tumor
Plasma Cell Neoplasm/Multiple Myeloma
Pleuropulmonary Blastoma
Pregnancy and Breast Cancer
Primary Central Nervous System Lymphoma Prostate Cancer

R

Rectal Cancer
Renal Cell (Kidney) Cancer
Renal Cell (Kidney) Cancer, Childhood
Renal Pelvis and Ureter, Transitional Cell Cancer
Respiratory Tract Carcinoma
Retinoblastoma
Rhabdomyosarcoma, Childhood

S

Salivary Gland Cancer
Salivary Gland Cancer, Childhood
Sarcoma, Ewing Family of Tumors
Sarcoma, Kaposi
Sarcoma, Soft Tissue, Adult
Sarcoma, Soft Tissue, Childhood
Sarcoma, Uterine
Sézary Syndrome
Skin Cancer (Nonmelanoma)
Skin Cancer, Childhood
Skin Cancer (Melanoma)
Skin Carcinoma, Merkel Cell
Small Cell Lung Cancer
Small Intestine Cancer
Soft Tissue Sarcoma, Adult
Soft Tissue Sarcoma, Childhoodv
Squamous Cell Carcinoma
Squamous Neck Cancer with Occult Primary, Metastatic
Stomach (Gastric) Cancer
Stomach (Gastric) Cancer, Childhood
Supratentorial Primitive Neuroectodermal Tumors, Childhood

T

T-Cell Lymphoma, Cutaneous
Testicular Cancer
Throat Cancer
Thymoma and Thymic Carcinoma
Thymoma and Thymic Carcinoma, Childhood
Thyroid Cancer
Thyroid Cancer, Childhood
Transitional Cell Cancer of the Renal Pelvis and Ureter
Trophoblastic Tumor, Gestational

U

Unknown Primary Site, Carcinoma of, Adult
Unknown Primary Site, Cancer of, Childhood
Unusual Cancers of Childhood
Ureter and Renal Pelvis, Transitional Cell
Cancer Urethral Cancer
Uterine Cancer, Endometrial
Uterine Sarcoma

V

Vaginal Cancer
Vaginal Cancer, Childhood
Visual Pathway and Hypothalamic Glioma, Childhood
Vulvar Cancer

W

Waldenström Macroglobulinemia Wilms Tumor
Women's Cancers

APPENDIX "C"

CANCER ORGANIZATIONS AND RESOURCES AVAILABLE TO YOU

There are many organizations, websites, chat groups, and resources that are easily located by searching the internet. Below are some organizations and websites that you may find to be useful resources for learning about cancer, symptoms, treatments, clinical trials, programs, and other important information.

CANCER ORGANIZATIONS/SITES/RESOURCES

Anderson Comprehensive Cancer Centers
http://www.mdanderson.org

American Association for Cancer Research (AACR)
615 Chestnut Street, 17th Fl.
Philadelphia, PA 19106
Phone: 215-440-9300
Toll Free: 866-423-3965
http://www.aacr.org

American Cancer Society 1599 Clifton Road, NE Atlanta, GA 30329-4251
Phone: 800-ACS-2345 http://www.cancer.org
American Cancer Society Cancer Action Network
1599 Clifton Road, NE
Atlanta, GA 30329-4251
Phone: 800-ACS-2345
http://www.acscan.org
American College of Surgeons: Cancer Programs

633 N. St. Clair Street
Chicago, IL 60611-3211
Toll Free: 800-621-4111
http://www.facs.org/cancer/index.html

American Institute for Cancer Research
1759 R Street, NW
Washington, DC 20009
Phone: 202-328-7744
Toll Free: 800-843-8114
http://www.aicr.org

American Psychosocial Oncology Society
2365 Hunters Way
Charlottesville, VA 22911
Phone: 434-293-5350
http://www.apos-society.org

American Society of Clinical Oncologists
http://www.asco.org

American Society of Hematology
2021 L Street NW, Suite 900
Washington, DC 20036
Phone: 202-776-0544
Fax: 202-776-0545
http://www.hematology.org

American Society for Therapeutic Radiology and Oncology
8280 Willow Oaks Corporate Dr., Suite 500
Fairfax, VA 22031
Phone: 1-800-962-7876
http://www.astro.org/patient

Association of Cancer Online Resources
173 Duane Street, Suite 3A
New York, NY 10013-3334
Phone: 212-226-5525

http://www.acor.org

Association of Community Cancer Centers (ACCC)
11600 Nebel Street, Suite 201
Rockville, MD 20852
Phone: 301-984-9496
http://www.accc-cancer.org

Association of Oncology Social Work (AOSW)
100 N. 20th Street, 4th Fl.
Philadelphia, PA 19103
Phone: 215-599-6093
http://www.aosw.org

Association of Pediatric Hematology/Oncology Nurses (APHON)
4700 W. Lake Ave.
Glenview, IL 60025
Phone: 847-375-4724
http://www.apon.org

CanCare
9575 Katy Fwy, Ste 428 Houston, TX 77024
Phone: (713) 461-0028
http://www.cancare.org

Cancer Hope Network
Two North Road, Suite A
Chester, NJ 07930-2308
Phone: 877-HOPENET
http://www.cancerhopenetwork.org
Cancer Information and Counseling Line (CICL)
AMC Cancer Research Center
1600 Pierce Street Denver, CO 80214
Phone: 800-525-3777 http://www.amc.org/counseling/CICL.pdf
Cancer News on the Net http://www.cancernews.com

Cancer Research Institute
One Exchange Plaza55 Broadway, Suite 1802

New York, NY 10006
Phone: 800-992-2627
http://www.cancerresearch.org

Cancer Trials Support Unit CTSU Data Operations Center 1441 W. Montgomery Ave. Rockville, MD 20850-2062 Phone: 888-823-5923
http://www.ctsu.org

Cancer.com
P.O. Box 6914
430 Route 22 East
Bridgewater, NJ 08807-0914
Phone: 888-227-5624
http://www.cancer.com

CancerCare
275 Seventh Ave.
New York, NY 10001
Phone: 800-813-HOPE (4673)
http://www.cancercare.org

Cancer411.org
15303 Ventura Blvd.
Sherman Oaks, CA 91403
Phone: 877-226-2741
http://www.cancer411.org

CancerQuest
2017 Rollins Research Center
1510 Clifton Rd., NE Atlanta, GA 30322
http://cancerquest.org

CancerSource
263 Summer Street,
5th Floor
Boston, MA 02210-1506
http://www.cancersource.com

CaringBridge
1995 Rahn Cliff Ct., St. 200
Eagan, MN 55122
Phone: 651-452-7940
http://www.caringbridge.org

Center to Advance Palliative Care (CAPC)
The Mount Sinai School of Medicine
1255 Fifth Ave., Suite C-2
New York, NY 10029
Phone: 212-201-2670
http://www.capc.org

Centers for Disease Control and Prevention (CDC)
1600 Clifton Road
Atlanta, GA 30333
Phone: 404-639-3311
Toll Free: 800-311-3435
http://www.cdc.gov

Chemo 101
Phone: 612-845-8769
http://chemo101.com

Exceptional Cancer Patients (ECaP)
522 Jackson Park Dr. Meadville, PA 16335
Phone: 814-337-8192
Fax: 814-337-0699
http://www.ecap-online.org

FDA Cancer Liaison Program
U.S. Food and Drug Administration (FDA)
Office of Special Health Issues
5600 Fishers Lane, HF-12, Rm. 9-49
Rockville, MD 20857
Phone: 888-INFOFDA
Fax: 301-443-4555
http://www.fda.gov/oashi/cancer/cancer.html

Fertile Hope
65 Broadway, Suite 603
New York, NY 10006
Phone: 888-994-HOPE (4673)
http://www.fertilehope.org

Fertile Action
Phone: 877-276-5951
http://www.Fertileaction.org

Gilda's Club Worldwide 322 Eighth Ave., Suite 1402
New York, NY 10001
Phone: 888-445-3248
Fax: 917-305-0549
http://www.gildasclub.org
Hippocratic Cancer Research Foundation
676 North S. Clair, Suite 1200
Chicago, IL 60611
Phone: 312-503-8306
info@hcrfwingstocure.org

Hippocratic Cancer Research Foundation
676 North St. Clair, Suite 1200
Chicago, IL 60611
info@hcrfwingstocure.org

Imerman Angels
400 W. Erie Street
Suite #405
Chicago, IL 60654
Phone: 877-274-5529
http://www.imermanangels.org

International Psycho-Oncology Society
C/O Custom Management Group
2365 Hunters Way
Charlottesville, VA 22911

Phone: 434-293-5350
Fax: 434-977-1856
http://www.ipos-society.org

Lotsa Helping Hands
365 Boston Post Rd., Suite 157
Sudbury, MA 01776
http://wwwlotsahelpinghands.com
Macmillan Cancer Support
89 Albert Embankment,
London, SE1 7UQ
Phone: 020 7840 7840
Fax: 020 7840 7841
http://www.macmillan.org.uk

Memorial Sloan-Kettering
http://www.mskcc.org

MUMS National Parent-to-Parent Network
150 Custer Court
Green Bay, WI 54301-1243
Phone: 877-336-5333
Fax: 920-339-0995
http://www.netnet.net/mums

National Cancer Institute (NCI)
Public Inquiries Office
6116 Executive Blvd., Room 3036A
Bethesda, MD 20892-2580
Phone: 800-4-CANCER
Fax: 301-402-0894
http://www.cancer.gov

National Center for Complementary and Alternative Medicine (NCCAM)
NCCAM Clearinghouse
P.O. Box 7923
Gaithersburg, MD 20898-7923
Phone: 888-644-6226

Fax: 866-464-3616
http://www.nccam.nih.gov

National Coalition for Cancer Survivorship (NCCS)
1010 Wayne Ave., Suite 770
Silver Spring, MD 20910-5600
Phone: 877-622-7937
Fax: 301-565-9670
http://www.canceradvocacy.org

National Comprehensive Cancer Network (NCCN)
500 Old York Rd., Suite 250
Jenkintown, PA 19046
Phone: 215-690-0300
Fax: 215-690-0280
http://www.nccn.org

National Library of Medicine
http://www.medlineplus.gov

National Organization for Rare Disorders (NORD)
55 Kenosia Ave.
P.O. Box 1968
Danbury, CT 06813-1968
Toll Free: 800-999-6673
Phone: 203-744-010
http://www.rarediseases.org

Northwestern Memorial Hospital
Comprehensive Cancer Center
Robert H. Lurie
251 E. Huron Street
Chicago, IL 60611
Phone: 312-926-2000
http://www.nmh.org

Patient Advocate Foundation (PAF)
700 Thimble Shoals Blvd., Suite 200

Newport News, VA 23606
Phone: 800-532-5274
Fax: 757-873-8999
http://www.patientadvocate.org

Patient Power
9220 SE 68th Street
Mercer Island, WA 98040-5135
Phone: 877-232-5445
http://www.patientpower.info

Patient Resource Publishing
6531 North National Dr.
Parkville, MO 64152
Phone: 816-584-8227
http://www.patientresource.net

Pregnant with Cancer Network P.O. Box 1243
Buffalo, NY 14220
Phone: 800-743-4471
http://www.pregnantwithcancer.org

Prepare to Live
http://www.preparetolive.org

Prevent Cancer Foundation 1600 Duke Street
Alexandria, VA 22314
Phone: 703-836-4412
Toll Free: 800-227-2732
http://www.preventcancer.org

Rare Cancer Alliance
1649 N. Pacana Way
Green Valley, AZ 85614 http://www.rare-cancer.org

Research Advocacy Network
309 E. Rand Rd., Suite 175
Arlington Heights, IL 60004

Phone: 877-276-2187 http://www.researchadvocacy.org

Rush University Medical Center
1653 W. Congress Parkway
Chicago, IL 60612
Phone: 312-942-5000
http://www.rush.edu

Stand Up 2 Cancer
http://www.standup2cancer.org

SuperSibs
4300 Lincoln Ave., Suite I
Rolling Meadows, IL 60008
Phone: 866-444-7427
Fax: 847-776-7084
http://www.supersibs.org

Teens Living With Cancer
Melissa's Living Legacy Foundation
245 Citation Dr.
Henrietta, NY 14467
Phone: 585-334-0858
Fax: 585-334-0858
http://www.teenslivingwithcancer.org

The Cancer Research Foundation
135 S. LaSalle Street
Suite 2020
Chicago, IL 60690
Phone: 312-630-0055
http://www.cancerresearchfdn.org/

The Ulman Cancer Fund for Young Adults
PMB 505
4725 Dorsey Hall Drive, Suite A
Ellicott City, MD 21042
Phone: 410-964-0202

Toll Free: 888-393-3863
Fax: 410-964-0402
http://www.ulmanfund.org

Vital Options and the Group Room Cancer Radio Show
4419 Coldwater Canyon Ave.,
Studio City, CA 91604-1479
Phone: 818-508-5657
Toll Free: 800-477-7666
Fax: 818-788-5260
http://www.vitaloptions.org

ORGANIZATIONS/SITES THAT FOCUS ON A PARTICULAR TYPE(S) OF CANCER

Adenoid

Adenoid Cystic Carcinoma Organization International
P.O. Box 15482
San Diego, CA 92175
http://www.accoi.org

Amyloidosis

Amyloidosis Foundation
7151 N. Main Street, Suite 208
Clarkston, MI 48346
Phone: 248-922-9610
Toll Free: 877-269-5463
http://www.amyloidosisresearchfoundation.org

Amyloidosis Support Groups, Inc. 232 Orchard Dr.
Wood Dale, IL 60191
Phone: 630-350-7539
Toll Free: 866-404-7539
http://www.amyloidosissupport.com

Amyloidosis Support Network
1490 Herndon Ln.
Marietta, GA 30062
Phone: 770-977-1500
Toll Free: 800-689-1239
http://www.amyloidosis.org

Bladder Cancer

American Urological Association
1000 Corporate Blvd.
Linthicum, MD 21090

Phone: 410-689-3700
Toll Free: 866-746-4282
http://www.urologyhealth.org
Bladder Cancer Advocacy Network
4813 St. Elmo Ave.
Bethesda, MD 20814
Phone: 301-215-9099
http://www.bcan.org

Bone Cancer

Bone and Cancer Foundation
120 Wall Street, Suite 1602
New York, NY 10005-4035
Phone: 888-862-0999
http://www.boneandcancerfoundation.org

Brain Tumor

American Brain Tumor Association
2720 River Rd.
Des Plaines, IL 60018
Phone: 800-886-2282
http://www.abta.org

Brain Tumor Society
124 Watertown Street, Suite 3-H
Watertown, MA
Phone: 800-770-8287
Fax: 617-924-9998

Children's Brain Tumor Foundation
274 Madison Ave., Suite 1004
New York, NY 10016
Phone: 866-228-4673
http://www.cbtf.org

National Brain Tumor Foundation
22 Battery Street, Suite 612
San Francisco, CA 94111
Phone: 800-934-2873
Fax: 415-834-9980
http://www.braintumor.org

Pediatric Brain Tumor Foundation
302 Ridgefield Ct.
Asheville, NC 28806
Phone: 800-253-6530
http://www.pbtfus.org

The Brain Tumor Foundation
1350 Avenue of the Americas, Suite 1200
New York, NY 10019
Phone: 212-265-2401
Fax: 212-489-0203
http://www.braintumorfoundation.org

The Childhood Brain Tumor Foundation
20312 Watkins Meadow Dr.
Germantown, MD 20876
Phone: 877-217-4166
http://www.childhoodbraintumor.org

Breast Cancer

American Society of Breast Disease
P.O. Box 140186
Dallas, TX 75214
Phone: 214-368-6836
http://www.asbd.org

Breast Cancer Network of Strength
212 W. Van Buren, Suite 1000
Chicago, IL 60607
Phone: 800-221-2141

Fax: 312-294-8597
http://www.networkofstrength.org
BreastCancer.Net
http://www.breastcancer.net

Breastcancer.org
111 Forrest Ave.,
1R Narberth, PA 19072
http://www.breastcancer.org

BreastCancerAdvisors.org
229 S. 18th Street
Philadelphia, PA 19103
http://www.breastcanceradvisors.org

HER2 Support Group Organization
6973 Mimosa Dr.
Carlsbad, CA 92009
Phone: 760-602-9178
http://www.her2support.org

Inflammatory Breast Cancer Research Foundation
321 High School Rd., NE, Suite D3, #149
Bainbridge Island, WA 98110
Phone: 877-786-7422
http://www.ibcresearch.org

Living Beyond Breast Cancer
10 E. Athens Ave., Suite 204
Ardmore, PA 19003
Phone: 610-645-4567
Toll Free: 888-753-5222
Fax: 610-645-4573
http://www.lbbc.org

Mothers Supporting Daughters with Breast Cancer
21710 Bayshore Rd.
Chestertown, MD 21620-4401

Phone: 410-778-198
http://www.mothersdaughters.org
National Breast and Cervical Cancer Early Detection Program
Centers for Disease Control and Prevention
Division of Cancer
Prevention and Control
4770 Buford Hwy., NE
Atlanta, GA 30341-3717
Phone: 800-292-4636
http://www.cdc.gov/cancer/index.htm

National Breast Cancer Coalition
1101 17th Street, NW,
Suite 1300 Washington, DC 20036
Phone: 800-622-2838
Fax: 202-265-6854

SHARE: Self-help for Women with Breast or Ovarian Cancer
1501 Broadway, Suite 704a
New York, NY 10036
Phone: 212-719-0364
Toll Free: 866-891-2392
http://www.sharecancersupport.org

Sisters Network, Inc.
8787 Woodway Dr., Suite 4206
Houston, TX 77063
Phone: 866-781-1808
Fax: 713-780-8998
http://www.sistersnetworkinc.org

Susan G. Komen for the Cure
5005 LBJ Freeway Suite 250
Dallas, TX 75244
Phone: 800-462-9273
http://www.komen.org
Young Survival Coalition 61 Broadway, Suite 2235
New York, NY 10006

Toll Free: 1-800-972-1011
Phone: 646-257-3000
http://www.youngsurvival.org

John W. Nick Foundation, Inc.
P.O. Box 4133
Vero Beach, FL 32963
Phone: 772-589-1440
http://www.johnwnickfoundation.org

Carcinoid Tumors

The Carcinoid Cancer Foundation, Inc.
333 Mamaroneck Ave., #492
White Plains, NY 10605
Phone: 914-683-1001
Toll Free: 888-722-3132
Fax: 914-683-0183
http://www.carcinoid.org

Cervical Cancer

Gynecologic Cancer Foundation (GCF)
230 W Monroe, Suite 2528
Chicago, IL 60606
Phone: 800-444-4441
Fax: 312-578-9769
http://www.thegcf.org

National Breast and Cervical Cancer Early Detection Program
Centers for Disease Control and Prevention
Division of Cancer
Prevention and Control
4770 Buford Hwy., NE
Atlanta, GA 30341-3717
Phone: 800-292-4636
http://www.cdc.gov/cancer/index.htm

National Cervical Cancer Coalition (NCCC)
6520 Platt Ave., #693
West Hills, CA 91307
Phone: 800-685-5531
http://www.nccc-online.org

Childhood Cancer

Alliance for Childhood Cancer
1900 Duke Street, Suite 200
Alexandria, VA 22314
Phone: 703-299-1050
Fax: 703-684-8364
http://www.childhoodcanceralliance.org

American Brain Tumor Association (ABTA)
2720 River Rd.
Des Plaines, IL 60018
Phone: 800-886-2282
http://www.abta.org

Bear Necessities Cancer Foundation
Chicago, IL
Phone: 312-214-1200
http://www.bearnecessitites.org

Beyond the Cure
1 South Memorial Dr., Suite 800
St. Louis, MO 63102
Phone: 800-532-6459
http://www.beyondthecure.org

Candlelighters Childhood Cancer Foundation
P.O. Box 498
Kensington, MD 20895-0498
Phone: 800-366-2223
Fax: 301-962-3521
http://www.candlelighters.org

Childhood Leukemia Center
http://www.patientcenters.com/leukemia

Children's Brain Tumor Foundation
274 Madison Ave., Suite 1004
New York, NY 10016
Phone: 866-228-4673 http://www.cbtf.org

National Childhood Cancer Foundation Children's Oncology Group
4600 East West Highway, #600
Bethesda, MD 20814-3457
Phone: 800-458-NCCF (6223)
Fax: 626-447-6359
http://www.curesearch.org

Make-A-Wish Foundation
3550 N Central Ave., Suite 300
Phoenix, AZ 85012-2127
Phone: 800-722-9474
Fax: 602-279-0855
http://www.wish.org

National Childhood Cancer Foundation
P.O. Box 60012
440 E Huntington Dr.
Arcadia, CA 91006-6012
Phone: 800-458-6223
Fax: 626-447-6359
http://www.nccf.org

National Children's Cancer Society
1 South Memorial Dr., Suite 800
St. Louis, MO 63102
Phone: 800-532-6459
http://www.nationalchildrenscancersociety.org

Neuroblastoma Children's Cancer Society P.O. Box 957672
Hoffman Estates, IL 60195

Phone: 800-532-5162
Fax: 847-605-0705
http://www.neuroblastomacancer.org

Outlook: Life Beyond Childhood Cancer http://www.outlook-life.org

Pediatric Brain Tumor Foundation
302 Ridgefield Ct. Asheville, NC 28806
Phone: 800-253-6530
http://www.pbtfus.org

Starlight Starbright Children's Foundation 5757 Wilshire Blvd., Suite M100
Los Angeles, CA 90036
Phone: 310-479-1212
http://www.slsb.org

The Childhood Brain Tumor Foundation 20312 Watkins Meadow Dr.
Germantown, MD 20876
Phone: 877-217-4166
http://www.childhoodbraintumor.org

The STARBRIGHT Foundation 1
850 Sawtelle Blvd., Suite 450
Los Angeles, CA 90025
Phone: 800-315-2580
Fax: 310-479-1235
http://www.starbright.org

Colorectal Cancer

Colon Cancer Alliance
5411 N. University Dr., Suite 202
Coral Springs, FL 33067
Phone: 877-422-2030
http://www.ccalliance.org

Colorectal Cancer Coalition
1225 King Street, 2nd Fl.

Alexandria, VA 22314
Phone: 877-427-2111
http://www.fightcolorectalcancer.org

The Susan Cohan Kasdas Colon Cancer Foundation
201 N Charles Street, Suite 2404
Baltimore, MD 21201
Phone: 410-244-1778
http://www.coloncancerfoundation.org

Esophageal Cancer

Cathy's EC Café
http://www.eccafe.org

Eye Cancer

The Eye Cancer Network Eye Care Foundation 115 E 61st Street
New York, NY 10021 Phone: 212-832-8170 http://www.eyecancer.com

Gastrointestinal Stromal Tumor (GIST)

GIST Support International
12 Bomaca Dr.
Doylestown, PA 18901
Phone: 215-340-9374
Fax: 215-340-1630
http://www.gistsupport.org

The Life Raft Group (LRG) 40 Galesi Dr., Suite 19
Wayne, NJ 07470
Phone: 973-837-9092
Fax: 973-837-9095
http://www.liferaftgroup.org

Head and Neck Cancer

Support for People with Oral, Head, and Neck Cancer (SPOHNC)
P.O. Box 53
Locust Valley, NY 11560-0053
Phone: 800-377-0928
Fax: 516-671-8794
http://www.spohnc.org
The Oral Cancer Foundation 3419 Via Lido, #205
Newport Beach, CA 92663 Phone: 949-646-8000
www.oralcancerfoundation.org

HIV/AIDS-Related Cancer

AIDSinfo
P.O. Box 6303
Rockville, MD 20849
Phone: 800-448-0440
http://aidsinfo.nih.gov

HIV InSite
UCSF Center for HIV Information
4150 Clement Street, Box 111V
San Francisco, CA 94121
http://hivinsite.ucsf.edu

Kidney Cancer

Action to Cure Kidney Cancer
150 West 75th Street, Suite 246
New York, NY 10023
Phone: 212-615-6404
http://www.ackc.org

American Urological Association
1000 Corporate Blvd.
Linthicum, MD 21090
Phone: 866-746-4282

http://www.UrologyHealth.org

Kidney Cancer Association
1234 Sherman Ave., Suite 203
Evanston, IL 60202
Phone: 800-850-9132
http://www.kidneycancer.org

VHL Family Alliance
2001 Beacon Street, Suite 208
Boston, MA 02135-7787
Toll Free: 800-767-4845
Phone: 617-277-5667
http://www.vhl.org

Laryngeal and Hypopharyngeal Cancer

The Oral Cancer Foundation
3419 Via Lido, #205
Newport Beach, CA 92663
Phone: 949-646-8000
www.oralcancerfoundation.org

Leukemia

American Society for Blood and Marrow Transplantation
85 W Algonquin Rd., Suite 550
Arlington Heights, IL 60005
Phone: 847-427-0224
Fax: 847-427-9656
http://www.asbmt.org

Blood and Marrow Transplant Information Network
2310 Skokie Valley Rd., Suite 104
Highland Park, IL 60035
Phone: 888-597-7674
Fax: 847-433-4599
http://www.bmtnews.org

Childhood Leukemia Center
http://www.patientcenters.com/leukemia

Leukemia Research Foundation
3520 Lake Ave., Suite 202
Wilmette, IL 60091
Phone: 888-558-5385
http://www.leukemia-research.org

National Bone Marrow Transplant Link
20411 West 12 Mile Rd., Suite 108
Southfield, MI 48076
Phone: 800-546-5268
http://www.nbmtlink.org

The National CML Society
130 Inverness Plaza #307
Birmingham, Alabama 35242
Phone: 877-431-2573
http://www.nationalcmlsociety.org

National Marrow Donor Program
3001 Broadway Street, NE, Suite 100
Minneapolis, MN 55413-1753
Phone: 800-627-7692
http://www.marrow.org

The Leukemia and Lymphoma Society
1311 Mamaroneck Ave., Suite 130
White Plains, NY 10605
Phone: 800-955-4572
http://www.lls.org

The Myelodysplastic Syndromes Foundation
P.O. Box 353
36 Front Street
Crosswicks, NJ 08515
Phone: 800-MDS-0839 (800-637-0839)

Fax: 609-298-0590
http://www.mds-foundation.org

Liver Cancer

LiverTumor.org
http://www.livertumor.org

Lung Cancer

American Lung Association
61 Broadway, 6th Fl.
New York, NY 10006
Phone: 800-586-4872
http://www.lungusa.org
It's Time to Focus on Lung Cancer
Phone: 877-646-5864
http://www.lungcancer.org

Lung Cancer Alliance
1747 Pennsylvania Ave. NW
Washington, DC 20006
Phone: 800-298-2436
http://www.lungcanceralliance.org

Lung Cancer Online
http://www.lungcanceronline.org

National Lung Cancer Partnership
222 N. Midvale Blvd., Suite 6
Madison, WI 53705
Phone: 608-233-7905
http://www.nationallungcancerpartnership.org

Lymphoma

CLL Topics
www.clltopics.org

Cutaneous Lymphoma Foundation
P.O. Box 374
Birmingham, MI 48012-0374
Phone: 248-644-9014
www.clfoundation.org

International Waldenstrom's Macroglobulinemia Foundation
IWMF Business Office
3932D Swift Road
Sarasota, FL 34231
Phone: 941-927-4963
www.iwmf.com
Lymphoma Coalition
http://www.lymphomacoalition.org

Lymphoma Research Foundation
8800 Venice Blvd., Suite 207
Los Angeles, CA 90034
Phone: 800-500-9976
Fax: 310-204-7043
http://www.lymphoma.org

Patients Against Lymphoma
3774 Buckwampum Rd.
Reigelsville, PA 18077
Phone: 610-346-8419
http://www.lymphomation.org

The Leukemia and Lymphoma Society
1311 Mamaroneck Ave., Suite 130
White Plains, NY 10605
Phone: 800-955-4572
http://www.lls.org

The Lymphoma Information Network
http://www.lymphomainfo.net

Melanoma

American Academy of Dermatology
P.O. Box 4014
Schaumburg, IL 60168-4014
Phone: 888-462-3376
Fax: 847-330-0050
http://www.skincarephysicians.com/skincancernet

Melanoma Center
http://www.melanomacenter.org

Melanoma International Foundation
250 Mapleflower Rd.
Glenmoore, PA 19343
Phone: 866-463-6663
www.melanomaintl.org
Melanoma Patients' Information Page
The Pattersons
P.O. Box 389
Cloverdale, CA 95425
http://www.mpip.org

Melanoma Research, Inc. (The Billy Foundation)
26203 Production Ave., 12-A/Zebra Suite
Haywood, CA 94545
Toll Free: 888-882-4559
Fax: 510-264-9079
http://www.bfmelanoma.com

National Council on Skin Cancer Prevention
5800 Wilson Ln.
Bethesda, MD 20817
http://www.skincancerprevention.org

SunWise Program
U.S. Environmental Protection Agency
1200 Pennsylvania Ave., NW

Washington, DC 20460
http://www.epa.gov/sunwise

The Skin Cancer Foundation
245 Fifth Ave., Suite 1403
New York, NY 10016
Phone: 800-754-6490
Fax: 212-725-5751
http://www.skincancer.org

Mesothelioma

Mesothelioma Applied Research Foundation
1609 Garden Street
Santa Barbara, CA 93101
Phone: 805-560-8942
Fax: 805-560-8962
http://www.marf.org

Myeloma

American Society for Blood and Marrow Transplantation
85 W Algonquin Rd., Suite 550
Arlington Heights, IL 60005
Phone: 847-427-0224
Fax: 847-427-9656
http://www.asbmt.org

Blood and Marrow Transplant Information Network
2310 Skokie Valley Rd., Suite 104
Highland Park, IL 60035
Phone: 888-597-7674
Fax: 847-433-4599
http://www.bmtnews.org

International Myeloma Foundation
12650 Riverside Dr., Suite 206
North Hollywood, CA 91607

Phone: 800-452-2873
Fax: 818-487-7454
http://www.myeloma.org

Multiple Myeloma Research Foundation
383 Main Ave., 5th floor
Norwalk, CT 06841
Phone: 203-229-0464
http://www.multiplemyeloma.org

National Bone Marrow Transplant Link
20411 West 12 Mile Rd., Suite 108
Southfield, MI 48076 Phone: 800-546-5268
Fax: 248-358-1889
http://www.nbmtlink.org

National Marrow Donor Program
3001 Broadway Street, NE, Suite 100
Minneapolis, MN 55413-1753
Phone: 800-627-7692
http://www.marrow.org

Oral and Oropharyngeal Cancer

Support for People with Oral, Head, and Neck Cancer
P.O. Box 53
Locust Valley, NY 11560-0053
Phone: 800-377-0928
Fax: 516-671-8794
http://www.spohnc.org
The Oral Cancer Foundation
3419 Via Lido, #205
Newport Beach, CA 92663
Phone: 949-646-8000
www.oralcancerfoundation.org

Ovarian Cancer

Conversations!
P.O. Box 7948
Amarillo, TX 79114-7948
Phone: 806-355-2565
Fax: 806-467-9757
http://www.ovarian-news.org

Facing Our Risk of Cancer Empowered
16057 Tampa Palms Blvd. West, PMB #373
Tampa, FL 33647
Phone: 866-288-7475
http://www.facingourrisk.org

Gilda Radner Familial Ovarian Cancer Registry
Roswell Park Cancer Institute
Elm and Carlton Streets
Buffalo, NY 14263-0001
Phone: 800-682-7426
http://www.ovariancancer.com

Gynecologic Cancer Foundation (GCF)
230 W Monroe, Suite 2528
Chicago, IL 60606
Phone: 800-444-4441
Fax: 312-578-9769
http://www.thegcf.org

National Ovarian Cancer Coalition (NOCC)
500 NE Spanish River Blvd., Suite 8
Boca Raton, FL 33431
Phone: 888-682-7426
http://www.ovarian.org

Ovarian Cancer National Alliance
910 17th Street, NW, Suite 1190
Washington, DC 20006

Phone: 866-399-6262
http://www.ovariancancer.org

SHARE: Self-help for Women with Breast or Ovarian Cancer
1501 Broadway, Suite 704a
New York, NY 10036
Phone: 866-891-2392
http://www.sharecancersupport.org

Pancreatic Cancer

Hirshberg Foundation for Pancreatic Cancer Research
2990 S. Sepulveda Blvd., Suite 300C
Los Angeles, CA 90064
Phone: 310-473-5121
http://www.pancreatic.org

Lustgarten Foundation for Pancreatic Cancer Research
1111 Stewart Ave.
Bethpage, NY 11714
Phone: 866-789-1000
Fax: 516-803-2303
http://www.lustgarten.org

Pancreatic Cancer Action Network (PanCAN)
2141 Rosecrans Ave., Suite 7000
El Segundo, CA 90245
Phone: 877-272-6226
Fax: 310-725-0029
http://www.pancan.org

Pancreatica.org
149 Bonifacio Place
Monterey, CA 93940
Phone: 831-658-0600
http://www.pancreatica.org

Prostate Cancer

American Urological Association
1000 Corporate Blvd.
Linthicum, MD 21090
Phone: 866-746-4282
http://www.UrologyHealth.org

National Prostate Cancer Coalition (NPCC)
1154 15th Street, NW
Washington, DC 20005
Phone: 888-245-9455
Fax: 202-463-9456
http://www.4npcc.org

Prostate Cancer Education Council (PCEC)
7009 S. Potomac Street, Suite 125
Centennial, CO 80121
Phone: 866-477-6788
http://www.pcaw.com

Prostate Cancer Foundation
1250 Fourth Street
Santa Monica, CA 90401
Phone: 800-757-2873
Fax: 310-570-4701
http://www.prostatecancerfoundation.org
The Prostate Net
P. O. Box 2192
Secaucus, NJ 07096-2192
Phone: 888-477-6763
Fax: 270-294-1565
http://www.prostate-online.com

US TOO Prostate Cancer Education and Support Network
5003 Fairview Ave.
Downers Grove, IL 60515
Phone: 800-808-7866

Fax: 630-795-1602
http://www.ustoo.org

Sarcoma

Sarcoma Alliance
775 E Blithedale, #334
Mill Valley, CA 94941
Phone: 415-381-7236
Fax: 415-381-7235
http://www.sarcomaalliance.org

Sarcoma Foundation of America
P.O. Box 458
Damascus, MD 20872
Phone: 301-253-8687
http://www.curesarcoma.org

Skin Cancer (Non-Melanoma)

American Academy of Dermatology
P.O. Box 4014
Schaumburg, IL 60168-4014
Phone: 888-462-3376
Fax: 847-330-0050
http://www.skincarephysicians.com/skincancernet

National Council on Skin Cancer Prevention
5800 Wilson Ln.
Bethesda, MD 20817
http://www.skincancerprevention.org

SunWise Program
U.S. Environmental Protection Agency
1200 Pennsylvania Ave., NW (6205J)
Washington, DC 20460
http://www.epa.gov/sunwise

The Skin Cancer Foundation
245 Fifth Ave., Suite 1403
New York, NY 10016
Phone: 212-725-5176
Toll Free: 800-754-6490
Fax: 212-725-5751
http://www.skincancer.org

Testicular Cancer

Testicular Cancer Resource Center
http://tcrc.acor.org

Uterine Cancer

Gynecologic Cancer Foundation (GCF)
230 W Monroe, Suite 2528
Chicago, IL 60606
Phone: 800-444-4441
Fax: 312-578-9769
http://www.thegcf.org

CAREGIVER ORGANIZATIONS/SITES

Center for Caregiver Training 1320 Divisadero Street
San Francisco, CA 94115
Phone: 415-563-9286
http://www.caregiving101.org

National Family Caregivers Association
10400 Connecticut Avenue, Suite 500
Kensington, MD 20895-3944
Phone: 301-942-6430
Fax: 800-896-3650
http://www.nfcacares.org

Well Spouse Association
63 W. Main Street, Suite H
Freehold, NJ 07728
Phone: 800-838-0879
Fax: 732-577-8644
http://www.wellspouse.org
Strength for Caring
http://www.strengthforcaring.com/

CLINICAL TRIAL INFORMATION

National Institutes of Health
http://www.clinicaltrials.gov

National Cancer Institute
http://www.cancer.gov/search/clinicaltrials

Coalition of National Cancer Cooperative Groups
http://www.cancertrialshelp.org

Emerging Med
http://www.emergingmed.com

CenterWatch
http://www.centerwatch.com

FINANCIAL ASSISTANCE/ TRANSPORTATION/LEGAL

Angel Flight
Central 500 Richards Road
Kansas City, MO 64116
Phone: 816-421-2300 or 866-569-9464
http://www.angelflightcentral.org

Cancer Financial Assistance Coalition
http://www.cancerfac.org

Cancer Legal Resource Center
Disability Rights Legal Center
Loyola Law School Public Interest Law Center
800 S. Figueroa St., Ste. #1120
Los Angeles, CA 90017
Phone: 866.843.2572
http://www.CancerLegalResourceCenter.org

Corporate Angel Network, Inc.
Phone: 866-328-1313
http://www.corpangelnetwork.org

Department of Veteran Affairs
Phone: 877-222-8387
http://www.va.gov

Healthwell Foundation
Phone: 800-675-8416
Hill-Burton Free Hospital Care
Phone: 800-638-0742
http://www.hrse.gov/hillburton

Joe's House
Phone: 877-563-7468
http://www.joeshouse.org

Medicare
http://www.medicare.gov

National Association of Hospital Hospitality Houses, Inc.
Phone: 800-542-9730
http://www.nahhh.org

National Children's Cancer Society
Phone: 800-532-6459
http://www.thenccs.org

National Foundation for Transplant
Phone: 800-489-3863
http://www.transplants.org

National Transplant Assistance Fund
Radnor Financial Center, Suite F-120
150 N. Radnor Chester Road
Radnor, PA 19087
Phone: 800-642-8399
Fax: 610-353-1616
http://www.transplantfund.org

Needy Meds
http://www.needymeds.org

Partnership for Prescription Assistance
1100 15th Street, NW
Washington, D.C. 20005
Phone: 888-477-2669
http://www.pparx.org

Patient Access Network
Phone: 866-316-7263

http://www.patientaccessnetwork.org
Patient Advocate Foundation
700 Thimble Shoals Boulevard, Suite 200
Newport News, VA 23606
Phone: 866-512-3861
Co-pay relief program:
866-512-3861
http://www.patientadvocate.org

Ronald McDonald House Charities
Phone: 630-623-7048
http://www.rmhc.org

Social Security Administration (SSA)
Office of Publication Inquiries
Windsor Park Building
6401 Security Boulevard
Baltimore, MD 21235-6401
Phone: 800-772-1213
http://www.ssa.gov

The Bone Marrow Foundation
Phone: 800-365-1336
http://www.bonemarrow.org

United Way of America
http://www.national.unitedway.org

MANY OF THE PHARACEUTICAL COMPANIES HAVE ASSISTANCE PROGRAMS
NUTRITION
American Dietetic Association
120 South Riverside Plaza, Suite 2000
Chicago, IL 60606-6995
Phone: 800-877-1600
http://www.eatright.org

American Institute for Cancer Research
1759 R Street, NW
Washington, D.C. 20009
Phone: 800-843-8114
http://www.aicr.org

Meals on Wheels Association of America
203 S. Union Street
Alexandria, VA 22314
Phone: 703-548-5558
http://www.mowaa.org

Cancer Nutrition Center
http://www.cancernutrition.com

PAIN MANAGEMENT

American Chronic Pain Association
P.O. Box 850
Rocklin, CA 95677
Phone: 800-533-3231
http://www.theacpa.org

American Pain Foundation
201 North Charles Street, Suite 710
Baltimore, MD 21201-4111
Phone: 888-615-7246
http://www.painfoundation.org

APPENDIX "D"

QUESTIONS TO ASK YOUR DOCTORS

Below is a listing of some questions that you can use as a resource for informing yourself about your condition, diagnosis, treatments, prognosis, and circumstances. This can be used for reference in conducting research, planning, speaking to other patients, as well as posing them directly to your doctors and healthcare providers. The financial and temporal realities require that you do as much research as possible in advance of undergoing a treatment or procedure or seeing a physician and that you determine which issues and questions you will raise with a particular doctor or healthcare provider. The list is far from exhaustive, but provides a good outline for areas of inquiry.

Questions To Ask About Tests

- What is the test?
- What should I do to prepare for the test?
- Any limitations on diet before the test?
- What will we learn from the test?
- Why is it important for me to have this test?
- Where will the test be taken (hospital or outpatient)?
- Any limitations on activities after the test (work, driving, etc.)?
- Describe how the test will be taken and what will be involved.
- How much will the test cost?
- What are the risks, complications, and side effects of the test?
- When and how will I get the results?
- What decisions will I have to make if the test is positive?
- What is the significance of the test being negative?
- What are the consequences if I do not have the test?

- Are there alternative tests available?
- What additional tests will I need?
- Notes: make sure the doctor is aware of prior tests to ensure that unnecessary tests are not conducted; verify time and place; confirm that test has been ordered and hospital or testing facilities are prepared to proceed before you arrive for the test.
- Obtain the test results and have the doctor review the results with you.

Questions To Ask About Diagnosis And Prognosis

- Do I have cancer (many tumors are benign and many patients with pre-cancerous conditions have left the doctor's office thinking they have cancer, when they do not)?
- What type of cancer do I have—specific type and all of the particulars (for example, you don't just need to know that you have blood cancer, lymphoma, or non-Hodgkin lymphoma—you need to know the exact type such as large, diffused, b-cell, non-Hodgkin lymphoma)?
- What is the basis for your diagnosis?
- Could it be something else?
- What else have we or should we rule out?
- How confident are you in the diagnosis?
- Is there any other test to confirm or rule out the diagnosis?
- What is my prognosis?
- What is the basis for the prognosis?
- What facts distinguish my case and suggest my chances are better?
- How advanced is my cancer?
- What stage is it and what is the basis for the staging?
- What are all of my treatment options?
- What treatments are best for me?
- How will I be followed after treatment and how often will I be checked?
- Can I go back to normal daily activities after treatment?
- Are there any clinical trials that might be beneficial?
- What has been your experience with cancer patients similar to me?
- Can you recommend any patient support groups in my area?
- Are there materials I can read about my cancer?

- Notes: you need to consider the confidence level that you have in the diagnosis, the confidence level that you have in the doctor and facility in terms of competence and approach, whether anything seems incorrect or questionable to you. You will want to obtain additional information and a second opinion, even if you are confident in the doctor and diagnosis.

Questions To Ask About Treatment

- What treatments are available?
- What treatment do you recommend?
- Why do you recommend it?
- Is this treatment necessary for me?
- Are there any alternatives?
- What are the alternatives and their relevant benefits and risks?
- Clinical trials?
- Are there potential treatments that you (or this institution) are not able to provide?
- What is the survival rate with the various alternative treatments?
- Why do you think this treatment is preferable?
- How many patients have you treated this way and what are the results in your experience?
- What does the literature or studies show about this treatment and the alternatives?
- Any factors unique to me that you think are important in recommending the treatment?
- What do you expect the results to be?
- How safe is the procedure?
- What are the side effects of the treatment?
- What can be done to eliminate or relieve the side effects?
- Can I be put on a treatment program that won't interfere with my work?
- How and when will we determine how well the treatment is working?
- Explain in detail the treatment, including preparations, how and when it is given, period of time, and all of the particulars?
- Cost and insurance issues?
- What options are available if the treatment does not work?

- By undergoing this treatment will other treatment options be limited or foreclosed?
- Where can I get additional information (written materials, organizations, and staff)?
- Note: if necessary, request a follow-up phone call or appointment during which you can ask more questions.

Questions To Ask About Surgery

- Why do you want to do the surgery?
- Exactly what will you do—in simple terms?
- Is it an outpatient procedure or is hospitalization required?
- How long will I be in the hospital?
- What are the chances of cure with surgery?
- What other treatments can be used instead of surgery?
- How many of these operations have you personally performed?
- What have the results been?
- How many of these operations have the hospital performed and what have the results been?
- Will the surgery be disfiguring (if so, how)?
- Are there any less extensive, less deforming, less painful operations than the one you are suggesting?
- What are the risks and side effects of the surgery?
- What are the risks of the other possible treatments?
- What is the risk of death or serious disability?
- Do you feel the benefits outweigh the risks? Why?
- What are the possible consequences of postponing the operation?
- What will happen if I don't have the surgery?
- Cost and insurance coverage?
- How long will my recovery take?
- Will I have to have drains, catheters, intravenous lines, transfusions?
- What are the possible after-effects?
- What medication will I be given before going into the operating room?
- Who will give me the medication and the anesthesia?
- What other medical procedures and medical devices will I require and why?
- How long will the operation take?

- How long will it be before I wake up?
- What preparation and tests are required?
- Am I a good candidate for surgery?
- What are the chances that surgery will remove all of my cancer?
- Will I undergo chemotherapy or radiation after surgery to make sure all the cancer is destroyed?
- What is the length of hospitalization and recovery?
- Will I need help at home after being discharged?
- When can I resume normal activities? Drive a car? Have sex? Play sports? Return to work?
- What limitations will there be on my activities and what accommodations will be required?
- Will I have to follow a special diet or regimen?
- What symptoms should I keep track of and report to you?
- What medications should I take?
- Request written information and resources.

Questions To Ask About Radiation Therapy

- Who will be responsible for my radiation treatment?
- Are there ways to minimize radiation to other areas?
- Can I work during the time I am receiving treatment?
- How long will each treatment take?
- How many sessions will there be?
- When and where will they take place?
- Can they be scheduled in a way that I can continue to work or have someone accompany me during the treatments?
- How much radiation will I receive?
- What areas will be radiated?
- Will I be fitted with a mold and how does that work?
- What are the risks?
- What side effects can I expect?
- What should I do if these side effects occur?
- Cost and insurance information?
- What are the benefits?
- What does the literature and studies prove in terms of benefits and risks?
- What are my alternatives?

- What is likely to happen if I don't have these treatments?
- Do I need to be on a special diet or regimen during these treatments?
- Do I need to put something special on my skin if I get "burned" by the treatments?
- What special attention do I need to pay to the area of my body that is being treated?
- Are there methods that would more effectively administer the radiation and limit the areas of radiation?
- What type of radiation will I be given and what machinery will be used to administer it?
- Is this state of the art equipment? How long has it been in use?
- How many patients have you treated with my type of cancer and what have the results been?

Questions To Ask About Chemotherapy

- Who will be giving me these treatments?
- What are the names of the drugs to be used?
- What are these drugs supposed to do?
- What are the possible side effects?
- What should I do if I have side effects?
- Anything to prevent or minimize the side effects?
- Which side effects should I report to the doctor immediately?
- How will the drugs be given to me?
- How often will the treatments be given?
- How long will each treatment take?
- How long will the whole series last?
- Is this a standard regimen?
- Are there other drugs or combination that could be used?
- Can I take other medications at the same time?
- Is there any special nutritional advice I should follow?
- Are there any special precautions I need to take while on chemotherapy?
- Cost and insurance questions?
- What are the risks involved?
- What are my alternatives?
- What are the likely consequences if I don't have this treatment?

- What do the studies and research show regarding benefits, effectiveness, and risks?
- How many patients have you treated with my type of cancer with this chemotherapy (and other treatments) and what have the results been?
- Explain the amount, cycle, and timing of the chemotherapy?
- What limitations will there be on my activities and ability to work during treatment?
- Will I be able to return to my normal activities after chemotherapy?
- Notes: obtain fact sheets on the various drugs. If necessary, request a follow up time to have questions answered.

Questions To Ask About Clinical Trials

- Why is this research being done?
- What is the purpose of the study?
- Who is sponsoring the study?
- Who has reviewed and approved this study?
- Why does the research team feel the treatment, drug, or medical device will work?
- How many hospitals or institutions are participating in the study and where did the study originate?
- Where is the study site?
- What kinds of therapies, procedures, and/or tests will I have during the trial?
- What treatment will I get?
- How will the tests in the study compare to tests I would have outside the study?
- How long will the study last?
- How often will I have to go to the study site?
- Who will provide my medical care after the study ends?
- Will I be able to take my regular medications during the trial?
- What medications, procedures, or treatments must I avoid while in the study?
- What are my responsibilities during the study?
- Will I have to be in the hospital during the study?
- Will the study researchers work with my doctor while I am in the study?

- Can anyone find out that I am participating in a study?
- Can I talk to other people in the study?
- Will I be able to find out the results of the trial?
- How do the possible risks and benefits of the study compare with approved treatments for me?
- What are the possible immediate and long-term side effects?
- Will the study or my insurance pay for the costs of any treatment or hospitalization I might need for side effects from the study?
- What other treatment options do I have?
- Will I have to pay anything to participate in the study?
- What are the charges likely to be?
- What are the odds of my getting a placebo or standard treatment?
- What risks do I run and what treatment opportunities will be lost by participating in the trial?
- What have the results been on the treatment being studied?

APPENDIX "E"

TIPS THE DOCTORS MAY FORGET TO TELL YOU

- **Fertility:** Cancer treatments can impact fertility of men and woman. If you are or may be interested in having children in the future be sure to ask your doctor about the potential impacts of the treatment and, where appropriate, take steps such as storing sperm, embryos, and eggs in advance of treatment.
- **Stem Cell Harvesting:** In some instances it may be beneficial to preserve stem cells prior to undergoing treatment.
- **Blood Donation:** In some instances it may be beneficial to donate blood for your own use in advance of surgery or treatment.
- **Adopt A Fighting Spirit:** A positive outlook is desirable, but no matter what adopt a fighting spirit and invoke a strong will to live.
- **Actively Participant In Your Treatment And Recovery:** This book tells you how to do this.
- **Become A Checker:** Double check things pertaining to your health and treatments. Ask questions when something does not seem right to you.
- **Adopt A Health Lifestyle:** Make positive changes in your lifestyle that will improve your outcome, such as quitting smoking, getting sleep and rest, incorporating exercise and proper diet, and avoiding exposures to carcinogens.
- **Laughter Is The Best Medicine:** Ask your sense of humor to work overtime, you will need it.
- **Arrange For Transportation And A Companion For Your Appointments:** Even though you may not want to be an imposition on people or lose some independence, often appointments, procedures, and treatments can make you tired or less than totally

effective. For your safety and comfort and that of others, have someone accompany you on appointments and treatments.
- **Take Notes:** You should take notes. You advocate or family member may help you remember and understand what your doctors are telling you and can watch over you to ensure you are getting the best care.
- **Participate In A Support Group Or Buddy System:** Support groups are important not only because of the emotional and psychological help they can provide, but also because of the information about treatments, side effects, remedies for side effects and other concrete information and suggestions you will receive. Other patients focus on things the doctors and nurses may not and will take the time to help you. If you are completely adjusted and knowledgeable and feel you do not need support, than provide it to someone who needs support.
- **Be A Warrior And Reach Out And Help Others Battling Illness:** This is as important for you as for other people because it forces you to step outside yourself, draw upon your better qualities, and will keep you positive, focused, and in control.
- **Get Up, Get Dressed, And Stay Well-Groomed:** There may be plenty of days that you do not feel like it and some days when you cannot, but force yourself to get out of bed, walk and move, talk to people, and get dressed and cleaned up whenever you can. It will help you physically and mentally.
- **Consider Ways To Nurture Or Pamper Yourself:** Try massage, aromatherapy, yoga, a new suit or dress, or something that makes you feel good or helps to relieve stress or discomfort.
- **Maintain Your Routine:** Continue to work, maintain your normal routine, and do "your thing" as much as possible, making appropriate allowances for your condition and treatments.
- **Keep A Journal:** Keep notes of your feelings and experiences. It will help you in developing your history, learning what works for you and what does not, and you will look back with amazement at what you were able to endure. Make it a point to note at least one positive thing from each day. We tend to focus on our pain, symptoms, and disease, yet it is important to remind ourselves of the good things in life. You can use Appendix "H" for this purpose.

- **Listen To Frank Sinatra Music, Read Scott's Law Books, And Watch "Curb Your Enthusiasm":** At least listen to music you enjoy, read uplifting books, and watch enjoyable movies or television programming.
- **Be Gentle On Yourself:** Remember that your memory, ability to concentrate, and energy level will fluctuate according to your treatment and medications.
- **Don't Be Too Gentle On Yourself:** It is important to be self-sufficient and to push to get better. But be smart about it and readily ask for help when needed.
- **If It Sounds Too Good To Be True, It Is:** Positive thinking is important, but use at least the same caution in selecting your treatments as in investing your money. There are many claimed panaceas—miracle cures and treatments—that are false and unproven.
- **Do Not Ignore Other Health Issues Or Symptoms:** While you are focused on cancer and cancer treatments, do not lose sight of other treatments and conditions. Make sure your oncologist and other doctors are informed of your other health conditions.
- **Don't Forget Your Bite:** Dental care is an important part of your overall health. Communicate with your dentist and oncologist. Your physician may advise you to complete any major dental procedures you need before beginning cancer therapy or suggest that you delay such procedures.
- **Get Your Vaccines And Shots:** Check with your oncologist and other doctors to ensure that you are getting the appropriate vaccines and shots. They may recommend that you get vaccines you otherwise would not get or forego ones you normally would get.
- **Second Opinions Are A Must:** Always obtain a second opinion regarding your cancer diagnosis and treatment options.
- **Childhood Cancers Raise Special Issues:** Although we have not addressed childhood cancers specifically in this book, children with cancer require special attention and care and consultation with doctors well-versed in pediatric cancer issues for a number of reasons, including proper consideration of long-term side effects of treatment.

- **Do Not Suffer In Silence:** There are medications, remedies, and things that you can to do to eliminate or minimize many symptoms and side-effects from treatment. Make sure you get the help you need. Appendix "K" addresses side effects from treatment.
- **Contact Information:** Make sure that you obtain meaningful contact information for your doctors and nurses, such as office numbers, pager numbers, cell phone numbers, and e-mail addresses. Do not settle for them telling you to contact or go to the emergency room. Communicate regarding the best way to communicate with your health care providers. Many physicians will respond quickly to emails. Appendix "I" provides space for contact information.
- **Understand Instructions:** Make sure you understand your discharge instructions and what you are supposed to look out for and do.
- **Ask Questions:** Do not be afraid to ask questions about your doctor's qualifications, your treatment, your symptoms, your choices, or anything you do not understand or believe to be correct. As patients we rely upon our doctors and feel that we are not in control. Remember as the patient you are the customer and the health care providers are there to serve you. When they forget this, remind them.
- **Research And Evaluate:** We have identified numerous sources of information in Appendix "C." In the internet age, it is important not only to find and review information relative to your disease and treatment options, but to evaluate the information and the source of the information. You need to consider the reliability of the source, any bias or financial interest, the foundation upon which the information is based, whether the information is current, and whether and to what extent the information is corroborated. Verify.
- **Do Not Become An Isolationist:** Do not isolate yourself. Try to have social interaction at least once a day with someone outside of the healthcare community.
- **Use The Patient Medical Information Notebook Found In Appendix "G":** It is important to understand, record, and have access to your key medical information.

APPENDIX "F"

INSURANCE AND LEGAL DOCUMENTS

The realities and limitations of life make it prudent to plan for illness, incapacity, and death. This book is not intended to provide legal or financial advice, but we include this checklist as a resource for people with cancer. Hopefully, you have made the appropriate arrangements long ago, but the diagnosis of cancer is an event that causes people to make arrangements and plans that have not been made before and review those plans and documents previously prepared to make sure that they are current and in accord with your current situation and wishes. Many documents and forms are available online and can be prepared by individuals. Nonetheless, everyone's portfolios, needs, desires, and circumstances are unique and laws vary from state to state. Accordingly, people should consult with their loved ones, legal counsel, accountants, and financial and other advisors as appropriate. Below are some of the documents that should be prepared and/or gathered for ready access.

- Health insurance policies, plans, and information (information regarding deductibles, in-service providers, co-pays, limits, coverage, and other requirements and limitations as well as the basic information such as insurer, employer, employee, and plan number, etc.).
- Medicare and Medicaid information.
- Short-term and long term disability insurance policies and documents.
- Life insurance policies and information.
- A living will (a document that provides instructions regarding such things as when life support should be provided or terminated). Living wills or advance directives can be downloaded for each

state from a variety of sources, including at: www.caringinfo.org/planning/advance-directives/by-state/.
- A durable power of attorney for health care designating someone of your choice and whom you trust to make health care decisions when you are unable to do so.
- Other powers of attorney (such as a general power of attorney to transact other business on your behalf), the scope of which and the person so designated must be carefully outlined and considered because these persons are legally authorized to act on your behalf and bind you.
- Wills, estate documents, trusts, property titles, guardianships, and estate planning (once again various assets and liabilities and legal issues are involved).
- Provisions and instructions for payment of bills during the period of time you may be hospitalized or incapacitated.
- Provisions and instructions for other transactions during the period of time you may be hospitalized or incapacitated.
- Provisions and instructions for care of children, pets, and running and maintaining the household.
- Provisions and instructions for work or business.
- Health information (including a listing of doctors, conditions, allergies, medications, prior medical history and conditions, and family medical history).
- Copies of recent medical tests, scans, and results.
- A list containing physician contact information.
- Information and wishes regarding funeral, burial, cremation, and final arrangements.
- Organ donation forms and information (if desired).
- Personal information, contact information of family members, employers, guardians, trustees, and attorneys.

State, federal, and local laws may impact you and may vest you with rights or provide assistance. A few examples are listed below:

- The Health Insurance Portability and Accountability Act (HIPAA) contains requirements regarding privacy and maintenance of health-related information by healthcare providers, healthcare

- clearing houses, and health insurance plans. http://www.hhs.gov/ocr/hipaa.
- The Americans with Disabilities Act (ADA) requires employers to make reasonable accommodations for employees with disabilities. http://www.ada.gov/.
- Under the Family Medical Leave Act (FMLA), eligible employees are entitled to a total of 12 weeks unpaid leave during any 12-month period for specified reasons including where the employee is unable to work due to a serious health condition or an immediate family member with a serious health condition. http://www.dol.gov/esa/whd/fmla.
- COBRA (Consolidated Omnibus Budget Reconciliation Act) provides continuation of group health coverage that might otherwise be terminated. It offers the right to temporary continuation of health coverage under certain conditions. http://www.dol.gov/ebsa/faqs/ faq_consumer_cobra.html.
- Affordable Care Act: http://www.healthcare.gov/law/index.html.

APPENDIX "G"

PATIENT MEDICAL INFORMATION NOTEBOOK

It is important to keep notes, write down questions, and have ready access to key medical information. We suggest this Patient Medical Information Notebook as a convenient way to keep this information for both the patient and the caregiver.

I. GENERAL CONTACT INFORMATION

Patients Full Name:

Address:
Home Phone:
Fax:
Cell Phone:
Social Security No.:

Contact 1 Full Name:

Relationship:
Address:
Home Phone:
Fax:
Cell Phone:

Contact 2 Full Name:

Relationship:
Address:
Home Phone:
Fax:
Cell Phone:

Contact 3 Full Name:

Relationship:
Address:
Home Phone:
Fax:
Cell Phone:

II. PHYSICIAN/HOSPITAL CONTACT INFORMATION

Internist:

Name:
Address:
Phone:

Oncologist:

Name:
Address:
Room:

Radiation-Oncologist:

Name:
Address:
Phone:

Surgeon:

Name:
Address:
Phone:

Other doctors:

Type:
Name:
Address:
Phone:

Hospital or treatment facility:

Name:
Address:
Room:
Phone:

Pharmacy:

Name:
Address:
Phone:
Fax:

III. EMPLOYMENT

Company:
Position:
Address:
Phone:
Fax:
Supervisor:
Benefits contact:

IV. INSURANCE *

Health Insurance:

Insurance company:
Address:
Phone:
Fax:
Company No.
Plan No.
Insurance card No.
Prescription card No.
Employee name (if not patient):
Employee No.
Summary of Key Terms:

*Copy of insurance card
*Copy of prescription card
*Copy of policy
*List of plan providers

Disability Insurance:

Insurance company:
Address:
Phone:
Fax:
Company No.
Plan No.
Employee name (if not patient):
Summary of key terms:

Life Insurance:

Insurer:
Address:
Policy No.:
Limits:
Beneficiary:
Inception date:

V. MEDICATIONS

Current prescription medications. For each list name; dosage; frequency; when taken; reason for taking; prescribing doctor; length of time on medicine:

1. _____
2. _____
3. _____
4. _____
5. _____
6. _____
7. _____
8. _____
9. _____
10. _____

Current non-prescription medications: For each list name; dosage; frequency; when taken; reason for taking; prescribing doctor; length of time on medicine:

1. _____
2. _____
3. _____
4. _____
5. _____
6. _____
7. _____
8. _____
9. _____
10. _____

VI. CANCER DIAGNOSIS *

Specific type of cancer (including subtype):
Location:
Date of diagnosis:
Stage:
Date(s) of relapse(s) if any:
Diagnosing doctor and institution:

Second Opinion:
Doctor and institution:
Diagnosis:
Date:

* Attach pathology reports; medical records containing diagnosis; X-ray, MRI, CT, and diagnostic test results; and blood test and blood marker reports

VII. SURGERY

Date of surgery:
Type of surgery:
Name and address of institution:
Telephone:
Surgeon's name:
Surgeon's telephone:
Results:
Any major complications:

* Attach discharge summary and pathology reports

VIII. CHEMOTHERAPY/IMMUNOTHERAPY

Name and address of institution:
Telephone:
Oncologist's name:
Oncologist's telephone:
Type of central line (if any):
Complications with central line (if any):
Name of treatment protocol or clinical trial:
For each specific drug in the protocol or trial:
Name of medication:
Dose per administration:
Number of doses:
Cumulative dose:
How administered:
Anti-nausea medications used:
Allergic reactions to any drugs:
Any adverse drug reactions:
Results:

IX. RADIATION THERAPY

Name and address of institution:
Telephone:
Name of radiologist-oncologist:
Physician's telephone:
Dates radiation given:
Type of machine or technology used:
Area treated
Amount per session:
Total dose of radiation:
Results:

X. STEM CELL OR BONE MARROW TRANSPLANT

Name and address of institution:
Telephone:
Name of physician:
Physician's telephone:
Date:
Type:
Donor:
Complications:
Results:
Meds:

XI. OTHER CANCER TREATMENTS AND NON-CANCER TREATMENTS

XII. GENERAL HEALTH/HEALTH HISTORY

Health history:
Other health conditions/diseases:
Other surgeries and procedures:
Limitations on activities:
Disabilities:
Family health history:
Other hospitalizations:
Allergies to medications:
Allergies to foods:
Other allergies:
Dietary restrictions:
Any implants or medical devises:

XIII. PATIENT'S QUESTIONS

PATIENT'S QUESTIONS (CONTINUED)

XIV. PATIENT'S NOTES

PATIENT'S NOTES (CONTINUED)

APPENDIX "H"

PATIENT'S WEEKLY SCHEDULE AND LOG

Week of Sunday,_____,___20, through Saturday _____,___20___

1. Medical Appointments (day, time, type, and result):

2. Medical Treatments (day, time, type, and result):

3. Other Appointments:

4. Weekly Medical Goals & Developments:

5. Weekly Non-Medical Goals & Developments:

6. Log of Key Statistics (*e.g.*, Blood Counts):

7. Dietary and Exercise Notes:

8. Key developments:

9. Side effects, complaints, and relief from symptoms:

10. Progress and positive notes:

11. To do list (task and timing):

PATIENT'S WEEKLY SCHEDULE AND LOG

Week of Sunday,_____,____20, through Saturday _____,____20____

1. Medical Appointments (day, time, type, and result):

2. Medical Treatments (day, time, type, and result):

3. Other Appointments:

4. Weekly Medical Goals & Developments:

5. Weekly Non-Medical Goals & Developments:

6. Log of Key Statistics (*e.g.*, Blood Counts):

7. Dietary and Exercise Notes:

8. Key developments:

9. Side effects, complaints, and relief from symptoms:

10. Progress and positive notes:

11. To do list (task and timing):

PATIENT'S WEEKLY SCHEDULE AND LOG

Week of Sunday,_____,____20, through Saturday _____,____20____

1. Medical Appointments (day, time, type, and result):

2. Medical Treatments (day, time, type, and result):

3. Other Appointments:

4. Weekly Medical Goals & Developments:

5. Weekly Non-Medical Goals & Developments:

6. Log of Key Statistics (*e.g.*, Blood Counts):

7. Dietary and Exercise Notes:

8. Key developments:

9. Side effects, complaints, and relief from symptoms:

10. Progress and positive notes:

11. To do list (task and timing):

PATIENT'S WEEKLY SCHEDULE AND LOG

Week of Sunday,_____,____20, through Saturday _____,____20____

1. Medical Appointments (day, time, type, and result):

2. Medical Treatments (day, time, type, and result):

3. Other Appointments:

4. Weekly Medical Goals & Developments:

5. Weekly Non-Medical Goals & Developments:

6. Log of Key Statistics (*e.g.*, Blood Counts):

7. Dietary and Exercise Notes:

8. Key developments:

9. Side effects, complaints, and relief from symptoms:

10. Progress and positive notes:

11. To do list (task and timing):

APPENDIX "I"

GIVING BACK TO HELP OTHERS SURVIVE AND TO CURE CANCER

I. IDENTIFY PEOPLE AND ORGANIZATIONS THAT HELPED YOU GET THROUGH AND DESCRIBE THE TYPE OF HELP THEY PROVIDED AND WHAT IT MEANT TO YOU:

II. DESCRIBE WHAT YOU CAN DO TO HELP OTHERS BATTLING CANCER AND WHAT YOU WILL DO TO HELP OTHERS AND TO CURE CANCER:

APPENDIX "J"

A COUPLE OTHER GOOD CANCER BOOKS

There are many good cancer books and many others that serve only to help patients defeat insomnia. Cancer books generally are not the best source for cancer diagnosis and treatment information. Patients usually will be better served by consulting physicians, websites, and non-profits for more comprehensive and more current information. Yet, a good cancer book can be wonderful source of information and inspiration.

Reading stories of survival and receiving tips from people who have battled the disease can be very helpful. Of course, everyone's experience as a person and "cancer patient" is different, but a good cancer book will provide: (1) stories and context that cancer patients and family members can relate to and appreciate; (2) accurate information and tips that doctors and health care providers do not have the time or the experience to provide; and (3) a healthy dose of inspiration so that readers know that they can beat cancer and some unique ammunition to help along the way.

Few cancer books are best sellers and those making the best seller list often do so because they are written or touted by stars. Many of the most helpful books, however, are not written by celebrities and often are only discovered by research or recommendation. Below are examples of a couple of the books that satisfy our good cancer book criteria.

The Emperor Of All Maladies: This book actually is a best seller. Siddhartha Mukherjee, a cancer physician and researcher at Columbia University, provides an interesting and informative "biography" of cancer—from its first documented appearances thousands of years ago through the present day efforts to understand, cure, control, and conquer cancer. Dr. Mukherjee recounts centuries of discoveries, setbacks, victories, and deaths and provides an interesting glimpse into the future of cancer treatments. Senator Durbin (D-IL) recommended the book to my wife this summer and it was a worthwhile book that will be of interest to people regardless of whether they are directly impacted by the disease.

The Web-Savvy Patient: An Insider's Guide to Navigating the Internet When Facing Medical Crisis: After being diagnosed with leukemia, Andrew Schorr (a medical journalist) emerged as one of the leading medical journalists and patient advocates, providing first-rate audio and video information to patients battling cancer and other diseases through PatientPower, which he founded several years ago. Mr. Schorr provides information, asks questions, and tells stories as only someone who has been through a serious personal health crises can. This book empowers patients and family members by providing important tips for taking advantage of the many benefits associated with obtaining information on the web and avoiding the dangers of misinformation and misapplication associated with using this unregulated resource. The step-by-step guide explores topics such as wading through search engine results, connecting with online communities, defining conditions, identifying the specialists, and organizing the outcome of your research so that doctors will listen. Mr. Schorr also includes inspiring stories of people with cancer and other diseases using the internet to their advantage. The web led Mr. Schorr to a physician and treatment that he believes saved his life and he shares his insights in this resource that should be on every family's book shelf.

APPENDIX "K"

MANAGING SIDE EFFECTS

Many times patients experience symptoms that can be attributable to their cancer or to their treatments. It is important to know that not all patients experience even the "common" side effects and the extent of the side effects vary considerable. Below are some of the side effects that some patients experience and some tips for addressing them. There are ways to treat or mitigate many of the side effects, so do not suffer in silence. The overriding point is to promptly advise your physicians or appropriate health care team member of any side effects and be vigilant in seeking ways to minimize them.

Chemo brain: Many patients experience some cognitive difficulties, which is now commonly referred to as chemo brain. For years, medical professionals did not acknowledge the existence of chemo brain, but in recent years this has received much greater attention. Symptoms can include fogginess, some difficulties with memory, concentration, finding the right words, or processing information. The cause is unknown, but generally the symptoms are relatively minor and usually dissipate after treatment and disappear over time. Only a small percentage of patients have long-term cognitive impairment. If you have trouble focusing or with your memory, write down reminders to yourself, place items such as house car keys, cell phones and planners in the same place, and allow some additional time to accomplish tasks. Discuss your symptoms with your health care team. Metformin, a drug used to treat diabetes and showing early promise as a cancer treatment (particularly in reducing relapse rates), may be a potentially useful drug in treating chemo brain.

Low blood counts: It is common for patients going through treatment to have low blood counts (red, white, and platelets). This sometimes is the intended result of chemotherapy. Years ago, more patients had to delay or interrupt their treatments because their counts were too low and more patients acquired infections. Fortunately, a category of drugs called growth factors can stimulate your bone marrow to make new blood cells. Commonly used growth factors include filgrastim (Neupogen), pegfilgrastim (Neulasta), G-CSF (granulocyte colony-stimulating factor), GM-CSF (granulocyte-macrophage colony-stimulating factor); and sargramostim (Leukine). In some instances, patients may require a blood transfusion.

Infection: As a result of low white counts and compromised immune systems, patients are particularly vulnerable to infection at least at some points during their treatment. Patients may be given antibiotics to prevent or treat infection. It is important to take all steps to avoid infection, including washing your hands regularly and thoroughly, making sure your health care providers and others you are in contact with wash their hands and, where appropriate, where masks and gowns. Avoid sick people, crowds, cuts, uncooked foods, and consider avoiding air travel. If you are receiving chemotherapy or other drugs through a central line or port, make sure catheters are cleaned meticulously. Watch for signs of infection such as a temperature, chills, persistent coughing, tenderness or redness, pain while urinating, or diarrhea. Notify your physician immediately. Ask your physician about which vaccines you should and should not receive.

Anemia: Anemia is caused by a low red cell count, potentially resulting in fatigue, shortness of breath, pale skin, gums or nails, light-headedness or dizziness, and/or a tendency to feel cold. Your health care team should monitor your counts and you should as well and adjust your diet. Red cell growth factors such as Epogen, Procrit, or Aranesp may be prescribed or a blood transfusion may be required. It is important to discuss with your physician the risks and benefits of this therapy.

Bleeding: Severally low platelet counts may cause excessive bleeding from cuts or bruises, pinhead-sized bleeding points in the skin (petechiae), black-and-blue spots on the skin from minor bumps without any apparent injury, reddish or pinkish urine, black or bloody bowel movements, bleeding from the gums or nose, headaches, weakness, and joint or muscle pain. Once the platelet count is restored these side effects usually rapidly fade. Certain medications can weaken the platelets and worsen bleeding problems as well. Ask your physician whether it is safe for you to take aspirin, acetaminophen, or ibuprofen. Avoid alcohol, use a soft toothbrush and brush gently, and avoid cuts and activities that might result in trauma or injury.

Hair loss: Hairy loss or alopecia is a common side effect of chemotherapy, but not all patients loss their hair. The extent to which patients experience hair loss or thinning depends upon the specific drugs, the dosages, and the individual patient. Hair loss does not occur with all drugs. Hair follicles are sensitive to chemotherapy because like cancer cells they multiple rapidly, but they will repair so the effects are temporary. Hair loss usually is not limited to the head and often takes place after the first cycle or two of chemotherapy and it will begin to grow back after completion of chemo and often before. Generally, the new hair looks like the old, but sometimes the color, texture, or curl may be a little different. Some patients have attempted to reduce hair loss by using tight bands or ice caps, with mixed results. During chemotherapy, some patients cut their hair short, wear wigs, or wear caps and scarves. This is a matter of personal preference. Remember to protect your scalp from exposure to the sun. The results of a small prospective cohort study suggest that wearing a scalp-cooling cap can reduce hair loss in women receiving chemotherapy for breast cancer. Among women who used the cooling headgear starting 20 minutes before chemotherapy and continuing for 60-90 minutes after the infusion, 24% did not wear a wig or headband upon completion of chemotherapy, compared with 4% of a control group that did not have access to the device. But additional research is needed to look at effectiveness as well as side effects from using the cooling devise.

Cancer-related fatigue: The majority of cancer patients experience fatigue to some extent. There is no panacea for fatigue, but many patients find that exercise, a good diet, drinking plenty of liquids (*e.g.*, water) to get rid of toxins helps reduce fatigue. Counseling, stress management, coping strategies, and other psychosocial interventions that reduce stress and increase support can help reduce fatigue and increase energy levels. Randomized trials have shown that cognitive behavioral strategies such as progressive muscle relaxation or relaxation breathing may reduce fatigue in those receiving radiation therapy or hematopoietic stem cell transplantation. Medications play a role in managing fatigue, but there is no consensus about which drugs are useful. Erythropoiesis stimulating agents (which stimulate the body to make red cells) may be prescribed for anemia; psychostimulants such as methylphenidate (Ritalin or Methylin) or dexmethylphenidate (Focalin); antidepressants, and corticosteroids are sometimes used depending upon the perceived caused and symptoms. All of these medications have potential side effects and the patient and physician must weigh the benefits and risks. Some useful coping strategies include: being flexible and set realistic goals factoring in the rigors of treatment and how you feel; prioritize and ask for help from family and friends; and schedule treatments for those times that will have the least effect on your job and activities. Fatigue among cancer survivors may be driven by changes in cytokines and stress hormones that contribute to inflammation. Thus, reducing inflammation in these patients could reduce fatigue. In a study of 633 breast cancer survivors, higher intake of omega-3 polyunsaturated fatty acids was linked with decreased inflammation (lower C-reactive protein levels) and decreased physical fatigue. Higher intake of omega-6 PUFA relative to omega-3 PUFA was significantly associated with higher CRP levels and greater likelihood of fatigue.

Diarrhea: Some anticancer drugs affect normal cells in the gastrointestinal tract by causing diarrhea. If diarrhea occurs, your doctor may prescribe antidiarrheal drugs, antibiotics, intravenous fluids or changes in diet. Drinking water may help. Avoid caffeinated beverages (coffee, tea and certain soft drinks), alcohol, and milk.

Constipation: Some drugs may cause or intensify constipation. Your physician may recommend laxatives, intravenous fluids, or changes in diet. Drinking warm or hot fluids may help.

Nausea and vomiting: Cancer treatment can irritate the gastrointestinal tract as well as stimulate an area of the brain that affects the gastrointestinal tract. The frequency and severity of nausea and vomiting vary among patients. Sometimes nausea and vomiting subside as you adjust to treatment. There are several medications available that help with nausea caused by chemotherapy treatments, including: Emend (aprepitant), Zofran (ondansetron), Reglan (metoclopramide), Kytril (granisetron), Anzemet (dolasetron), and Aloxi (palonosetron). However, a 2012 clinical trial showed that the antipsychotic drug olanzapine (Zyprexa) performed much better than the standard treatments for chemotherapy-induced nausea and vomiting. In the double-blind phase III study, 30 (71%) of 42 patients, who received olanzapine had no emesis (vomiting) compared with 12 (32%) of 38 patients who received metoclopramide (Reglan) during a 72-hour observation period after chemotherapy. In addition, 28 (67%) of patients on olanzapine had no nausea, compared with nine (24%) of those patients on metoclopramide. Temporary weight gain may be associated with olanzapine. Some patients find that acupuncture and therapeutic massage can help manage or relieve nausea and vomiting. A steroid called Dexamethasone has been shown to prevent radiation-induced vomiting, especially in treatment of cancers of the abdomen.

Mouth sores and other mouth symptoms: The lining of your mouth and throat are particularly susceptible to damage from cancer treatment. Mouth sores (ulcers) or cold sores; a burning sensation or pain in the mouth or throat (stomatitis); a decrease in saliva during treatment; a red and swollen tongue; a stinging sensation in the throat or difficulty swallowing (dysphagia), a white coating or patches on the tongue, inside of the cheeks or floor of the mouth (candidiasis), which may suggest a yeast infection; and dry, cracked, sore or bleeding lips are among the potential mouth-related symptoms. Xerostomia is a chronic dry-mouth condition caused by damage from radiation therapy to the salivary glands. Amifostine is a radiation protector and the only drug that has been approved by the FDA for xerostomia in patients receiving radiation therapy for cancers of the head and neck. The topical agent sucralfate may protect mucous membranes and is often used during and after radiation therapy to prevent and treat mucositis or mouth sores. Topical antiseptics, such as chlorhexidine and benzydamine, have been used for the prevention of mucositis, but recent studies suggest these may not be effective. In one German study, patients treated with chlorhexidine actually seemed to have more problems with inflammation, resulting in mucositis.

Difficulty swallowing: Here are some things that may help with difficulty swallowing: gargle with baby aspirin pills dissolved in lukewarm water which can reduce inflammation in your throat and esophagus; drink hot honey and lemon tea which can soothe the throat while trying to swallow pills or food; use lozenges, gels, sprays and rinses to replace saliva where lack of saliva is making swallowing difficult; eat soft, smooth foods, such as yogurt, pudding, or ice cream; mash or blend foods, or moisten dry foods with broth, sauce, butter, or milk and avoid dry foods and bread; thicken liquids by adding gelatin, tapioca, baby rice cereal, or commercial thickening products; use a straw to drink liquids and soft foods; eat foods that are cold (to help numb pain) or at room temperature; take extra small and chew slowly and thoroughly; drink with meals; and sit upright when eating or drinking.

Pain: Bone and muscle pain may be related to your cancer, its treatment, or other coexisting diseases such as arthritis. The proper approach depends upon the cause, severity, and frequency of the pain as well as balancing the benefits and side effects of treating the pain. Pain assessment is an important part of any medical evaluation, and pain management is an important part of care. Left untreated, pain can suppress the immune system, delay healing and lead to depression. Many patients experience partial relief from pain though a variety of non-drug therapies. Some of these include: physical therapy and rehabilitation; meditation, hypnosis, electrical nerve stimulation guided imagery, herbs, special diets, vitamins; massage, chiropractic manipulation, acupuncture, exercise (such as walking or pool therapy); and hot or cold packs. There are a range of medications, including non-steroidal anti-inflammatory drugs, acetaminophen, opioid analgesics, antidepressant and anticonvulsant drugs, nerve blocks, corticosteroids, anesthetics; specialized injections, infusions, topical creams and skin patches. Talk to your health care providers regarding your pain and ways to reduce it.

Depression, anxiety, and stress: These not only normal responses to a cancer diagnosis and treatment, someone would have to be crazy not to experience some level of depression, anxiety, and stress under these circumstances. You may feel overwhelmed by your cancer and that your life has been overtaken by treatment. Certain anticancer medications may contribute to feelings of anxiety and symptoms of depression. Where your experience with any of these conditions is prolonged or severe, make sure you get help. These conditions are no less harmless and no less worthy or treatment than pain.

Peripheral neuropathy: Cancer treatment or sometimes the disease itself can cause peripheral neuropathy, which is damage to nerves of the peripheral nervous system, which transmits information from the brain and spinal cord to other parts of the body. Chemotherapy-induced peripheral neuropathy affects between 30% and 40% of patients receiving cancer treatment. Chemotherapy agents most commonly linked to peripheral neuropathy are taxanes (paclitaxel, docetaxel), platinum agents (carboplatin, cisplatin, oxaliplatin), vinca alkaloids (vincristine, vinblastine), bortezomib (velcade), and thalidomide. It can manifest in numbness, tingling, burning, coldness, weakness, and/or temperature sensitivity especially in the fingers, toes, hands, and feet. Individuals at greatest risk of peripheral neuropathy associated with chemotherapy are those with preexisting peripheral neuropathy from conditions such as diabetes or immune disorders and people who previously have received chemotherapy. The patient's age, duration of treatment, dosage, and administration of other neurotoxic drugs also are factors. It is critical that you let your physician know if you are experiencing neuropathy as it must be closely monitored and adjustments to treatments such as changing agents or dosages may be required. Your physician may prescribe certain medications and vitamins to help prevent or lesson neuropathy. Tricyclic antidepressants and anticonvulsants showed some initial promise, but further investigations have failed to demonstrate that these agents cause any alleviation of painful symptoms. Most drugs that have been effective for diabetic neuropathy have not proven to be effective for chemotherapy-induced peripheral neuropathy. Several other treatments currently being investigated suggest some benefit for patients, although additional larger trials are needed. Some of these drugs include: baclofen, amitriptyline, and ketamine in a pluronic lecithin, venlafaxine (Effexor) and duloxetine (Cymbalta). Scrambler therapy is a novel approach to pain control that attempt to relieve pain by providing "non-pain" information via cutaneous nerves to block the effect of pain information. It has shown effectiveness in some patients. Electrostimulation and acupuncture have been reported by some patients to lesson symptoms. In terms of prevention, intravenous administration of calcium and magnesium, before and after oxaliplatin-based treatment regimens, has been shown in several studies to prevent neurotoxicity. Other agents that may prove beneficial in preventing chemotherapy-induced neuropathy are acetyl-L-carnitine, glutamine, glutathione, and N-acetylcysteine, but additional research is needed. Chemotherapy induced neuropathy may gradually decrease after you complete therapy. Many people recover fully from neuropathy, but in some cases symptoms may persist.

APPENDIX "L"

YOUR KEY CONTACTS

NAME	PHONE	EMAIL

ABOUT THE AUTHORS

(WE DID NOT SET OUT TO BE CANCER WARRIORS)

SCOTT SEAMAN is a partner at the law firm of Hinshaw & Culbertson LLP. He is a business and corporate litigator and trial lawyer with more than 33 years of experience. He is a member of the firm's Executive Committee and serves as Co-Chair of the firm's Global Insurance Services Practice Group. At the time of his cancer diagnosis and treatment, he was a member of the law firm Meckler, Bulger & Tilson LLP. He has successfully represented companies in trial courts, appellate courts, and arbitrations across the country in a variety of high stakes matters, including cases and cessions involving insurance coverage, reinsurance, international disputes, professional liability issues, torts and product liability, and business and commercial cases (including corporate control, contract disputes, business torts, misappropriation, cyber/data breach, and other matters).

Scott is rated AV-Preeminent (5.0/5.0) by Martindale & Hubbell (highest rating for legal ability and ethics) and has been an Illinois Super Lawyer since that selection process began in Illinois. He is a fellow of the American College of Coverage Counsel, the American Bar Foundation, and the Litigation Counsel of America. In addition to numerous individual awards and recognitions, he is included in Chambers USA (Band 1): America's Leading Lawyers for Business, Best Lawyers in America, Leading Lawyers, Euromoney Legal Media Group, Expert Guides: "World's Leading Insurance and Reinsurance Lawyers," and Who's Who Legal Thought Leaders – Insurance & Reinsurance. Scott was named by the *American Lawyer* in its inaugural list of Midwest Trailblazers. The list recognizes 50 professionals from 12 Midwestern states "who have moved the needle in the legal industry" and "are truly agents of change." He was selected for his "high-profile, complex insurance coverage cases nationwide, which resulted in precedent setting rulings that have altered insurance law. Scott is a frequent speaker and prolific author on legal, business, and litigation matters.

Scott graduated first in his law school class, served as a law journal editor, and has received numerous awards including: Illinois Lawyers Auxiliary Scholarship; Loyola Leadership and Service Award; Chief Justice Roger B. Taney Award; Judge John C. Hayes Award; Thomas L. Owens Award; and Judge John V. McCormack Award.

Scott is a 23-year survivor of non-Hodgkin lymphoma. He co-founded the Chicago Chapter of the Lymphoma Research Foundation. He is a champion for people with cancer through his fundraising, public policy advocacy, patient advocacy, and cancer awareness and media appearances. Scott has forged numerous partnerships to promote public awareness, education, and community outreach. Scott served as a member of the National Board of Selectors of the Jefferson Awards for Public Service. Scott delivered the Keynote address at the 2006 North American Forum on Lymphoma in Los Angeles. He is a Founding Board Member of the Hippocratic Cancer Research Foundation. He has co-hosted a radio show and television series on cancer and served as the National Cancer Examiner and Chicago Cancer Examiner.

CHARLENE SEAMAN served as a Member of the National Board of Selectors of the Jefferson Awards for Public Service and was involved in launching a landmark national program to promote health, physical activity, and well-being in students. Charlene was part of a delegation to report to the White House and US Senate on the state of volunteering in America. She also helped lead a student leadership and philanthropy program.

Charlene is a Founding Board Member of the Hippocratic Cancer Research Foundation and has been active in events benefiting children with cancer. She co-hosted the *Battling and Beating Cancer* radio show on the Blog Talk Radio Network and a television series bearing the same name. Previously, she co-founded and was past president of the Chicago Chapter of the Lymphoma Research Foundation, which was the first chapter formed by the organization. The Chicago Chapter raised over $3 million and served as a blueprint for other chapters across the country during its formative years. Charlene spearheaded and chaired the Lymphomathon 5K walk and run which began in Chicago (raising millions of dollars in Chicago alone in the first six years) and has become an annual event at numerous cities across the country. Charlene is a tireless advocate for cancer patients and has helped many patients and family members through her amazing referral network that includes the numerous charitable organizations she works with, doctors and healthcare providers, websites and blogs, and people she has helped in the past. She is active in public policy advocacy on health and cancer issues.

As NBC 5 Chicago noted, Charlene's "activities and efforts in organizing charitable organizations, educational events, and fundraisers have had a tremendous impact of the lives of countless patients and families living with cancer in the Chicagoland area and on a national basis." Charlene is a Jefferson Award Recipient and a Chicago Woman of the Year first place winner.

Charlene helped organize the first Livestrong Day in Chicago and launched the Chain of Life. She has served on the board of numerous non-profit organizations and numerous committees and has chaired numerous fundraising and educational events.

Charlene is a former corporate executive who served as President and Chief Executive Officer of a consulting firm and Vice President and Chief Operating Officer of a financial services company. She earned her Bachelor of Science in Psychology. Charlene has brought her leadership skills and more than 35 years of corporate experience, along with her knowledge and passion, to the front lines in the battle against cancer.

CHARLENE AND SCOTT
THE CANCER WARRIORS

"Warren Buffet once said, 'Someone's sitting in the shade today because someone planted a tree a long time ago.' That person was Scott Seaman, a Bartlett resident who was recently honored for planting trees for cancer patients throughout Chicago. Seaman and his wife, Charlene . . ., were recently honored at a dinner for starting the first Chicago chapter of the Lymphoma Research Foundation."

Bartlett Press

"Lymphoma Research Foundation is pleased to announce that Charlene . . . has been awarded a 2008 Jefferson Award for Public Service. Charlene is founding member and past president of the Chicago Chapter and has spearheaded the Lymphomathon effort. Charlene was honored for being a champion for lymphoma and other cancer patients through her patient advocacy, public policy and fundraising activities. The prestigious Jefferson Awards were founded in 1972 by Jacqueline Kennedy Onassis, U.S. Senator Robert Taft, Jr. and Sam Beard to establish a Nobel Prize for public and community service. Once again, congratulations to Charlene."

Lymphoma Today

"Scott and Charlene not only share their wisdom and resources for dealing with the difficult challenges of cancer, but they also share their experiences from the heart, and inspire people to fight and believe. They are truly a living example of how positive attitude, gratitude, and giving back, are all part of the healing."

**Sergio Rojas
NBC 5 Fitness Expert
Corporate And Community Fitness Expert**

"I believe everything happens for a reason. Charlene came into my life and made me part of hers. She gave more support, knowledge, and help than I ever could have hoped for from someone who I met by chance. She and Scott both helped to literally save my mother's life for more than 2 years and they did so unconditionally. For this, I could never repay them. They helped us because that is how they are. They will always be an inspiration to me. They will always be my family. The world would be a better place with more people like Scott and Charlene. I love them. I am not unique because people know, if you need help, knowledge, information, and most of all support, you go straight to Charlene. Many people I personally know have since needed her help, she is always there. Thanks to both of them."

Lisa DeBlasio

Charlene "helped start the Lymphoma Research Foundation's first local chapter outside New York . . . . The Cardinal event to catch on elsewhere has been the Lymphomathon, a 5K walk-run Charlene spearheaded in 2003. What began as 400 people at Montrose Harbor has turned into an annual event in 16 cities. Charlene is devoted to helping patients and families with health problems . . . . Her activities and efforts in organizing charitable organizations, educational events, and fundraisers have had a tremendous impact of the lives of countless patients and families living with Cancer in the Chicagoland area and on a national basis."

NBC 5 Chicago

"Seaman and his wife helped start the first one in Chicago. Since then, the Chicago chapter has served as a blueprint for 22 others that followed. [Seaman] is a leader in the truest sense, creating excitement, inspiring people to raise money and making them feel good about their involvement and contributions. And his wife Charlene is right there alongside of him, doing the same thing. They work really well together."

Lymphoma Today

"Scott Seaman is witty, compassionate, self-deprecating and, given all of his accomplishments in life, commendably humble. I first met Scott, a pre-eminent commercial trial lawyer and corporate problem-solver with a nation-wide practice, when he and his lovely wife Charlene had me on their *Battling and Beating Cancer* radio show on the Blog Talk Radio Network (they're also co-authors of a book and co-host a television series of the same name). Scott, a [23]-year survivor of NHL, and Charlene are true champions for people battling blood cancer. . . . Scott is doing as much as anyone I know to increase lymphoma awareness, to help patients, and find a cure."

Jamie Reno
Award-winning journalist, longtime Newsweek correspondent, singer-songwriter, and patient advocate

"Astounded by the lack of information available to them at the time, the Bartlett couple began a crusade with the mission to eradicate lymphoma and educate people along the way."

Daily Herald

"[A]long with her husband, Scott Seaman, Charlene's enthusiasm and dedication helped the chapter reach new heights in 2007 through their record-breaking Lymphomathon, which raised nearly $425,000 and the addition of chapter staff—a first for LRF. Her commitment to patient education and maintaining strong relationships with healthcare professionals led to LRF's ability to expand its programming . . ."

Chicago Daily Law Bulletin

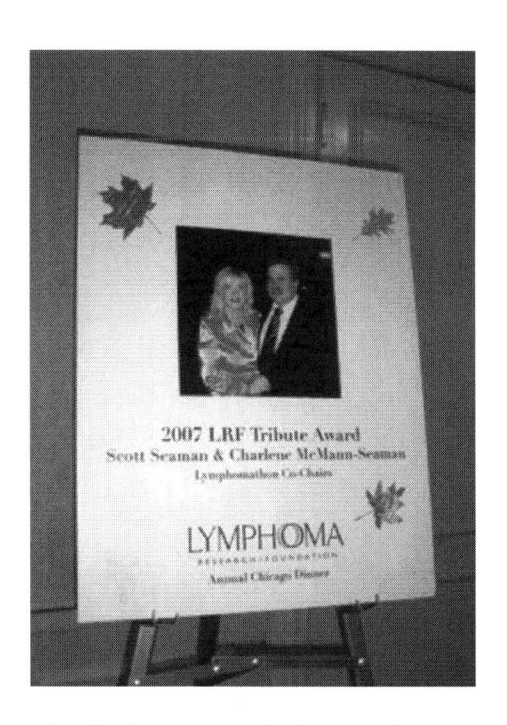

If you would like to contact Charlene or Scott, have them speak at an event, or if you would like to become involved in their cancer educational, advocacy, or fundraising activities or join their non-profit mission, please visit www. charleneandscott.org.